REDUCING THE RISK OF CANCERS

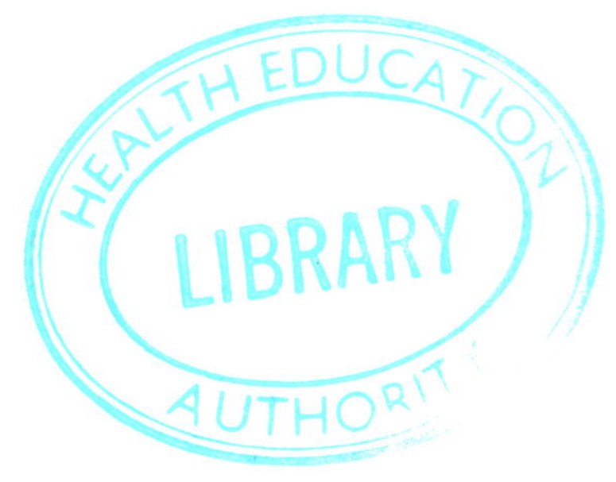

Reducing the Risk of CANCERS

Edited by Tom Heller, Basiro Davey and Lorna Bailey

Hodder & Stoughton
LONDON SYDNEY AUCKLAND TORONTO

IN ASSOCIATION WITH THE OPEN UNIVERSITY AND THE EUROPEAN COMMISSION

AS PART OF THE EUROPE AGAINST CANCER PROGRAMME

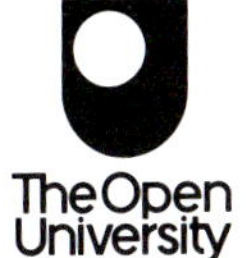

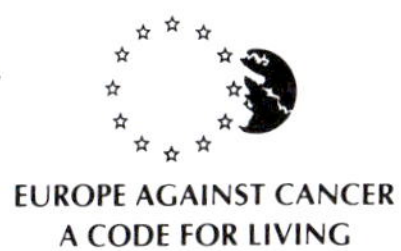

Academic Editors: Tom Heller, Basiro Davey, Lorna Bailey

Project Manager: Ghislaine Adams

Editor: Kathy Eason

Designers: John Bradley, Siân Lewis

Graphic Artist: Janis Gilbert

This book is based on the commissioned papers and deliberations of the Lisbon Colloquium *The Prevention of Cancers: Spreading the Message* held in February 1989. The Colloquium, for European cancer specialists and health education experts, was funded by the European Commission's Europe Against Cancer programme and organized by The Open University, UK, with the local assistance of the Portuguese Open University and members of the Portuguese Europe Against Cancer team.

Colloquium planning team

The European Commission's Europe Against Cancer programme: Michel Richonnier, Coordinator of the Europe Against Cancer programme, and David Sweet

The Open University, UK: Professor Malcolm Johnson, Director of the Department of Health and Social Welfare

OU Academic Team: Lorna Bailey, Dr. Basiro Davey and Dr. Tom Heller

with the assistance of: Dr. Beverley Littlepage and Professor James McEwen; Dr. Jack Winkler as Colloquium moderator; and Jean Mossman and Dr. Elizabeth Skinner of the United Kingdom Coordinating Committee for Cancer Research (UKCCCR).

OU Administration: Peter Leppard and Caroline Malone

Open University of Portugal: Professor Armando Rocha Trindade and Dr. Judite Nozes

Portuguese Committee of Cancer Experts: Professor José Condé

ISBN 0 340 51827 8

First published in Great Britain 1989.

Produced by the Open University for the educational publishing division of Hodder and Stoughton Ltd, Mill Road, Dunton Green, Sevenoaks, Kent.

Printed by M & A Thomson Litho Ltd, East Kilbride, Scotland.

CONTENTS

HOW THIS BOOK CAME TO BE MADE

The Lisbon Colloquium

This book has been prepared from the material generated before and during a Colloquium held in Lisbon in February 1989. The European Commission funded this meeting as one of the first events of Europe Against Cancer Year (1989) in order to further developments in reaching its target of 15 per cent fewer deaths from cancer by the year 2000.

The meeting was organized and hosted by the Open University of the United Kingdom. Academics from the Departments of Health and Social Welfare, Biology, and Community Education at the Open University were responsible for the planning of the Colloquium, for the collection of the outcomes, and for the production and editing of this book.

The Colloquium brought together a range of experts so that knowledge derived from medical research, epidemiology and health education could be combined in an integrated statement on the avoidance and early detection of cancers. A full list of those attending the Colloquium appears at the end of this book.

At the Colloquium all the participants worked together in small groups with a variety of specialist skills and expert knowledge. The groups had specific tasks and subjects to tackle during the various sessions of the Colloquium. The outcome of these discussions and deliberations was recorded, and forms the basis of the introductory sections to each chapter in this book.

The organizers who acted as rapporteurs and editors are aware that it is impossible, in the recording and editing of each of these sessions, to be totally objective in the selection of material that is reported as the conclusions of each of the group discussions. However, we have attempted to convey the vital essence of all the group discussions and to condense and formulate the information and views that were expressed during the Colloquium. Not every participant will agree with every statement that is recorded in this book. However, we are confident that the final report conveys the most important themes and messages that were the outcome of the Colloquium.

Every participant was asked to contribute a paper on their specialized subject for distribution to all the other participants before the Colloquium. This method ensured that the Colloquium itself was full of informed debate and discussion. We are reproducing a selection of the papers that were prepared for the Colloquium. Unfortunately space does not allow us to print all the articles that were prepared*, and some editing has been undertaken on the papers that are reproduced here; the selection and editing of the papers has been the responsibility of the academic team from the Open University.

The papers we reproduce in this book represent a selection of the views, research and examples of positive action that are under way throughout Europe. The final book represents an important record of the outcomes of the Colloquium and a unique review of the state of the art of cancer prevention throughout Europe during Europe Against Cancer Year.

---

*A complete set of all the unedited papers that were written for the Colloquium is available from the Cancer Project Co-ordinator, Department of Health and Social Welfare, the Open University, Walton Hall, Milton Keynes MK7 6AA.

Chapter 1

THE PREVENTION OF CANCERS: SPREADING THE MESSAGE

Introduction

There is increasingly good evidence to show that the majority of all cancers are potentially avoidable diseases and that they could be largely prevented using knowledge that is already available. These facts do not seem to have entered the general public's consciousness, and indeed many health workers and health policy makers similarly regard cancers as inevitable and caused by factors outside human control. Action is needed to change this false impression and to ensure that effective cancer-prevention programmes are initiated and maintained.

Certain cancers are known to be potentially preventable diseases, but the exact causes are not yet identified. For example, the cancers associated with dietary factors are known to make up a major proportion of preventable cancers, but the exact dietary causes for particular cancers are still being established. For this group of cancers, there is sufficient evidence to be able to advocate dietary changes for communities and for individuals, while scientific research continues to establish more exact causality.

On an individual level, there is much people can do to reduce their risks of developing a cancer. The 'ten commandments' for individual action promoted by the European Commission (see Figure 1.1) represent a simple summary of the current state of knowledge about how best to reduce personal risk factors. However, action and positive change is also required at many other levels to create the conditions under which individuals can realistically make changes to reduce the risks they currently take. For example, it is useless to exhort people to change their diets if the healthy components of diet are not available or are too expensive, or to present themselves for screening, if screening services are not easily available. In addition, controls must be introduced to regulate the activities of those organizations that directly or indirectly increase the risks we are exposed to.

This book seeks to take the debate further by discussing the ways in which action might be taken at all levels to reduce the incidence of cancers. The components of the book are largely taken from the outcome of discussions at the European Commission Colloquium, organized by the British Open University in Lisbon during February 1989, during which a range of experts from all over Europe met to discuss the ways in which action is required to prevent cancers, and to bring about a reduction in the death rates from cancers in member states. This book includes a selection of the background papers that were prepared for the Colloquium and summaries of much of the discussion and conclusions from the working groups that met to consider particular topics.

Most cancers can be prevented

Sir Richard Doll, in his opening address to the Colloquium, stated that:

> All who have studied the subject agree that the age-specific risks that are common throughout Europe are, for the most part, potentially capable of being reduced by at least four-fifths and that much of this reduction could be brought about by using the knowledge that we already have. (Keynote Address)

EUROPEAN CODE AGAINST CANCER

CERTAIN CANCERS MAY BE AVOIDED:

1. **Do not smoke**
   Smokers, stop as quickly as possible and do not smoke in the presence of others
2. **Moderate your consumption of alcoholic drinks,**
   beers, wines or spirits
3. **Avoid excessive exposure to the sun**
4. **Follow health and safety instructions,**
   especially in the working environment concerning production, handling, or use of any substance which may cause cancer.

Your general health will benefit from the following two commandments which may also reduce the risks of some cancers:

5. **Frequently eat fresh fruits and vegetables and cereals with a high fibre content**
6. **Avoid becoming overweight**
   and limit your intake of fatty foods

MORE CANCERS WILL BE CURED IF DETECTED EARLY

7. **See a doctor if you notice a lump or observe a change in a mole or abnormal bleeding**
8. **See a doctor if you have persistent problems,**
   such as a persistent cough, a persistent hoarseness, a change in bowel habits or an unexplained weight loss

For women:

9. **Have a cervical smear regularly**
10. **Check your breasts regularly**
    and, if possible, undergo mammography at regular intervals above the age of 50

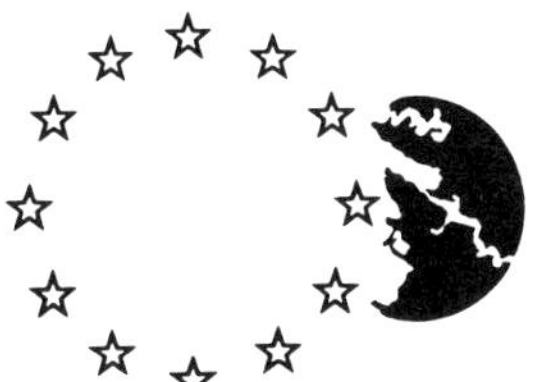

EUROPE AGAINST CANCER

Figure 1.1 The European Code Against Cancer

In a previous publication (Doll and Peto, 1981), he estimated the proportions of cancer deaths attributed to various risk factors. These are shown in Figure 1.2 below.

The available knowledge is highly reliable for some of the risk factors—for example, the relationship between tobacco use and certain cancers. For others, we are less certain. The specific changes in diet that would be required to bring about a reduction in the 30 to 35 per cent of cancers that seem to be related to dietary factors is yet to be determined, but nevertheless it is still possible to give useful general advice.

Although particular risk factors might be relatively unimportant on a national or international scale, they are, of course, of major importance to individuals or to communities exposed to that particular risk. For example, the cancers that are caused by industrial or occupational exposure to carcinogens are numerically of minor importance in population terms, but will be of vital importance to people involved in hazardous industries. It would, therefore, seem appropriate that action should be undertaken to reduce all the known hazards that produce cancers, and not simply to concentrate on the most common ones.

Public knowledge about cancers

The general public throughout Europe seem to have a very imperfect knowledge about the preventability of cancers. In a major survey carried out throughout the European Community (EC, 1987), 11 600 people were asked their opinion as to the proportion of cancers that could be prevented. Almost two-thirds (62%) either didn't know, or thought that cancers could only be prevented in a quarter of cases or less. An alarming 8 per cent thought cancers could never be prevented. The survey showed that there were differences in knowledge and perception in the various European countries and amongst different groups within countries. Some groups were far more pessimistic in their estimations than the average values quoted above.

This general lack of knowledge about the preventability of cancers seems also to be reflected in the low priority given by policy makers, politicians and even health-care workers to action to bring about a reduction of the risk factors for cancers.

The consensus from the Lisbon Colloquium was that governments, policy makers at all levels, and the entire range of health-care workers require much more information and education

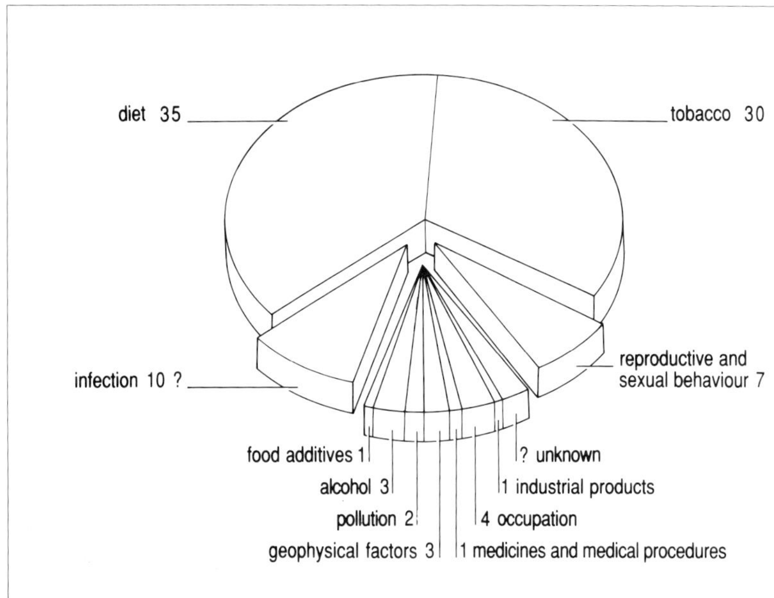

Figure 1.2 Estimated percentage of cancer deaths attributed to various factors

about the preventability of cancers before additional resources will be allocated and positive action will be taken. Where good plans are being developed and exciting initiatives are under way to tackle the problems of cancer prevention, more action is required to 'spread the message' about these projects to areas where plans are less well developed. We have produced this book to help educate all health workers and health policy makers throughout Europe on how the risk factors for cancers can be reduced.

Taking action to prevent cancers

Action is required at many different levels to get across the positive message of the preventability of most cancers, and to bring about changes that will ensure a falling death rate from cancers in the future.

The levels at which activity needs to be undertaken were identified and discussed at the Colloquium and are reported in full in later chapters of this book. In brief, the levels were as follows:

Supragovernmental organizations The Commission of the European Communities has an active role to play in the provision of suitable information and education to prevent cancers throughout Europe. In the first instance, this activity was spearheaded by the widest possible dissemination of the European Code Against Cancer, and is now being followed up with more detailed work about the ways in which the recommendations of the Code can be implemented in practice. Improved training for all health workers will be encouraged by financial support for individual schemes in all countries on this subject. Research and collaboration will be supported throughout Europe to find out more about the exact causes of all the cancers and how they can be prevented.

Government Action is required by governments in all countries to create the setting in which cancer-prevention activities can take place. The major activities that governments can undertake were discussed at the Colloquium and are reported in more detail in Chapter 6. In brief, these are:

- improved cancer registration and statistics;
- setting a good example in their own establishments;
- coordination of messages and activities between relevant organizations;
- control measures over harmful products and their advertising;
- taxation and fiscal controls over harmful products and the promotion of healthy ones;
- positive screening policies for early detection, where appropriate;
- development of research policy;
- health service development;
- international and intergovernmental coordination;
- control over the export of hazards to other countries.

Businesses and commercial producers
These have a duty both to their own workforce and to wider society, including their customers, to produce safe products in such a way that their own workers are not put in jeopardy. The group discussing these issues reports the outcome of their discussions in Chapter 5 of this book, and uses examples from the tobacco and food industries to show how direct influence might be brought to bear on companies and businesses to work towards the prevention of particular cancers.

Commercial companies exist to make profits from their activities. They are, however, susceptible to pressure from below (the consumers), from above (governments and legislation) and from within (the workforce and trades unions).

The main points of action discussed at the Colloquium were:

- It may not be relevant to spread specific preventive messages to all businesses and commercial concerns, but more appropriate to target specific businesses and industries where the health effect will be greatest. These will obviously include those businesses who expose their workforce to occupational hazards, either directly through specific carcinogens in the production process, or indirectly via tobacco smoke in the workplace.

- Special activities should be directed at those businesses producing substances that could potentially be harmful.

- Businesses whose products do not have a direct effect on health may, however, indirectly influence health and preventive activities, and so may need special targeting. In particular, the media have an important role to play in portraying either positive or negative health messages. Also, the insurance and finance industries can provide financial incentives and penalties in such a way as to promote a healthy life style.

- Negative messages to the business sector are unlikely to be effective. Greater potential can be achieved through positive educational effort. Diversification for companies away from the production of harmful products into other commercial areas needs supporting.

- Businesses can be persuaded that there may be considerable profit to be made from the production of products that can then be marketed with a 'healthy-life-style' image attached.

- Businesses may need reminding that if their workforce remains healthy, it is likely to become more efficient. Less absenteeism and more positive attitudes to production will be the result.

Health workers and health policy makers

At present, these groups seem to give preventive activity (specifically activities intended to prevent cancers) a low priority. There is considerable status attached to careers in high technology medicine and in curative and surgical specialities, but often low status and poor career prospects for those specializing in preventive medicine. Throughout Europe, the teaching and training of health workers on cancer-related subjects, and particularly about the preventive aspects, has been described in a recent survey (EORTC, 1988) as 'inadequate in terms of lack of clear objectives, curriculum design and coordination ... with clear inadequacies in many schools for health workers.'

Health policy makers themselves need more educating to recognize the importance of the prevention of cancers. At present, their efforts are often sporadic and unplanned and insufficient funds are designated to make their efforts effective in any realistic way. However, there are substantial opportunities for health workers to take the lead in pursuing positive changes in health policy and to influence the behaviour of people who come to them seeking help.

The majority of the population are in contact with health establishments, such as hospitals and clinics, in some way or other every year. These health establishments are also major employers. A 'healthy health service' would therefore provide a wonderful demonstration project for the general public and show the resolve of health policy makers to put important theory into practice. This would include the provision for all employees, patients and visitors to benefit from a smoke-free environment and the availability of healthy meals. A more detailed description and discussion of these policies, and ways of implementing them, are contained in Chapter 4.

Cancer education for individuals and communities

The message that needs to be transmitted is that prevention of cancers is one component of a healthy life-style approach. It is unlikely that people will be motivated to change their risk-factor behaviours for a single, apparently remote cause, such as the possible reduction of risk of cancers in the future.

Discussions at the Colloquium concluded that:

- Messages about cancer prevention should not conflict with other health messages—for example, with those designed to promote a healthy life style in order to reduce the risk of coronary heart disease.

- Health messages about cancer prevention and a healthy life style are needed from an early age, and should probably be incorporated into many areas of the syllabus in schools.
- All messages need to be tailored to suit the particular culture of the group whose behaviours the educators are trying to influence.
- In most cases, individuals are best reached through groups already established within each community. Working with the community at local level—for example, with womens' groups, voluntary organizations, community groups, minority group organizations—is more likely to be effective than untargeted, 'blanket' campaigns.
- Using a community development model of health promotion, working at a local level, it is possible to involve many local opinion leaders in implementing the necessary changes.
- All changes need to be clearly designed in small steps and in full consultation with the community groups.
- Other, more traditional, types of health-education work with individuals or groups should not be excluded. These might be in the workplace or as opportunistic programmes when people are attending clinics for other health-related reasons.
- It is essential to build in an element of evaluation and research in order that the most effective ways of changing people's risk-related behaviours can be assessed, and so that modifications can be made to future programmes if necessary.

Planning for integrated action

Integrated action at all the levels described above is necessary to be most effective in reducing the incidence of cancers in the future. A framework for coordinated action is needed at national, regional and local level. Discussion of this complex task and some examples of planning integrated action from different European countries are included in Chapter 7.

References

European Commission (1987), survey, *Europeans and the prevention of cancer. A working document of the services of the European Commission*, Brussels.

EC/EORTC (European Organization for Research and Treatment of Cancers) (1988) *A curriculum in oncology for medical students in Europe*, May 1988.

Doll, R. and Peto, R. (1981) *The Causes of Cancer*, Oxford University Press, Oxford.

Keynote Address

THE PREVENTION OF CANCER: OPPORTUNITIES AND CHALLENGES

Sir Richard Doll

Imperial Cancer Research Fund, Cancer Epidemiology and Clinical Trials Unit, Radcliffe Infirmary, Oxford, England

Introduction

Cancer, like death, will be with us always. It is an inevitable part of the biological process that has led to the evolution of Man and the risk of developing cancer is part of the price we pay for the privilege of life. It is inevitable, too, that the risk will increase with age, once childhood is past, as the increased risk reflects the wear and tear on cells associated with their continued multiplication and exposure to potentially damaging agents in the environment. The size of the risk at any given age is, however, to a large extent in our own hands, either as individuals or corporatively through the governments that act on our behalf. How far we can control the size of the risk is still uncertain; but all who have studied the subject agree that the age-specific risks common throughout Europe are, for the most part, potentially capable of being reduced by at least four-fifths and that much of this reduction could be brought about by using the knowledge that we already have.

The public lecture on possibilities for the prevention of cancer that was given at the Royal Society (Doll, 1986a) forms the background to this keynote address. In that lecture, various measures were listed that would help to reduce the risk, classified according to the size of the effect they might be expected to have. The lecture concluded with a discussion of the prospects for the future, which pays particular reference to the potential for preventing cancer by immunization against viral infection and by the modification of the diet. Screening was not considered, because shortness of time made some selection of topics necessary and because the two applications that had been shown to be effective (examination of cervical smears to detect premalignant lesions of the cervix, and mass mammography to pick up early lesions of the breast) partook as much of the character of curative medicine as of prevention.

In this paper I shall again omit screening, apart from saying that both methods referred to have been proved to save life, and I shall concentrate on the practical means by which our knowledge of the causes of cancer can be used to reduce the risk of developing the diseases. These are essentially the same throughout Europe, but the emphasis in different countries will inevitably be different due to differences in the prevalence of the various carcinogenic agents, and in particular in the stage of development of the epidemic of cancer caused by smoking. This is illustrated in Figures 1 and 2, which show the trends in mortality from cancer in men and women in Britain and France over the past 35 years. In one country, the mortality is stable or decreasing in men and increasing in women, while in the other it is increasing in men and decreasing in women.

No new major causes have been discovered for any of the cancers that are prevalent in Europe since the public lecture was delivered, but advances in knowledge have changed, to some extent, our estimate of the relative importance of different causes of cancer (for example, the emerging importance of pollution as a potential cause of increased exposure to ultraviolet light) and have strengthened our confidence in the value of several prophylactic measures.

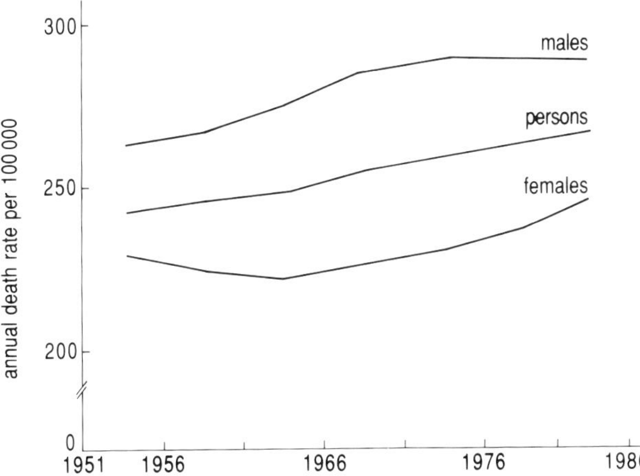

Figure 1 Trends in mortality from all neoplasms, England and Wales, 1951–55 to 1981–85, by sex: annual mortality per 100 000 standardized for age on the population of England and Wales in 1980 (IARC, 1982).

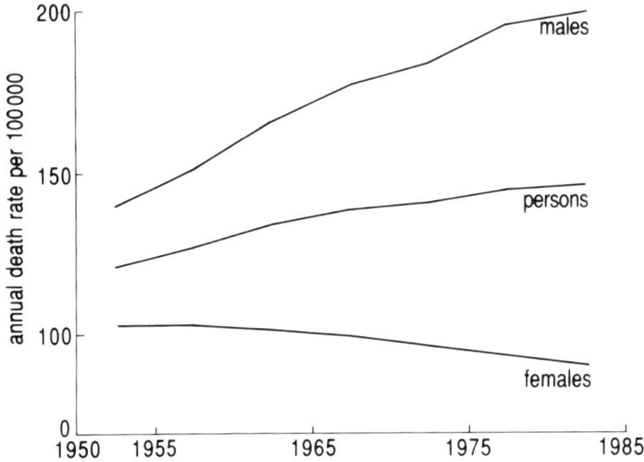

Figure 2 Trends in mortality from all cancers, France, 1950–4 to 1980–4, by sex: annual mortality per 100 000 standardized for age in the standard world population (International Agency for Research on Cancer, 1982).

Immunization

From the public's point of view, two methods of prevention stand out as the methods of choice, as neither require any alteration in people's accustomed behaviour: namely, immunization against oncogenic viruses, and the elimination of carcinogenic agents from the environment to which people are involuntarily exposed. On present knowledge, however, neither seems likely to be able to have much effect on the current incidence of cancers in Europe.

A vaccine against one oncogenic virus (the hepatitis B virus or HBV) is already available and should greatly reduce the risk of liver cancer in high risk areas; but the disease is so uncommon in Europe, with the exception of some parts of Greece, that we should probably wait to see the results of the experiments in prophylaxis that are now being carried out in high risk areas in the Gambia and the Far East before deciding how to use the vaccine here. Another vaccine should also be available within two or three years (namely, one against the Epstein–Barr virus or EBV), and this may help to prevent nasopharyngeal cancer in China and Burkitt's lymphoma in Africa; but it could not be expected to prevent more than a handful of cases of non-Hodgkin's lymphoma in Europe.

The position would be very different if it proves possible to produce vaccines against the specific types of the human papilloma virus (HPV) that seem to be necessary for the development of most cancers of the cervix, vulva, penis, and anus, and of some cancers of the skin. At present, however, such vaccines are only gleams in the eyes of research workers and the only recommendation we can make with regard to them is the recommendation for intensified research.

Involuntary exposure to environmental carcinogens

Elimination, by prohibition or voluntary agreement, of agents that have been proved to cause cancers in humans has been an important means of reducing occupational hazards and has contributed to the reduction of risk in the general population when people have been exposed to smaller amounts of the same agents in industrial products or industrial waste. This has been possible in the cases of 2-naphthylamine, 4-aminobiphenyl, and benzidine. More often, however, because the agents have had valuable social uses and no effective substitutes have been to hand, their use has been continued and the extent to which individuals are exposed has been controlled, as in the cases of ionizing radiation, the combustion products of fossil fuels, asbestos, 2-chloromethyl ether, vinyl chloride, benzene and some inorganic compounds of arsenic, nickel and chromium.

The practical question that has to be answered is, therefore, whether efforts need to be made to reduce further the trace amounts in the environment of these agents and of the many others in use that have not been shown conclusively to cause cancers in humans, but which have been shown to cause cancers in animals or which lead to the production of carcinogenic substances *in vivo*.

Much publicity has been given to the exposure of the public to these proven and suspected carcinogenic agents and there is often great pressure on governments to ban their use or reduce still further the extent to which individuals are likely to be exposed. The cost of so doing may, however, be large in social or economic terms and, it may be argued, greater than the benefit. In a few instances, however, the need for action is clear.

Ionizing radiation

One instance is the risk of cancer associated with exposure to radon in the air of domestic buildings, which may be responsible for 1 per cent or so of all lung cancers in Europe. The long-term carcinogenic effect of ionizing radiation is now thought to be some two to five times greater than it used to be (United Nations Scientific Committee on the Effects of Atomic Radiation, 1988), as a result of revised estimates of the dose received by the survivors of the Hiroshima and Nagasaki explosions and the continuation of observations on the survivors for a longer period. But it is by no means certain that these higher estimates apply to the effect of exposure to the very small doses to which people are constantly exposed from the ubiquitous sources of natural radioactivity.

Whether or not they do should be determined over the course of the next few years, when we have the results of the international study of nuclear energy workers that is being organized by the International Agency for Research on Cancer in Lyon. This, however, will not affect the need to deal with the radon in the air of those houses scattered throughout many parts of Europe that have an unusually high concentration of radon, even 100 times greater than average, as a result of their structure and the nature of the ground on which they are built.

Concentrations of more than 400 Bq m^{-3}, like those which, it is thought, occur in one in 1000 British houses, will give rise to a dose of about 20 mSv y^{-1} and are estimated to cause a lifetime risk of fatal cancer in the order of 10 per cent: that is, nearly half the normal risk of death from cancers due to all other causes combined. Fortunately these high levels can be reduced relatively easily by modifying the floors of the buildings or by putting in exhaust fans, but this can be done only after the buildings have been identified. Large-scale surveys to identify such houses are therefore an urgent need.

Ultraviolet light

Another case where action is certainly required arises from the destruction of the ozone layer of the earth's atmosphere with the resultant increase in the amount of ultraviolet light that reaches the earth's surface. Several agents may be contributing to this destruction, including the nitrogen oxides in the exhaust fumes of cars, but the principal agents are the chlorofluorocarbons (CFCs) that are widely used as propellants in aerosol sprays, refrigerants, blowing agents in the production of plastic foams, and solvents in the manufacture and cleaning of electronic equipment, and the related halons that are used primarily as fire suppressants.

The current rate of production of CFCs is estimated to deplete the ozone layer by 5 per cent, but the demand has been so great that production has been growing by 8 per cent a year. The effect of an increase in the flux of ultraviolet light on agriculture may be more important economically than the effect on health; but increases of the order expected would certainly have a substantial effect on the risk of cancers of the skin, including, of course, the risk of fatal melanoma. The Montreal agreement for freezing consumption of CFCs at the 1986 level, and reducing that by half by 1998, goes some way to meeting the problem; but the long-term effects of the destruction of the ozone layer are too serious for us to be content merely with their diminution and the use of CFCs for all but the most essential purposes needs to be eliminated.

Asbestos

A third case is the use of asbestos, which has been of enormous benefit to society in many ways, most particularly in preventing the spread of fire and providing motor vehicles with effective brakes. The continued use of asbestos would seem to be undesirable, however, because it is so resistant to destruction, which is, of course, the very characteristic that has made it such a valuable material. This indestructibility means that fibres released into the atmosphere remain in the environment, like lead, virtually for ever. Today there is no justification for the continued use of crocidolite and amosite, which are persistent *in vivo* and are the principal causes of pleural and peritoneal mesotheliomas. Chrysotile, however, is less persistent *in vivo* and seldom causes mesothelioma, and a case can be made for its continued use under controlled conditions until the efficacy and safety of its substitutes have been proved.

In this respect, it is reassuring that the mortality from lung cancer in non-smokers of both sexes has remained virtually constant in the United States over the past 25 years, as is shown by the results of the American Cancer Society's massive cohort studies, which are summarized in Table 1. Evidently, the enormous increase in the use of asbestos in the first half of the century and the resulting pollution of the atmosphere with asbestos fibres has not produced any detectable change in the mortality from this disease—nor, for that matter, does it appear that any other form of atmospheric pollution introduced in the same period can have done so either.

Other pollutants

It is less clear what other measures should be taken to prevent or diminish involuntary exposure to agents that are suspected of increasing the risk of cancer, other than a requirement to test for potential carcinogenicity any new chemical that is intended to be used on a large scale. Several need to be considered, such as the diminution of trihalomethanes in chlorinated drinking water, because they may contribute to the risk of bladder cancer (Cantor *et al.*, 1987), but I know of none, other than those to which I have already referred, that would clearly produce a benefit greater than the social cost.

Tobacco

What then are the causes of cancer that we can usefully seek to remove? Head and shoulders above all others is the smoking of tobacco, the total effect of which is only just beginning to be appreciated in some countries. That it has sometimes taken so long to appreciate the effect is because tobacco is generally much more harmful when smoked in the form of cigarettes than when smoked in pipes or cigars, and because tobacco smoke is a weak carcinogen which causes cancer in a high proportion of smokers only after regular exposure for 30 or 40 years. It is not, therefore, until cigarette smoking has been prevalent in young people for two generations that the most specific type of tobacco-induced cancers (namely, cancer of the lung) begins to cause major concern. This is illustrated in Figure 3, which shows the increase in cigarette consumption and the corresponding increase in lung cancer in England and Wales, and in France.

The many types of cancer which, according to the International Agency for Research on Cancer (1986), are caused by tobacco, and the proportions of each that are attributable to smoking, were described in the Royal Society lecture (Doll, 1986a). The corresponding proportions for the United States as estimated last month by the US Surgeon General (1989) are summarized in Table 2. To these, recent research now suggests that we probably need to add a small proportion of deaths from leukaemia and from cancers of the nose, stomach and cervix uteri (Doll, 1988). In total, the habit of smoking has become responsible for one in three of all cancer deaths in some countries and Peto has estimated, in a paper

Table 1 Trends in mortality from lung cancer in non-smokers: USA 1959–86

Sex	Authors of study	Annual mortality per 100 000 standardized for age			
		1960–64	1965–68	1969–72	1982–86
Women	Garfinkel & Stellman, 1988[1]	11.7	12.4	12.2	12.1
	US Surgeon-General, 1989[2,3]	10.3	–	–	11.4
Men	US Surgeon-General, 1989[2,4]	15.5	–	–	13.6

1 Standardized on US female population in 1970; numbers of deaths 176, 186, 205 and 174 respectively.
2 Standardized on US white population in 1965.
3 First period 1959–65; 95% confidence limits first period 8.9 and 11.9, second period 9.8 and 13.3.
4 First period 1959–65; 95% confidence limits first period 12.5 and 19.3, second period 10.8 and 17.0.

presented to a meeting organized by the European Office of the World Health Organization in Madrid last November (Peto, 1988), that already 400 000 Europeans die from cancer due to smoking every year. Reduction in smoking must, therefore, be a central plank in any programme aimed seriously at the prevention of cancer.

Prohibition of tobacco is out of the question. It would certainly lead to a black market and an increase in crime, quite apart from any philosophical consideration of the impropriety of enforcing health on people against their will. Effective measures can be introduced only with public support, so public opinion must first be prepared. A programme of prevention requires, therefore, first and foremost public education. This, however, can be expected to be effective only if the educators themselves set the example—'Do what I say, not what I do' has never cut much ice. Secondly, it needs government support in the ways set out in Table 3: the first to show that governments accept that tobacco constitutes a serious hazard; the second to provide a financial incentive to stop smoking; the third to establish that non-smoking is regarded as the norm and to reduce the small but real risk due to exposure to other people's smoke; and the fourth and fifth to reduce the risk for the significant proportion of people who must be expected to continue to smoke for at least some years to come.

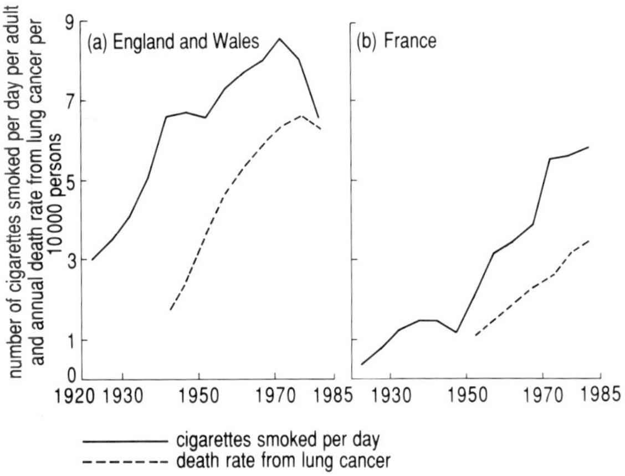

Figure 3 Trends in consumption of cigarettes per adult per day and mortality from lung cancer per 10 000 persons per year, (a) in England and Wales, and (b) in France, 1920 to 1985. Data standardized for age on the standard world population (International Agency for Research on Cancer, 1982).

Table 2 Cancer deaths due to smoking: USA 1985 (Surgeon General, 1989)

Type of cancer	Per cent of deaths attributable to smoking Men	Women	Estimated number of deaths attributable to smoking per year (1000s)
lung	90	79	106
lip, oral cavity, pharynx	92	61	7
oesophagus	78	75	7
bladder	47	37	4
kidney	48	12	3
larynx	81	87	3

The importance of reducing tar levels has been established not only by case-control studies of the type of cigarettes that people with and without lung cancer have tended to smoke (Lubin *et al.*, 1984), but also by the dramatic reduction in the mortality from lung cancer in young men who have mostly smoked only low-tar cigarettes compared with their predecessors in countries where low-tar cigarettes have become the norm. This latter reduction has occurred sooner and to a much greater extent than could be explained by changes in the amounts smoked (Doll, 1986b). It should not be expected, however, that low-tar cigarettes will necessarily have any effect on the incidence of cancers that result from the absorption of carcinogens into the bloodstream or on the incidence of such other tobacco-induced conditions as myocardial infarction, as people tend to inhale the smoke from low-tar, low-nicotine cigarettes more deeply to obtain increments of nicotine in the blood equal to those obtained with cigarettes delivering larger amounts of nicotine in their smoke.

Table 3 Measures to reduce the risk of cancers produced by smoking

- prohibit advertising of tobacco
- increase taxation
- prohibit smoking in public vehicles and most parts of public buildings
- reduce tar levels in smoke (by setting limits or differential taxation)
- establish clinics for nicotine addicts.

Alcohol

Second only in importance to smoking as a proven cause of cancer in Europe is the consumption of alcoholic drinks which, in some countries, may be responsible, in conjunction with smoking, for as much as 10 per cent of all cancer deaths. Alcohol itself is not carcinogenic in animals and the experimental evidence of a synergistic effect with any proven carcinogen is weak (International Agency for Research on Cancer, 1989). The human evidence, however, is overwhelming. All types of alcoholic drink have a similar effect. The observational evidence that the risks of several types of cancer increase sharply with the amount drunk to more than ten times that in lifelong non-drinkers, combined with observations of high risks in occupations associated with high consumption and low risks in social groups that abjure alcohol, and reduced risks in ex-drinkers, point incontrovertibly to a carcinogenic effect of alcohol in humans.

Table 4 Cancers produced by consumption of alcohol

Certainly produced		
	cancers of the	mouth
		pharynx
		oesophagus
		larynx
		liver
Possibly produced		
	cancers of the	breast
		rectum

The types of cancer caused in part by alcohol are listed in Table 4, along with two others for which the evidence is inconclusive, one of which (cancer of the rectum) is specifically related only to beer, if it is related to alcohol at all. Policies for prevention have to take into account four facts: (i) that the consumption of alcohol has been common for centuries and is regarded by many as a pleasurable activity; (ii) that its carcinogenic effect is synergistic with smoking and possibly with some aspects of malnutrition, so that the risk associated with moderate consumption in the well nourished non-smoker is very small; (iii) that moderate consumption, of the order of two to three units a day, seems to be associated with a reduced risk of coronary thrombosis; and (iv) that heavy consumption has many other deleterious social effects other than the production of cancer. In these circumstances, the most appropriate preventive measure may well be public education, including in particular the importance of the interaction with smoking, increased taxation (which hitherto has proved the most effective means of reducing heavy consumption), and specific measures (such as legal limits on blood alcohol when driving) that are designed to diminish each individual deleterious social effect.

Diet

Promisingly, but still inconclusively, there is accumulating evidence that the risk of cancer can be materially reduced—possibly by a third or more—by the modification of diet in a way that has already proved acceptable to many. That diet can influence the incidence of cancer to some extent is abundantly clear from experimental studies in animals, which have shown that it can do so in many different ways: not only by introducing into the body carcinogens or substances from which carcinogens are formed *in vivo*, but also by affecting the metabolism of carcinogens and the body's reaction to them. In the last way, diet might, for example, reduce the risk of lung cancer from cigarette smoking, but more importantly it might, in one or other way, hold the key to the control of cancers of the stomach, large bowel, and breast—the causes of which are still uncertain or unknown—but which constitute three of the four most common lethal cancers throughout the world.

Many practicable modifications of diet that the US National Research Council (1982) suggested might reduce the risk of cancer were listed in the Royal Society lecture (Doll, 1986a) and are reproduced in Table 5. For several, however, the evidence is theoretical or based on animal experiments of dubious relevance, and the human evidence is either contradictory or, in my opinion, too weak to justify specific intervention. These include reducing the consumption of saccharin and smoked and grilled food, and, in my opinion, nitrates—though this I recognize is controversial.

Table 5 Dietary measures suggested for the prevention of cancer

Measure	Type of cancer affected
reduce:	
calories (avoid obesity)	gall bladder, body of uterus, possibly breast
fat	breast, possibly colon and rectum
smoked and grilled food	stomach, possibly others
salt-cured food	stomach
nitrates	stomach, possibly others
saccharin	bladder
increase:	
fibre	colon and rectum
vegetables	colon and rectum
fruit	stomach
vitamins A, C, E	many sites
beta-carotene	many sites
selenium	many sites

Increasingly, too, the evidence that saturated fat is a cause of breast cancer, which seemed to be so reasonable on the basis of intercommunal correlations, has become progressively less tenable with the increasing amount of information about the fat consumption of individuals. This may be, as Goodwin and Boyd (1987) suggest, because the correlation studies have been able to examine populations with a wide range of fat consumption, while studies of individuals in developed countries have not.

It is difficult, however, to dismiss altogether, on these grounds, the negative results of two recent cohort studies in the USA, which have found the lowest risks to be in the groups with the highest consumption (Willett *et al.*, 1987; Jones *et al.*, 1988). There is slightly stronger evidence that fat consumption may increase the risk of cancers of the prostate and large bowel. But taken all in all, the evidence does not justify recommending specific measures to reduce the consumption of fat, whether saturated or not, just to reduce the risk of cancer—although, of course, the reduction of saturated fat is amply justified to reduce the risk of myocardial infarction.

Nor is it, in my opinion, as yet strong enough to recommend the specific addition of vitamins A and E, beta-carotene, or selenium, despite some suggestive experimental evidence and the frequent finding in case-control studies that patients with a wide variety of cancers give dietary histories of lower intakes of these nutrients than are given by controls. Twelve cohort studies, in which measurements were made of serum levels in apparently healthy people, showed no difference between the concentration of serum retinol in individuals who subsequently developed cancer and those who did not, and the idea that vitamin A is protective can, I think, be ruled out.

The position is different, however, with regard to beta-carotene, selenium and vitamin E. All have been consistently lower, on average, in the future cancer group than in controls, as is shown in 11 studies in Table 6. The differences are mostly small, but substantial differences in risk of the order of two- or threefold have commonly been observed when individuals with the lowest values are compared with those with the highest. This is illustrated by the findings in a recent Finnish study in which nearly 800 cancers were observed in 36 000 men and women, who were followed for a mean of eight years. The results in relation to alpha-tocopherol are summarized in Table 7. It may be, too, that greater differences occur for some types of cancer than for others; but in this respect we are still in the stage of hypothesis forming and consistent differences have not yet been demonstrated in different studies. The strongest evidence relates to beta-carotene, which has been shown experimentally to reduce the proportion of micronucleated cells in buccal smears from tobacco chewers (Stich *et al.*, 1988). Its value as an antipromoter is currently being tested by Stampfer *et al.* (1985) in 23 000 US doctors who have been allocated at random a regular dose of beta-carotene or a placebo.

The qualitative effects of the other measures suggested by the US National Research Council (1982) are shown in Table 8. The quantitative effects that might be possible are unclear, but they might amount to halving the total risk of the six types of cancer listed in the table. Only the effect of obesity is established beyond dispute. The accumulating evidence from case-control and cohort studies is, however, in my opinion, sufficiently strong also to justify public education about the desirability of increasing the consumption of fruit, green vegetables, and fibre.

Table 6 Levels of serum beta-carotene, vitamin E and selenium predictive of cancer in cohort studies

Country	Study	Type of cancer	Number of cancers	Serum level of cases expressed as a percentage of the level in controls		
				Beta-carotene	Vitamin E	Selenium
USA	1	all	111		92	96*
	2	5 sites	284	82*	100	99
	3	lung	99	87*	88*	103
		colon	72	96	92	96
UK	4	all	271	90*	98	
	5	breast	39	72	78	
Finland	6	all	51		98	88*
	7	all	109		95	
	8	all	766	89	97	97
Netherlands	9	all	69		85*	96
Sweden	10	all	35		90	93
Switzerland	11	all	115	79	94	

*$P<0.05$

References: 1 Willett *et al.* (1984), 2 Nomura *et al.* (1985 & 1987), 3 Menkes *et al.* (1986) and Schober *et al.* (1987), 4 Wald *et al.* (1987a, b), 5 Wald *et al.* (1984), 6 Salonen *et al.* (1985), 7 Virtamo *et al.* (1987), 8 Knekt *et al.* (1988) and Knekt (1988), 9 Kok *et al.* (1987a, b), 10 Fex *et al.* (1987), 11 Stahelin *et al.* (1984).

Table 7 Relative risk of cancer for different levels of serum alpha-tocopherol†

Sex	Type of cancer	Risk relative to that in highest quartile of serum level*				
		1	2	3	4	5
Male	related to smoking	1.00	1.03	0.72	0.91	0.90
	other	1.00	1.37	1.45	0.74	0.71
Female	arising from reproductive organs	1.00	0.82	0.51	0.74	0.60
	other epithelial	1.00	0.59	0.59	0.49	0.54

*Adjusted for smoking.
(†after Knekt *et al.*, 1988; Knekt, 1988)

In the case of fibre, the evidence has been confused by the complexity of the material and uncertainty about the specific compounds that exert the beneficial effect. These, it seems, are nutrients that reach the large bowel, where they serve as substrates for the growth of bacteria. They are not limited to the components of what has been defined as fibre in the past, but include a proportion of dietary starch, which may exist in a resistant form as, for example, in cold potatoes. Classical fibre, however, is an important component of the undigested carbohydrate that reaches the large bowel and, from the point of view of public education, we can still specifically recommend an increased consumption of unrefined cereals and green vegetables, in which it principally occurs.

Whether anything can be done to encourage increased consumption of these beneficial foods by government intervention will, I hope, be discussed later in this Colloquium. I am, however, too ignorant of government policies regulating agricultural production to be able to make any constructive suggestions personally.

Table 8 Dietary measures to reduce the incidence of cancer

Measure	Type of cancer affected
reduce calorie intake	
to reduce obesity	gall bladder body of uterus
increase consumption of:	
fruit	stomach, possibly oesophagus
green vegetables	colon, rectum
fibre and resistant starch	colon, rectum

Other preventive measures

Two other practical means of prevention also depend largely on changes in personal behaviour, and the responsibility of oncologists and governments is principally to see that the public is informed of the nature and size of the specific hazards.

Exposure to ultraviolet light

I have referred earlier to the need for action by governments to prevent an increase in the risk of cancers due to an increased flux of ultraviolet light, but the increase in the incidence of melanoma that has occurred in all developed countries since the First World War must be attributed to the change in life style that has caused many people to expose untanned skin in a manner that was inconceivable at the beginning of the century. That ultraviolet light causes the easily curable squamous and basal cell carcinomas has long been obvious, but the fact that melanomas commonly occur in parts of the body that are rarely exposed to the sun, and that, in some countries, they tend to be more common in office workers than in outdoor workers, has made the relationship difficult to understand. It now seems, however, that the risk of melanoma is characteristically produced when the untanned skin is exposed to intensive radiation. Public education should, therefore, aim at encouraging indoor workers to use sunscreen ointments during periods of unusual exposure and not to sunbathe in the middle of the day when the ultraviolet flux is at its maximum.

Sexually transmitted diseases

Lastly, it is now widely appreciated that sexually transmitted viruses commonly initiate the lesions that precede and give rise to cancer of the cervix. It is gradually coming to be realized that the behaviour of the male is just as relevant to the spread of infection as the behaviour of the female, and that the types of cancer that these viruses may cause also include cancers of the penis and anus. Education, however, has so far failed to get across the prophylactic value of condoms, even though there is the added threat of infection with the human immunodeficiency virus (HIV). In the absence of a vaccine, the possibility of a government subsidy to reduce the cost of condoms may be worth consideration.

Research

In this brief review, I have said very little about occupational hazards or about cancers of the breast and prostate, which are two of the six most common lethal cancers in Europe. Occupational hazards, when known, have been controlled to different extents in different countries and it is to be hoped that the unification of Europe will level the standards of control upwards rather than down. It is doubtful, however, whether all such hazards have been detected, and there is a continuing need for industry to check that no hazard has been overlooked. That I have said very little about cancers of the breast and prostate is for the simple reason that we still know very little about their causation, and what we do know about the factors that affect the incidence of cancer of the breast (namely, age at menarche, nulliparity, age at first full-term delivery, and the use of oestrogens and oral contraceptives) does not offer any practicable means of control. The

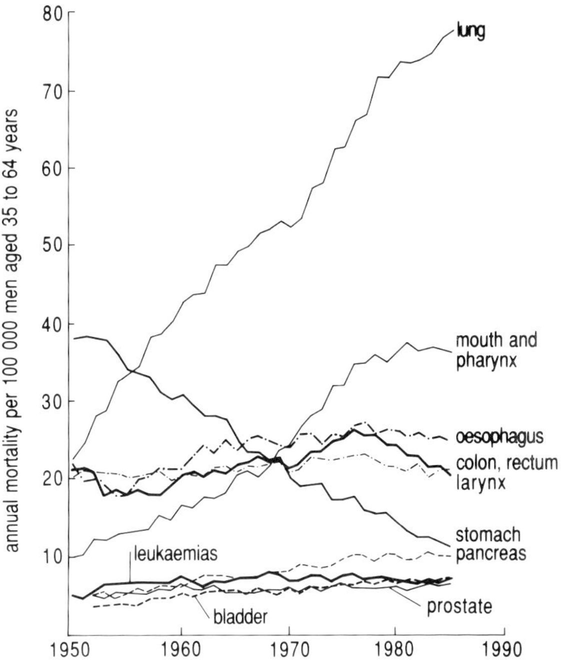

Figure 4 Trends in mortality from principal cancers in France: annual mortality per 100 000 men aged 35 to 64 years, standardized for age on the population of Europe (Hill *et al.*, 1988).

reasons for the variation in the incidence of both diseases in different communities, and for the small increases in mortality in recent years that have been attributed to them, are still largely, or in the case of cancer of the prostate completely, unknown. The only practical recommendation we can make, apart from the more widespread provision of mass mammography, is for support for further research into their aetiology.

Research is also urgently required into the causes of three other types of cancer that have become more common for unknown reasons, as the increases are presumably due to new agents or to new forms of behaviour that could be removed or altered, and which might cause major epidemics if their spread went unchecked. These are: cancer of the testis, which has become steadily more common throughout the developed world for the last 50 years; non-Hodgkin's lymphoma, which has doubled in incidence in many countries since the Second World War and has been attributed, in some studies, to chemicals used in agriculture and forestry; and cancers of the mouth and pharynx which, as Figure 4 shows (Hill *et al.*, 1988), have become very much more common in France. The last have increased to some extent in many countries due to an increased consumption of tobacco and alcohol but, unlike lung cancer, they are not specifically related to the consumption of cigarettes, and tobacco and alcohol alone are insufficient to account for the fourfold increase in mortality since 1950 that has been attributed to them.

Conclusion

Biological science, it is clear, still has much to do before cancer can be relegated to the position of a minor cause of death. It has, however, given us confidence that this is a reasonable objective and has pointed to fields where research might be hoped to provide quick returns. More importantly, it has already indicated the means by which mortality rates could be largely reduced. In a few cases these require government action to control hazards to which people are involuntarily exposed. In most, however, they depend on changes in personal behaviour that experience has shown are capable of being brought about. They cannot be forced, in any country in which I would like to live, but they can be assisted by government action after public education has made that action acceptable. By a combination of such means we could, I believe, reasonably expect to see the age-specific death rate from cancer halved over the next two or three decades.

References

Cantor, K.P., Hoover, R., Hartge, P., Mason, T.J., Silverman, D.T. *et al.* (1987) Bladder cancer, drinking water source, and tap-water consumption: a case-control study, *JNCI* **79**, 1269–79.

Doll, R. (1986a) *Possibilities for the Prevention of Cancer*, Royal Society, London.

Doll, R. (1986b) *Lung cancer: observed and expected changes in incidence from active and passive smoking*, proceedings of the 14th International Cancer Congress, Karger, Budapest.

Doll, R. (1988) Tobacco related disease, in *Tobacco or Health: the Way Ahead*, proceedings of the First European Conference on Tobacco Policy, Madrid, 7–11 November, 1988, WHO Regional Office for Europe, Copenhagen.

Fex, G., Pettersson, B., Akesson, B. (1987) Low plasma selenium as a risk factor for cancer death in middle-age men, *Nutr. Cancer* **10**, 221–29.

Garfinkel, L. and Stellman, S. D. (1988) Smoking and lung cancer in women: findings in a prospective survey, *Cancer Res.* **48**, 6951–55.

Goodwin, P. J. and Boyd, N. R. (1987) Critical appraisal of the evidence that dietary fat intake is related to breast cancer risk in humans, *JNCI* **79**, 473–85.

Hill, C., Benhamou, E., Doyon, F. and Flamant, R. (1988) *Evolution de la mortalité par cancer en France, entre 1950 et 1985*, Les Editions INSERM, Paris.

International Agency for Research on Cancer (1982) *Cancer Incidence in Five Continents*, vol. iv, J. Waterhouse, C. Muir, K. Shanmugaratriam, J. Powell (eds.) IARC, Lyon.

International Agency for Research on Cancer (1986) *IARC Monographs on the Evaluation of the Carcinogenic Risk of Chemicals to Humans: Tobacco Smoking*, IARC, Lyon.

International Agency for Research on Cancer (1989) *IARC Monographs on the Evaluation of the Carcinogenic Risk of Chemicals to Humans: Alcoholic Beverages*, IARC, Lyon (in press).

Jones, D. Y., Schatzkin, A., Green, S. B., Block, G., Brinton, L. A. *et al.* (1987) Dietary fat and breast cancer in the national health and nutrition examination survey: epidemiologic follow-up study, *JNCI* **79**, 465–71.

Knekt, P. (1988) Serum vitamin E level and risk of female cancers, *Int. J. Epidemiol.* **17**, 281–86.

Knekt, P., Aromaa, A., Maatela, J., Ritva-Kaarina, A., Nikkari, T. *et al.* (1988) Serum vitamin E and risk of cancer among Finnish men during a 10-year follow-up, *Am. J. Epidemiol.* **127**, 28–41.

Kok, F. J., de Bruijn, A. M., Hofman, A., Vermeeren, R., Valkenburg, H. A. (1987a) Is serum selenium a risk factor for cancer in men only? *Am. J. Epidemiol.* **125**, 12–16.

Kok, F. J., van Duijn, C. M., Hofman, A., Vermeeren, R., de Bruijn, A. M. *et al.* (1987b) Micronutrients and the risk of lung cancer, *New Engl. J. Med.* **316**, 1416.

Lubin, J. H., Blot, W. J., Berrino, F., Flamant, R., Gillis, C.R. *et al.* (1984) Patterns of lung cancer according to type of cigarette smoked, *Int. J. Cancer* **33**, 569–76.

Menkes, M. S., Comstock, G. W., Vuilleumier, J. P., Helsing, K. J., Rider, A. A. *et al.* (1986) Serum beta-carotene, vitamins A and E. selenium, and the risk of lung cancer, *New Engl. J. Med.* **315**, 1250–54.

Nomura, A., Heilbrun, L. K., Morris, J. S., Stemmermann, G. N. (1987) Serum selenium and the risk of cancer, by specific sites: case-control analysis of prospective data, *JNCI* **79**, 103–8.

Nomura, A., Stemmermann, G. N., Heilbrun, L. K., Salkeld, R. M., Vuilleumier, J. P. (1985) Serum vitamin levels and the risk of cancer of specific sites in men of Japanese ancestry in Hawaii, *Cancer Res.* **45**, 2369–72.

Peto, R. (1988) The future effects caused by smoking, in *Tobacco or Health: the Way Ahead*, proceedings of the First European Conference on Tobacco Policy, Madrid, 7–11 November, 1988, WHO Regional Office for Europe, Copenhagen.

Salonen, J. T., Salonen, R., Lappeteläinen, R., Mäenpää, P. H., Alfthan, G. *et al.* (1985) Risk of cancer in relation to serum concentrations of selenium and vitamins A and E: matched case-control analysis of prospective data, *Brit. Med. J.* **290**, 417–20.

Schober, S. E., Comstock, G. W., Helsing, K. J. et al. (1987) Serologic precursors of cancer, I, Prediagnostic serum nutrients and colon cancer risk, *Am. J. Epidemiol.* **126**, 1033–41.

Stahelin, H. B., Rosel, R., Buess, E., Brubacher, G. (1984) Cancer, vitamins, and plasma lipids: prospective Basel study, *JNCI* **73**, 1463–68.

Stampfer, M. J., Buring, J. E., Willett, W., Rosner, B., Berlein, K. (1985) The 2 x 2 factorial design: its application to a randomized trial of aspirin and carotene in US physicians, *Stats. in Med.* **4**, 111–16.

Stich, H. F., Rosin, M. P., Hornby, A. F., Mathew, B., Sankaranarayanan, R. *et al.* (1988) Remission of oral leukoplakias and micronuclei in tobacco/betel quid chewers treated with beta-carotene and with betacarotene plus vitamin A, *Int. J .Cancer* **42**, 195–99.

Surgeon General (1989) *Reducing the Health Consequences of Smoking: 25 Years of Progress*, Report of the Surgeon General, 1989, US Department of Health and Human Services, Maryland.

United Nations Scientific Committee on the Effects of Atomic Radiation (1988) *Sources, Effects and Risks of Ionizing Radiation*, United Nations, New York.

US National Research Council (1982) *Diet, Nutrition and Cancer*, National Academy Press, Washington, D.C.

Virtamo, J., Valkeila, E., Alfthan, G., Punsar, S., Huttunen, J. K. et al. (1987) Serum selenium and risk of cancer, a prospective follow-up of nine years, *Cancer* **60**, 145–48.

Wald, N. J., Boreham, J., Hayward, J. L., Bulbrook, R. D. (1984) Plasma retinol, beta-carotene and vitamin E levels in relation to the future risk of breast cancer, *Brit. J. Cancer* **49**, 321–24.

Wald, N. J., Thompson, S. G., Densem, J. W., Boreham, J., Bailey, A. (1987a) Serum vitamin E and subsequent risk of cancer, *Br. J. Cancer* **56**, 69–72.

Wald, N. J., Thompson, S. G., Densem, J. W., Boreham, J., Bailey, A. (1987b) Serum beta-carotene and subsequent risk from cancer: results from the BUPA study, *Br. J. Cancer* **57**, 428–33.

Willett, W. C., Polk, F., Underwood, B. A., Stampfer, M. J., Pressel, S. *et al* (1984) Relation of serum vitamins A and E and carotenoids to risk of cancer, *New Engl. J. Med.* **310**, 430–34.

Willett, W. C., Stampfer, M. J., Colditz, G. A., Rosner, B. A., Hennekens, C. H. et al (1987) Dietary fat and the risk of breast cancer, *New Engl. J. Med.* **316**, 22–28.

Chapter 2

CURRENT KNOWLEDGE ABOUT CANCER PREVENTION

Summary

Cancer experts from the fields of epidemiology, health education and medicine met in four parallel working groups at the Colloquium in order to review each of the major cancers that currently affect Europeans. Their recommendations concerning primary and secondary prevention strategies and key research areas for the future have been re-analyzed for this chapter, and are grouped according to principal causes. The discussion is presented as a commentary on the Ten Points of the European Code Against Cancer.

Paper 2.1: *The Cancer Burden with Special Reference to Europe and the EC Countries* Dr. Calum Muir

Paper 2.2: *Radiation and Cancer: Overview and Implications for Prevention* Dr. Elisabeth Cardis and Dr. John Kaldor

Paper 2.3: *The Role of Occupation in the Causation of Cancer and its Prevention* Dr. Elsebeth Lynge

Paper 2.4: *Diet and Cancer: A Sobering Look* Dr. Eyvind Thorling

Paper 2.5: *Cancer Prevention and the New Biology* Dr. Graham Currie

Introduction

Action is urgently needed if the European Commission's target is to be met of reducing mortality from cancers in member states by 15 per cent by the year 2000. The paper by Muir (Paper 2.1) predicts that the total burden of cancers in EC member states will *rise* by the year 2000, even though certain specific cancers are declining in prevalence. The background papers (some of which are reproduced at the end of this chapter) and the working group discussions concluded that immediate progress could be made in reducing the incidence of several types of cancer by disseminating and explaining the ten points of the European Code Against Cancer.

However, it was recognized that the Code is aimed at educating *individuals* about positive action to reduce their cancer risks. In addition, other initiatives and strategies should also be incorporated into a coordinated European approach to cancer prevention. Such a programme would have the following features:

A. Governments, businesses, health policy makers, health care workers and educators, as well as the lay population of EC member states, require more detailed information about the causes of particular cancers and hence the most effective strategies for prevention.

B. Areas of uncertainty about the effectiveness of certain strategies should not be concealed. Neither should these uncertainties immobilize us from taking positive steps to ensure that the best information and advice currently available is disseminated to all the groups listed in A, even if that advice requires modification in the future.

C. Research is urgently needed to overcome the lack of very basic knowledge in many areas of molecular biology, medical oncology and epidemiology. In particular, we need to know more about the natural history of cancer development, the carcinogenicity of certain compounds and energy sources, and the efficacy of preventive strategies.

The Keynote Address by Professor Sir Richard Doll stresses the preventability of most cancers. The variation in the incidence of specific cancers between and within European countries (as elsewhere in the world) is reviewed by Muir (Paper 2.1), and gives reason for optimism that avoidable causes could be identified in addition to those for which causality has already been established. However, it is essential that all members of the European Community develop compatible systems of data collection to ensure that cancer registration and mortality statistics are complete and comparable across member states.

The discussion papers and the consensus statements from the four working groups who reviewed the current state of knowledge about cancer prevention provide a fund of information about present and future policy directions. In addition to the papers circulated at the Colloquium, the editors of this book have commissioned a paper on the current state of knowledge about cancer biology, with particular emphasis on the contribution that advances in molecular genetics and genetic engineering may have on the preventability of cancers in the future (Currie, Paper 2.5).

Smoking-related cancers

Point 1 of the European Code Against Cancer states:

DO NOT SMOKE.

SMOKERS, STOP AS QUICKLY AS POSSIBLE AND DO NOT SMOKE IN THE PRESENCE OF OTHERS.

Sir Richard Doll points to the 'epidemic of cancer caused by smoking' that has occurred in every country in Europe (Keynote Address). Data reported by Muir (Paper 2.1) show that, in the male population of the whole of Europe, lung cancer is the most common malignancy and cancer of the bladder is among the five most common cancers. In Northern European women, lung cancer ranks third in frequency, although it is not yet in the five commonest cancers in Southern Europe. It has been calculated that 400 000 Europeans currently die from smoking-related cancers every year (Peto, 1988).

Doll's public lecture to the Royal Society of London (1986) places the problem of smoking-related cancers at the top of the list of priorities for cancer prevention in the whole of the industrialized world:

> when tobacco is smoked it is responsible for the vast majority of all cancers of the lung throughout the world. ... Moreover, when chewed, it is responsible for the vast majority of the cancers of the mouth that are common throughout much of South East Asia.

Several participants in the discussion emphasized the worrying increase in smoking-related cancers among young people and in particular among young women, and pointed to the rising tide of lung cancer in developing countries such as China.

The Lisbon Colloquium reached widespread agreement that tobacco products are the most prevalent source of carcinogens in Europe and the most clearly proven primary or contributory cause of several major lethal cancers. A reduction in smoking rates could be expected to have a major impact on death rates from cancers of the lung and upper respiratory tract, the bladder and kidney and the oesophagus. Other sites may also be affected to a lesser degree, for example, the pancreas and the uterine cervix.

Primary prevention strategies are, without doubt, those that enable current smokers to quit smoking and reduce the numbers of people who start smoking. Help should be targeted particularly at young people in all member states and at women (at least in Northern Europe). Strategies for the primary prevention of smoking-related cancers are discussed in more detail in later chapters of this book, but a few key points can be stated briefly here.

Effective education programmes are needed urgently, especially in schools and other settings where young people meet. Quit-smoking clinics must be adequately funded and supported. Action could be taken at government level to reduce the direct and indirect advertising of tobacco products (note, for example, that in the UK in the financial year from 1987–88, the tobacco companies spent almost £6 million on sports sponsorship, according to government figures.) Taxation on tobacco could be regulated to act more effectively as a disincentive to smoke, or to change over to a brand with a lower tar content. In addition, action should be taken to reduce passive smoking—that is, exposure of non-smokers to smoke in enclosed spaces such as workplaces, public buildings and on public transport—and to raise awareness of the dangers of passive smoking to children in domestic situations.

Secondary prevention strategies pose a far greater problem, since currently available screening methods for early detection of most smoking-related cancers are either inadequate or are rendered inappropriate because of the lack of effective treatments. Screening programmes for lung cancers have been abandoned because their effect was simply to bring forward the date of diagnosis without altering the date of death. However, some progress may be made in the early detection of bladder cancer, but further evaluation is necessary. Oral cancers might be detected earlier if better training in surveillance techniques is offered to dentists.

Key recommendations for research focused on the need for:

• basic research into the natural history of lung cancers. Efforts to intervene through early detection and effective treatment are hampered by lack of knowledge about the delay between the first exposure to a carcinogen and the transformation of lung cells to the malignant state, and about the subsequent delay (if any) before metastasis occurs.

• thorough evaluation of currently available cytology screening methods for early detection of bladder cancers.

• development of new screening methods for early detection of cancers. Examples currently under investigation include the use of monoclonal antibodies as diagnostic tools, or the detection of genetic lesions or cancer-related proteins in the body fluids of those at risk (see Currie, Paper 2.5, for a review of progress in this field).

• clarification at the molecular and the epidemiological level of the interaction between carcinogens in tobacco and other primary carcinogens, such as alcohol, radiation, arsenic, asbestos, aromatic amines, etc.

• identification of factors that promote or enhance the progression of smoking-related cancers, possibly derived from elements in the diet.

Alcohol-related cancers

Point 2 of the European Code Against Cancer states:

MODERATE YOUR CONSUMPTION OF ALCOHOLIC DRINKS, BEERS, WINES OR SPIRITS.

Excessive intake of alcohol is considered by Doll (Keynote Address) to be 'second only in importance to smoking as a proven cause of cancer in Europe'. Alcohol is clearly implicated either as the primary carcinogen, or in concert with smoking, as a cause of cancers of the upper respiratory tract, oesophagus and liver, and may contribute to the incidence of cancers of the breast and rectum.

Like tobacco, the use of alcohol is strongly influenced by cultural factors, which complicate attempts to change patterns of consumption. The association of alcohol with certain cancers is not so widely known as the association between lung cancer and tobacco, and this may partly explain why there has not been a reduction in the higher rates of consumption even in European countries where tobacco use is declining in certain sections of the population.

Primary prevention strategies are, without doubt, to enable individuals to moderate their intake of alcohol. Advice about safe limits on alcohol consumption should be clearly stated; dissatisfaction was expressed by some participants in the Lisbon working groups that the European Code simply exhorted alcohol drinkers to *moderate* their consumption. Nonspecific advice is easy to ignore if a person considers that their alcohol consumption is already, in cultural terms, moderate and therefore acceptable, when it may in fact be hazardous to health. Individuals must also be made far more aware of the significant interaction between alcohol and smoking in cancer causation.

Secondary prevention strategies currently face the same problems as those described above for smoking-related cancers. Early detection methods for cancers of the mouth, oesophagus and liver are currently either non-existent or inadequate. Patients frequently present with advanced disease for which there is no effective treatment.

Key recommendations for research focused on:

- major gaps in current knowledge about how alcohol may exert its carcinogenic effect given the very weak carcinogenicity of alcohol in experimental animals in contrast to its effect in humans (Doll, Keynote Address).
- interaction with other carcinogens, principally those derived from tobacco. Thorling (Paper 2.4) reports the suggestion that alcohol may act as a solvent for other carcinogens.
- investigation of the rising trend in liver cancer incidence in Scandinavian countries. Further epidemiological research is needed to evaluate whether this trend is due to rising alcohol consumption or is an artefact of better rates of diagnosis and reporting.
- better evaluation of the 'safe limits' on alcohol consumption for individuals; for example, we need to know more about the effect of body weight and the effect of consistency of consumption (i.e. is it more harmful to drink a small number of alcohol units every day for prolonged periods, or the same number of units in a single day once a week?)
- improving knowledge about alcohol addiction and about educational strategies aimed at helping 'social' drinkers to reduce their consumption to a safe level.

Ultraviolet radiation and skin cancers

Point 3 of the European Code Against Cancer states:

AVOID EXCESSIVE EXPOSURE TO THE SUN.

The incidence of malignant melanoma has increased in the northern hemisphere more than 600 times since 1935. The dramatic recent trend in one part of Northern Europe is illustrated in Figure 2.1. The rising trend may be attributed to changes in the life style of Caucasians who now frequently expose themselves to intermittent periods of sunburning radiation. This view is borne out by the relationship between age at registration and per cent change in incidence. Young adults—who have the spending power to afford yearly or twice-yearly holidays in Southern Europe—show a marked increase in incidence over recent decades.

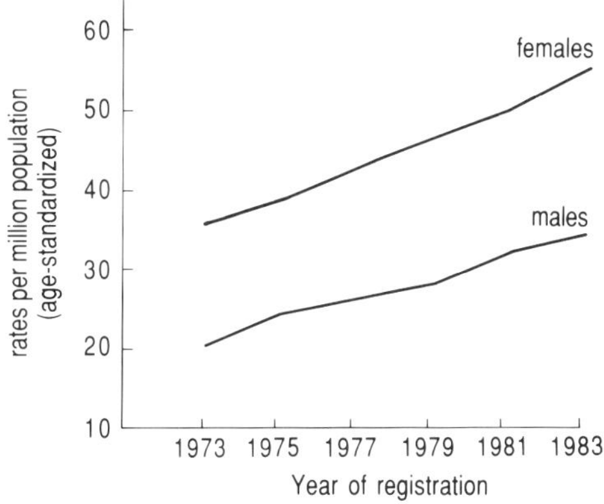

Figure 2.1 The rising trend in incidence rates of malignant melanoma in England and Wales, 1973–1983, age-standardized (Cancer Research Campaign, 1987).

Cardis and Kaldor (Paper 2.2) review the sources of ultraviolet radiation and their effects on the incidence of skin cancers, particularly malignant melanoma. They stress the difficulties in interpreting the results of epidemiological research into sunbathing and melanoma induction, a point made also by Doll (Keynote Address). Currie (Paper 2.5) reminds us that the transformation of melanocytes to malignancy may require only one or two genetic lesions to be inflicted on the cell, in contrast to the multi-stage process required for malignant transformation in many other cancers. This may explain, in part, the prevalence of this cancer in younger age groups.

Primary prevention strategies are, without doubt, to recommend moderation in exposure to ultraviolet radiation, the use of protective creams and, in particular, the avoidance of intermittent sunburning. This advice should be targeted effectively at fair-skinned Northern Europeans, in particular those who work indoors for most of the year. We must avoid giving unnecessary alarm to outdoor workers, who seem to be at lower risk than indoor workers in some countries, possibly due to the regularity of their exposure to ultraviolet radiation.

In the Keynote Address, Doll takes the issue of primary prevention on to the global stage. He draws attention to increases in exposure to ultraviolet radiation that may occur as a result of damage to the ozone layer by avoidable chemical pollution, particularly from the burning of fossil fuels and the release of chlorofluorocarbon compounds (CFCs).

Secondary prevention strategies are referred to in point 7 of the European Code Against Cancer, which states:

SEE A DOCTOR IF YOU NOTICE A LUMP OR OBSERVE A CHANGE IN A MOLE OR ABNORMAL BLEEDING.

More information should be given to individuals about the changes to moles that require a medical check. In addition, screening is recommended in high-risk families where hereditary predisposing factors exist; this policy might increase the curability of melanomas that are detected early (see Currie, Paper 2.5).

Key recommendations for research focused on:

- quantifying the risks to individuals of different skin types and with different patterns of exposure.

- evaluating the effectiveness of sunscreen creams in preventing skin cancers.

Occupational carcinogens

Point 4 of the European Code Against Cancer states:

FOLLOW HEALTH AND SAFETY INSTRUCTIONS, ESPECIALLY IN THE WORKING ENVIRONMENT, CONCERNING PRODUCTION, HANDLING OR USE OF ANY SUBSTANCE WHICH MAY CAUSE CANCER.

The working group discussions of occupational carcinogens tended to stress the obligation of the employer (rather than the worker) to protect the workforce by provision of a safe working environment, adequate education about hazards and safe working practices, correct labelling of carcinogens and immediate action to curtail any breaches in safety. Exposure to sources of ionizing radiation at work are reviewed by Cardis and Kaldor (Paper 2.2) and Lynge offers a comprehensive discussion of chemical carcinogens in occupational settings (Paper 2.3).

Cancers for which rates are known to be affected by occupational exposures to radiation and to chemical carcinogens are primarily those of the upper respiratory tract, the lung, thorax, bladder, and the leukaemias.

A relatively small proportion of these cancers are primarily caused by occupational exposures, although occupational carcinogens may interact with other causal factors (for example, tobacco smoke) to elevate incidence rates. However, although the contribution of occupational exposures to national cancer mortality rates may be very small, it can be *locally* very significant.

Exposure to occupational carcinogens over a prolonged period may be necessary to cause malignant transformation. Any reduction in sources of carcinogens *currently* contaminating the workplace can only be expected to reduce mortality rates in the *next* generation of workers. Therefore, it is unrealistic to expect that there will be a 15 per cent reduction in the incidence of occupationally related cancers by the year 2000.

Lynge (Paper 2.3) makes the additional point that the workplace may also contribute *indirectly* to cancer causation, for example through exposure of workers to tobacco smoke, to an unhealthy diet in canteens, and via sedentary working practices. The contribution of workplace environments to cancer risks is discussed at length in Chapter 5 of this book.

Primary prevention strategies should focus on reducing the use of carcinogens where possible—Doll points out that safe alternatives may not exist (Keynote Address)—and reducing the exposure of workers to carcinogens that remain in production. A consistent labelling policy should be implemented so that workers are adequately warned of the hazards to which they may be exposed. At present, there are still inconsistencies in labelling practice, which may compromise the effectiveness of workplace safety measures.

Secondary prevention strategies involve regular screening of all at-risk workers for early detection of occupational cancers, where suitable screening methods exist. Accidental exposures must be followed up rigorously to evaluate their long-term effects on cancer rates. Data should be collected about high-risk workers long after they have left the workforce.

Key recommendations for research focused on:

- identification of new carcinogens and further research on the effects of those we already know about.
- developing adequate screening methods to detect workers who have been exposed to carcinogens (molecular biology is expected to supply new methods for detecting carcinogen-induced genetic damage in the near future; see Currie, Paper 2.5).
- the continued evaluation of safety limits on exposure levels.

Diet-related cancers

Points 5 and 6 of the European Code Against Cancer state:

FREQUENTLY EAT FRESH FRUITS AND VEGETABLES AND CEREALS WITH A HIGH FIBRE CONTENT.

AVOID BECOMING OVERWEIGHT AND LIMIT YOUR INTAKE OF FATTY FOODS.

This is the area of most uncertainty in current knowledge about the prevention of cancers. Two papers emphasize the central paradox of diet-related cancers (see Doll, Keynote Address, and Thorling, Paper 2.4)—namely, that epidemiological evidence points overwhelmingly to diet as a major factor in cancer causation, but we are far from certain about precisely which elements of the diet are implicated in which cancers. Moreover, certain elements of the diet may be protective against certain cancers, but again the evidence is indirect or inconclusive. Research findings have often been shown to be contradictory, and there is considerable dispute between experts on the value of reducing certain components (for example, salt, saccharin, nitrates, smoked food and even saturated fats) or increasing others (for example, beta-carotene, selenium and vitamin E).

However, the data available indicate that a diet that is high in fibre and low in certain fats could be expected to have a beneficial impact on the incidence of cancers of the colon and rectum, the breast, stomach (and possibly also) the body of the uterus, the prostate and the lung (although the reduction in lung cancers is likely to be very small).

Obesity is implicated by epidemiological evidence in cancers of the breast and uterus. The cancers listed above are among the most common in most European countries (see Muir, Paper 2.1). Breast cancer is the most common cancer among women in all parts of Europe, and mortality has shown a consistently rising trend in recent decades, as Figure 2.2 illustrates. Similar mortality trends have been demonstrated for older women.

The trend in incidence of cancer of the prostate is also rising throughout Europe and it ranks third or fourth in frequency in male cancer rates (Muir, Paper 2.1). The strong association between trends in the incidence of breast cancer and prostate cancer strengthen the possibility that there is some common causal factor, such as fat intake. However, Doll (Keynote Address) refers to two recent studies

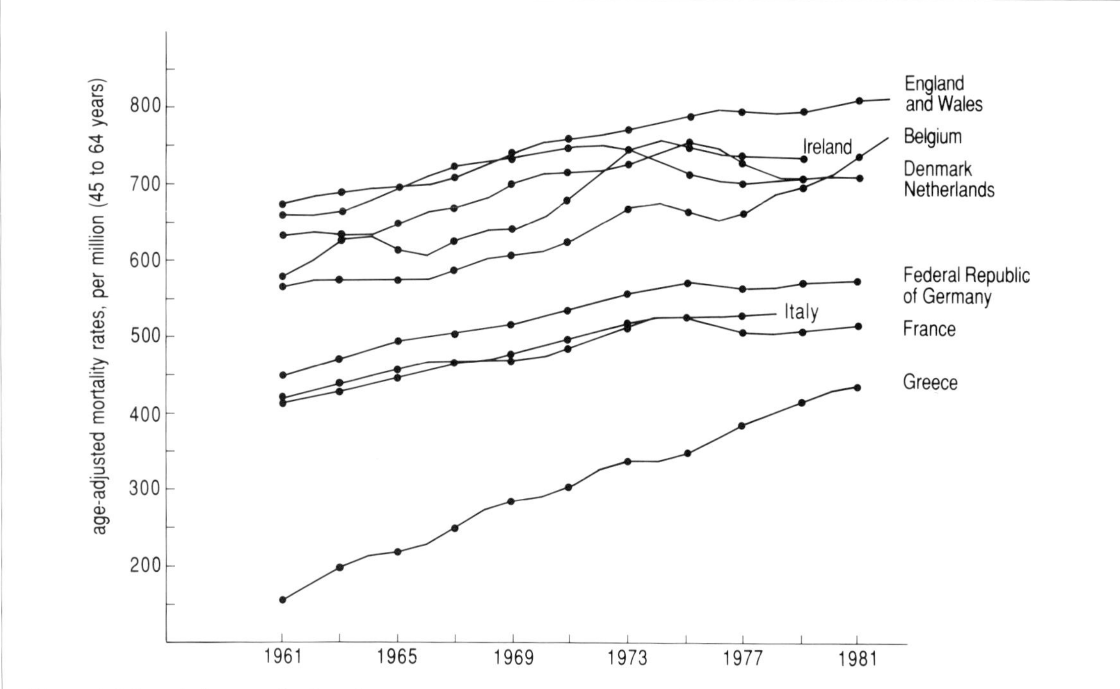

Figure 2.2 Trends in mortality from breast cancer among women aged 45 to 64 years in nine European countries; age-adjusted death rates per million (Joossens and Geboers, 1984).

in the USA, which failed to find an association between fat consumption and the incidence of breast cancer.

By contrast, the incidence of cancer of the body of the uterus has undergone a marked decline (see Figure 2.3), although it still ranks in frequency in the top five cancers among Southern European women (Muir, Paper 2.1).

Primary prevention strategies for diet-related cancers are, at present, restricted to making suitable recommendations about a healthy diet and about avoiding obesity. Specific recommendations about diet in relation to cancer prevention are premature in the view of most—but not all—participants to the discussion. Fortunately, the recommendations for a healthy diet, as opposed to one that is aimed specifically at reducing cancers, are consistent with the recommendations of the European Code.

More detailed dietary recommendations are given in the consensus statement emerging from the European conference in Århus, Denmark in 1985 (quoted by Thorling, Paper 2.4). Such a diet is also recommended for the reduction of cardiovascular disease, maturity-onset diabetes and non-malignant conditions of the alimentary tract, such as diverticular disease and ulcerative colitis. We may therefore advocate increasing the fibre content of the diet, particularly by the consumption of fruits, vegetables and cereals, and reducing the total intake of fats to an agreed level without fear of causing harm and in the expectation of doing good. Similarly, we may freely advertise the importance of avoiding obesity, whatever its dietary cause.

However, particular aspects of the European Code's recommendations for cancer prevention aroused debate in the working groups. For example, a minority of participants felt strongly that the Code should recommend limiting the intake of *salt*. Others were unhappy with the wording relating to *fresh* fruits and vegetables; it was argued that an increase in the intake of frozen or tinned fruits and vegetables would not only be beneficial, but more available to large sections of the population whose access to fresh produce is restricted by geography or

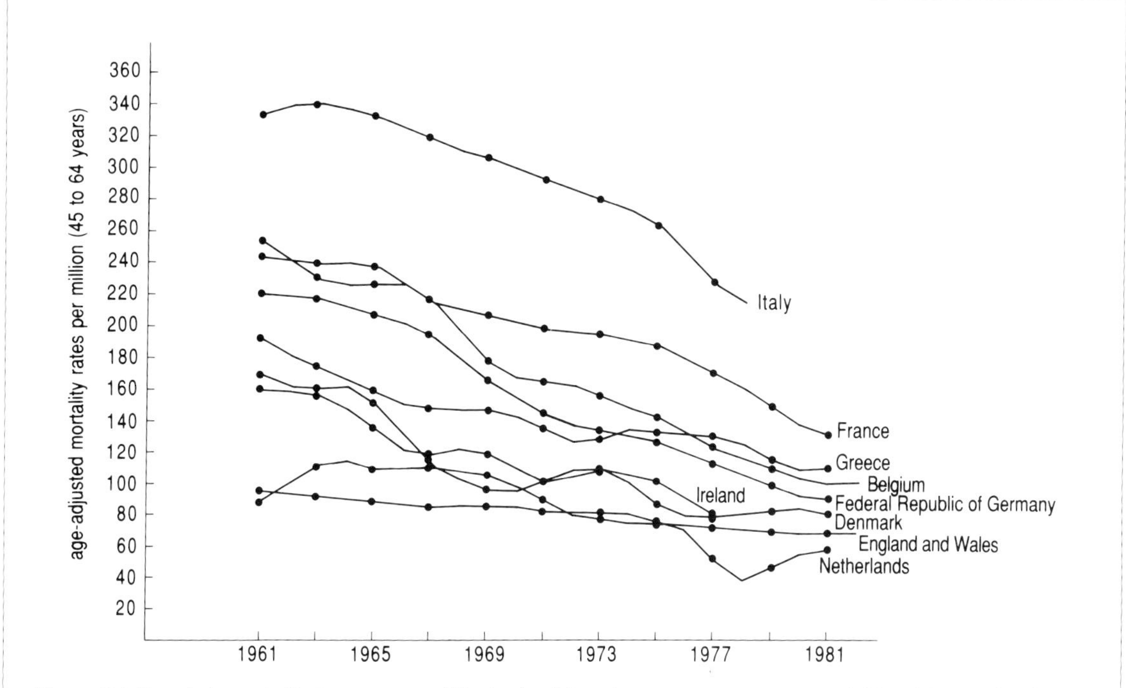

Figure 2.3 Trends in mortality from cancer of the body of the uterus among women aged 45 to 64 years in nine European countries; age-adjusted death rates per million (Joossens and Geboers, 1984).

price. Several contributors wanted more detail to be given about the meaning of *fatty foods*, since the data about saturated and even polyunsaturated fats is equivocal. Moreover, the fat intake of the population in southern European countries is overwhelmingly poly- or mono-unsaturated (principally, olive oil); there is no evidence to suggest that this should be reduced. In this context, obesity or total calorie intake may be more important than the elements of the diet that contribute to it.

In addition, a sedentary life style may contribute to the incidence of cancer of the colon and, indirectly by promoting obesity, to cancers of the breast and uterus. Therefore, the advocacy of regular exercise may be beneficial in preventing certain cancers and is consistent with general health messages.

Secondary prevention strategies involve recommendations relating to specific cancers:

• screening for early detection of breast cancer by mammography in women over 50 years of age, and (with far less agreement) the education of women in the technique of breast self-examination or regular palpation by a physician. These recommendations are consistent with point 10 of the European Code, which states:

CHECK YOUR BREASTS REGULARLY AND, IF POSSIBLE, UNDERGO MAMMOGRAPHY AT REGULAR INTERVALS ABOVE THE AGE OF 50.

However, the emphasis placed by the Code on breast self-examination was the subject of an unresolved debate.

• screening for early detection of cancers of the colon should be undertaken in high-risk families or individuals, i.e. those with a history of familial polyposis or ulcerative colitis. More widespread screening for colorectal cancers by detecting occult blood in stool samples was also advocated by some participants and is currently being evaluated in several major trials.

• the unopposed use of oestrogens for treatment of menopausal symptoms should be avoided where possible. Similarly, prolonged use of high-dose, oestrogen-based contraceptives is not recommended in younger women. The contribution of hormone status to the incidence of these cancers is accepted, at least for some women, and there may be an interaction between dietary and hormonal factors.

Key recommendations for research focused on the following:

- resolution of major uncertainties about the biochemical and physiological mechanisms by which dietary factors or obesity might exert an effect on cancer rates. The current state of knowledge about causal mechanisms is reviewed briefly by Thorling (Paper 2.4).

- clarification of the multi-stage nature of the malignant transformation in diet-related cancers (see Currie, Paper 2.5, for a discussion of sequential lesions in the aetiology of colorectal cancers).

- the interaction of diet, obesity and hormone levels with particular respect to cancers of the breast, uterus and (possibly) the prostate. Thorling (Paper 2.4) refers to the association between the age of menarche, menopause and first childbirth with the incidence of breast cancer.

- evaluating the contribution of a sedentary life style to cancer rates.

- investigating the age relationship with fat intake; participants were intrigued by data reported verbally at the Colloquium by Dr. Berrino that there may be a 'window' around the years of menarche in which the level of fat intake might correlate with the incidence of breast cancer in later life.

- evaluating the possible protective effect of certain dietary factors (such as selenium or vitamin E) and of certain life-style factors (such as breast feeding and regular exercise).

- evaluating the long-term consequences on mortality from breast cancer of regular breast self-examination, or palpation by a physician, and the psychological and financial costs of extensive screening by mammography.

Virus-related cancers

Cancers for which there is good evidence of a viral aetiology are rare in Europe, but represent a major health problem in other parts of the world. Doll (Keynote Address) mentions liver cancer caused by hepatitis B virus (HBV) in the Gambia and Far East; Burkitt's lymphoma caused by Epstein–Barr virus (EBV) in Africa; and nasopharyngeal cancer in China, also caused by EBV. Currie (Paper 2.5) adds T cell leukaemia caused by HTLV-1 in the Caribbean and rural Japan. Currie describes the biological mechanisms by which cancer-causing viruses are thought to exert their malignant effect on cells and discusses the development of genetically engineered vaccines in the future.

Both Doll and Currie refer to the far greater impact that could be expected on European cancer rates if a vaccine against human papilloma virus (HPV) could be developed. Although the evidence for an involvement of HPV in cancers of the cervix, vulva, penis, anus and possibly certain skin cancers is not conclusive, it is nonetheless compelling. Cancer of the uterine cervix ranks fifth in incidence among cancers developed by women in Southern Europe (Muir, Paper 2.1). Although trends in mortality have been falling in some Northern European countries during recent decades (for example, Denmark), they have risen in others (for example, Greece), as Figure 2.4 shows.

The influence on mortality rates of screening programmes for the early detection of pre-cancerous and malignant changes in the cervix is, as yet, unclear in many European countries. Currie (Paper 2.5) points to the future impact of molecular biology on cervical cytology screening, which could be made far more systematic if the detection of genetic lesions caused by HPV were incorporated into the screening test.

Primary prevention strategies aimed at reducing the incidence of cervical cancer should involve the education of young people of both sexes about the likelihood that it is (at least partly) due to a sexually transmitted infection. Therefore, recommendations about 'safer sex' currently being promoted in relation to HIV infection (i.e. reduction in numbers of sexual partners and the use of barrier methods of contraception), might also reduce the incidence of cervical cancer in future generations.

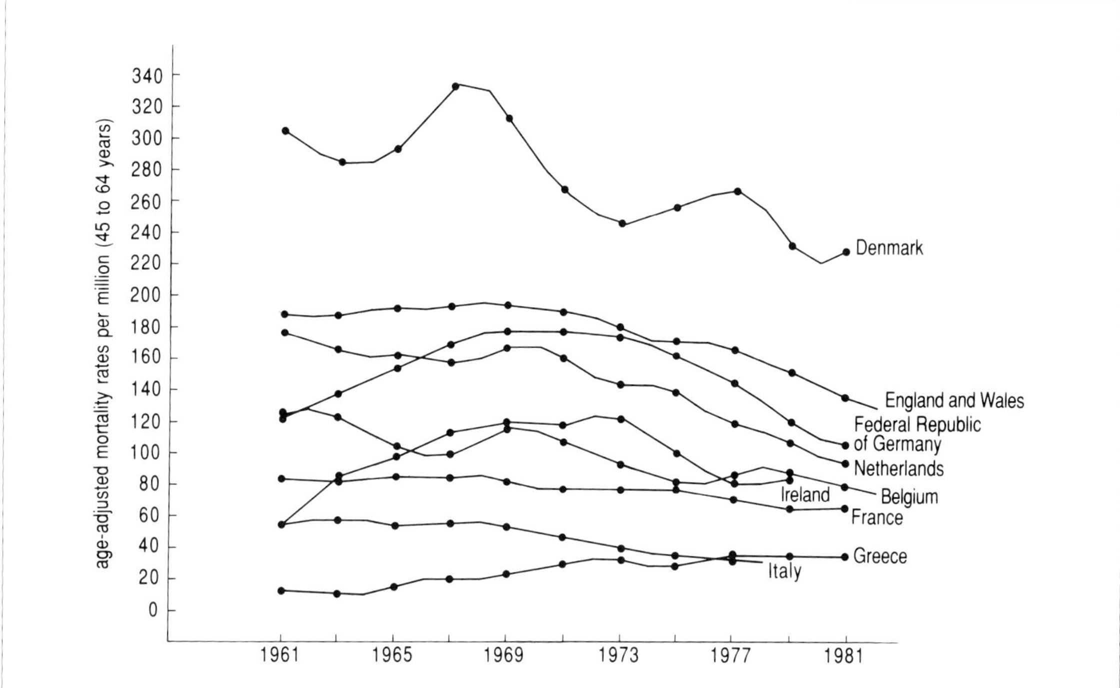

Figure 2.4 Trends in mortality from cancer of the uterine cervix in nine European countries among women aged 45 to 64 years; age-adjusted death rates per million (Joossens and Geboers, 1984).

Secondary prevention strategies aimed at reducing the incidence of cervical cancer are, without doubt, the recommendation contained in point 9 of the European Code Against Cancer, which states that women should:

HAVE A CERVICAL SMEAR REGULARLY.

However, the view was expressed that the wording of the Code should specify a lower age limit for screening, i.e. *after the age of 25 years*. Moreover, the availability and reliability of the screening test must be improved and systematic invitation and recall methods must be applied across the whole population at risk.

Key recommendations for research focused on:

- the development of a vaccine with protective effect against HPV and its evaluation in cancer prevention trials.
- better evaluation of the diagnostic value of colposcopy.
- better identification and evaluation of behavioural factors in the aetiology of cancers of the cervix (and possibly also the penis). In particular, interest was expressed in epidemiological evidence from the UK showing a possible link between husband's occupation in certain trades with increased rates of cervical cancer in their wives (Office of Population Censuses and Surveys, 1986). This effect *may* be mediated by the sexual behaviour of men whose work takes them away from home for days at a time, but it may also indicate that a carcinogen is being transported home from work. Other studies have shown stronger associations between smoking rates (Trevathan *et al.*, 1983) and the use of oestrogen-based contraceptive pills independently of sexual behaviour (Vessey *et al.*, 1983) in the aetiology of cervical cancer. These factors require further investigation.

Radiation-induced cancers

Cancers induced or promoted by occupational exposures to ionizing radiation were mentioned earlier in this chapter, but exposures at the workplace are insufficient to account for the rates of several cancers in Europe that are known to be affected by radiation. Radiation-induced cancers are reviewed by Cardis and Kaldor (Paper 2.2) and include cancers of the lung, breast, thyroid, gastrointestinal tract, liver, bone, and the leukaemias.

The major sources of ionizing radiation in the environment are naturally occurring and are often difficult to eliminate (see Figure 2.5). However, exposures arising from medical diagnosis and treatment, the nuclear industries, from the explosion of nuclear weapons or plants and from radon gas collecting in houses could be reduced. A significant contribution to lung cancer rates from exposure to radon gas has been claimed in a recent report in the UK (National Radiological Protection Board, 1988).

Primary prevention strategies should focus on reducing avoidable exposures to ionizing radiation, especially those caused by a build-up of radon gas in particular houses (Doll, Keynote Address). The case was argued that the radiation protection boards have set adequate standards for safe limits on exposures and have rigorously enforced them over many years; we must be vigilant in maintaining those standards against economic pressures to reduce them.

Secondary prevention strategies There is nothing to add to the recommendations made earlier in this chapter for the secondary prevention of specific cancers in the list of those to which radiation may contribute.

Key recommendations for research focused on:

• clarification of the molecular biology of radiation-induced lesions in DNA and the consequences of this for malignant transformation. Currie (Paper 2.5) reviews current knowledge and the prospects for DNA repair techniques in the future.

Cancers for which causal factors are in serious doubt

There was general agreement that there are very serious gaps in current knowledge about the aetiology of cancers of the prostate, ovary, testis and stomach, despite evidence that dietary factors may be associated with prostatic and stomach cancers (see earlier discussion). Therefore, no recommendations for primary or secondary prevention strategies can yet be made.

Key recommendations for research focused on:

• detailed investigation of the molecular biology of these cancers (see the discussion of oncogenes by Currie, Paper 2.5).

• further epidemiological investigation to ascertain why rates of stomach cancer are decreasing in all countries in the absence of

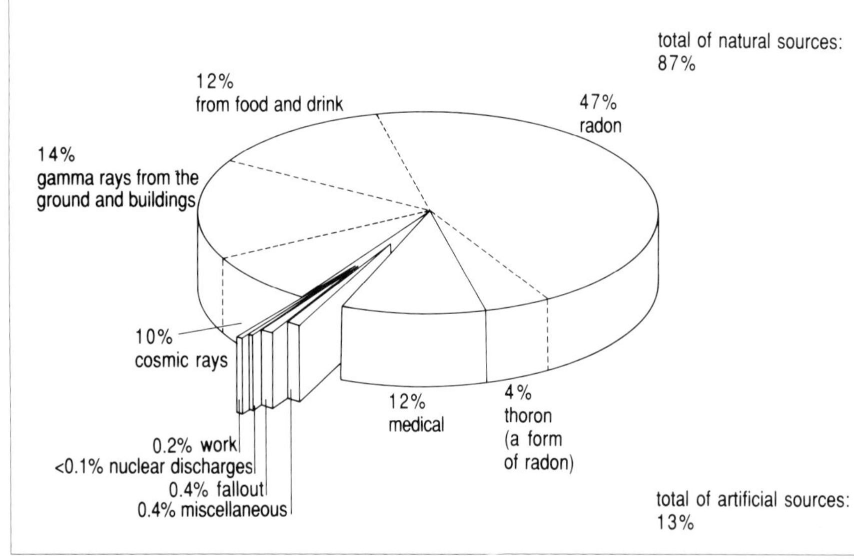

Figure 2.5 Sources of radiation exposure in the UK population, 1988 (based on data supplied by the National Radiological Protection Board).

any planned intervention and, conversely, why rates of cancer of the testis are increasing.

- evaluation of the effectiveness of screening for cancer of the prostate, but no intervention should currently be made outside a properly controlled trial.

Conclusion

The knowledge that is currently available about the causation of cancers is adequate to make a major impact on mortality rates in Europe. Despite the very great need for further research at even the most basic level, we could begin to reduce deaths from cancers of the lung, upper respiratory and gastrointestinal tract, bladder, kidney, breast, cervix and liver, by implementing the recommendations reported above for primary and secondary prevention strategies. Such a goal has been within our grasp for many years, since none of the key data are new. The central problem remains to persuade governments, businesses, health workers, educators, lay and voluntary organizations, local communities and individuals that cancers can be prevented on a massive scale by the actions that we could take now.

References

Cancer Research Campaign (1987) *Malignant Melanoma*, Factsheet No. 4.1; **2**, Carlton House Terrace, London SW1Y 5AR.

Doll, R. (1986) Possibilities for the Prevention of Cancer, Lecture for the Public given at the Royal Society of London, 13 November 1986.

Joossens, J.V. and Geboers, J. (1984) Epidemiological and mortality trends of sex-related cancers, in *Hormones and Sexual Factors in Human Cancer Aetiology*, J.-P. Wolff and J. S. Scott (eds.), Elsevier Science Publishers, Barking, Essex, UK.

National Radiological Protection Board (1988) *Radiation Exposure of the UK Population - 1988 Review*, HMSO, London, UK.

Office of Population Censuses and Surveys (1986) *Occupational Mortality, 1979–1980, 1982–83*, HMSO, London, UK.

Peto, R. (1988) The future effects caused by smoking, in *Tobacco or Health: the Way Ahead*, proceedings of the First European Conference on Tobacco Policy, Madrid 7–11 November, 1988, WHO Regional Office for Europe, Copenhagen.

Trevathan, E., Layde, P., Webster, L.A., Adams, J. B. and Benigno, B. B. (1983) Cigarette smoking and dysplasia and carcinoma in situ of the uterine cervix, *J. Am. Med. Assoc.*, **250**, 499–502.

Vessey, M.P., Lawless, M., McPherson, K. and Yeats, D. (1983) Neoplasia of the uterine cervix and contraception: a possible adverse effect of the pill, *Lancet*, **2**, 930–934.

Paper 2.1

THE CANCER BURDEN WITH SPECIAL REFERENCE TO EUROPE AND THE EC COUNTRIES

Dr. Calum Muir
International Agency for Research on Cancer, Lyon, France

Leading cancer sites

Estimates of the burden of cancer in Europe and other parts of the world in 1980 have recently been published by Parkin *et al.* (1988). These estimates, based on a variety of sources, were presented for the 24 demographic regions recognized by the United Nations. As far as Europe is concerned, these regions are: Western Europe (Austria, *Belgium*, *France*, *Federal Republic of Germany*, *Luxembourg*, *Netherlands*, Switzerland); Southern Europe (Albania, *Greece*, *Italy*, Malta, *Portugal*, *Spain*, Yugoslavia); Northern Europe (*Denmark*, Finland, Iceland, *Ireland*, Norway, Sweden, *United Kingdom of Great Britain and Northern Ireland*); and Eastern Europe (Bulgaria, Czechoslovakia, German Democratic Republic, Hungary, Poland, Romania). EC countries (those in italics) are thus to be found in all but Eastern Europe.

The rank orders are given in Tables 2.1 and 2.2: the principal sites of cancer in males are lung, stomach and colon-rectum in Eastern and Southern Europe; and lung, colon-rectum and prostate in Northern and Western Europe; in females, breast, colon-rectum and stomach occupy the first three places in rank order, with lung displacing stomach to fourth rank in Northern Europe. The 'top five' sites account for about 60 per cent of all cancers in each of the four regions of Europe.

Table 2.1 The most frequent cancers in Northern and Southern Europe around 1980*

Northern Europe	Sex	Rank	Site	No. (000)	%	Southern Europe	Sex	Rank	Site	No. (000)	%
	Males	1	Lung	39.4	27.0		Males	1	Lung	43.8	19.9
		2	Colon/Rectum	18.7	12.8			2	Stomach	29.0	13.2
		3	Prostate	17.7	12.1			3	Colon/Rectum	23.1	10.5
		4	Stomach	11.3	7.8			4	Prostate	19.5	8.9
		5	Bladder	10.5	7.2			5	Bladder	16.1	7.3
			Total:		66.9**				Total:		59.8**
	Females	1	Breast	35.4	24.7		Females	1	Breast	45.2	24.8
		2	Colon/Rectum	20.4	14.2			2	Colon/Rectum	21.4	11.7
		3	Lung	12.4	8.6			3	Stomach	19.2	10.5
		4	Stomach	7.6	5.3			4	Corpus uteri	13.1	7.2
		5	Ovary	7.6	5.3			5	Cervix	8.4	4.6
			Total:		58.1**				Total:		58.8**

* Source: Parkin *et al.*, 1988 ** Percentage of all cancers

Table 2.2 The most frequent cancers in Western and Eastern Europe around 1980*

Western Europe	Sex	Rank	Site	No. (000)	%	Eastern Europe	Sex	Rank	Site	No. (000)	%
	Males	1	Lung	64.5	23.2		**Males**	1	Lung	32.6	25.2
		2	Colon/Rectum	36.6	13.2			2	Stomach	19.4	15.0
		3	Prostate	31.6	11.4			3	Colon/Rectum	12.6	9.7
		4	Bladder	18.3	6.6			4	Prostate	9.3	7.2
		5	Oral	17.7	6.4			5	Bladder	6.4	4.9
			Total:		60.8**				Total:		62.0**
	Females	1	Breast	68.4	26.1		**Females**	1	Breast	23.3	19.6
		2	Colon/Rectum	39.2	15.0			2	Colon/Rectum	13.0	10.9
		3	Stomach	16.5	6.3			3	Stomach	12.0	10.1
		4	Corpus uteri	16.1	6.1			4	Cervixi	11.7	9.8
		5	Cervix	15.4	6.1			5	Corpus uteri	7.6	6.4
			Total:		59.6**				Total:		56.8**

* Source: Parkin *et al.*, 1988 ** Percentage of all cancers

Table 2.3 gives the burden of cancer for Northern, Southern, and Western Europe for the major sites. For completeness and contrast, combined data for the six countries of Eastern Europe are also provided.

Table 2.3 Estimated numbers of new cancer cases (thousands) in 1980, by site, sex and area*

ICD code**		All cancers	**140–149**		**150**		**151**		**153–154**		**155**	
Region		No.	No.	%	No.	%	No.	%	No.	%	No.	%
Northern Europe	Male	145.8	3.8	2.6	3.2	2.2	11.3	7.8	18.7	12.8	1.3	0.9
	Female	143.4	1.9	1.3	2.4	1.7	7.6	5.3	20.4	14.2	1.0	0.7
	Both	289.2	5.7	2.0	5.6	1.9	18.9	6.5	39.1	13.5	2.3	0.8
Southern Europe	Male	219.8	12.4	5.6	4.7	2.1	29.0	13.2	23.1	10.5	5.5	2.5
	Female	182.4	2.1	1.2	0.9	0.5	19.2	10.5	21.4	11.7	4.1	2.2
	Both	402.2	14.5	3.6	5.6	1.4	48.2	12.0	44.5	11.1	9.6	2.4
Western Europe	Male	278.3	17.7	6.4	8.2	2.9	21.1	7.6	36.6	13.2	4.0	1.4
	Female	261.9	3.1	1.2	1.5	0.6	16.5	6.3	39.2	15.0	2.1	0.8
	Both	540.2	20.8	3.9	9.7	1.8	37.6	7.0	75.8	14.0	6.1	1.1
Eastern Europe	Male	129.3	6.4	4.9	1.8	1.4	19.4	15.0	12.6	9.7	3.7	2.9
	Female	119.1	1.7	1.4	0.4	0.3	12.0	10.1	13.0	10.9	2.8	2.4
	Both	248.4	8.1	3.3	2.2	0.9	31.4	12.6	25.6	10.3	6.5	2.6

Table 2.3 (continued) Estimated numbers of new cancer cases (thousands) in 1980, by site, sex and area*

ICD code**		161		162		174		180		182	
Region		No.	%	No.	%	No.	%	No.	%	No.	%
Northern Europe	Male	2.3	1.6	39.4	27.0	–	–	–	–	–	–
	Female	0.5	0.3	12.4	8.6	35.4	24.7	6.4	4.5	6.4	4.5
	Both	2.8	1.0	51.8	17.9	35.4	12.2	6.4	2.2	6.4	2.2
Southern Europe	Male	10.8	4.9	43.8	19.9	–	–	–	–	–	–
	Female	0.6	0.3	6.3	3.5	45.2	24.8	8.4	4.6	13.1	7.2
	Both	11.4	2.8	50.1	12.5	45.2	11.2	8.4	2.1	13.1	3.3
Western Europe	Male	7.4	2.7	64.5	23.2	–	–	–	–	–	–
	Female	0.7	0.3	9.7	3.7	68.4	12.7	15.4	2.9	16.1	6.1
	Both	8.1	1.5	74.2	13.7	68.4	12.7	15.4	2.9	16.1	3.0
Eastern Europe	Male	5.4	4.2	32.6	35.2	–	–	–	–	–	–
	Female	0.4	0.3	5.7	4.8	23.3	19.6	11.7	9.8	7.6	6.4
	Both	5.8	2.3	38.3	15.4	23.3	9.4	11.7	4.7	7.6	3.1

Table 2.3 (continued) Estimated numbers of new cancer cases (thousands) in 1980, by site, sex and area*

ICD code**		183		185		188		202–203		204–208	
Region		No.	%	No.	%	No.	%	No.	%	No.	%
Northern Europe	Male	–	–	17.7	12.1	10.5	7.2	6.3	4.3	3.8	2.6
	Female	7.6	5.3	–	–	3.9	2.7	5.5	3.8	3.1	2.2
	Both	7.6	2.6	17.7	6.1	14.4	5.0	11.8	4.1	6.9	2.4
Southern Europe	Male	–	–	19.5	8.9	16.1	7.3	8.9	4.0	6.3	2.9
	Female	7.8	4.3	–	–	3.4	1.9	6.2	3.4	5.2	2.9
	Both	7.8	1.9	19.5	4.8	19.5	4.8	15.1	3.8	11.5	2.9
Western Europe	Male	–	–	31.6	11.4	18.3	6.6	9.4	3.4	6.9	2.5
	Female	12.7	4.8	–	–	5.3	2.0	8.4	3.2	6.2	2.4
	Both	12.7	2.4	31.6	5.8	23.6	4.4	17.8	3.3	13.1	2.4
Eastern Europe	Male	–	–	9.3	7.2	6.4	4.9	4.1	3.2	3.6	2.8
	Female	6.9	5.8	–	–	1.7	1.4	3.3	2.8	3.0	2.5
	Both	6.9	2.8	9.3	3.7	8.1	3.3	7.4	3.0	6.6	2.7

* Source: Parkin *et al.*, 1988

** The ICD codes are those of the 9th Revision of the International Classification of Diseases (WHO, 1977)

140–149 Oral cavity and pharynx
150 Oesophagus
151 Stomach
153–154 Colon and rectum
155 Liver
161 Larynx
162 Lung
174 Breast (females)
180 Cervix uteri
182 Corpus uteri
183 Ovary
185 Prostate
188 Bladder
202–203 Malignant lymphoma, myeloma
204–208 Leukaemia

Cancer mortality patterns in EC countries

Although the rank order of the major cancer sites is much the same—the first five accounting for about 60 per cent of all cancer (Tables 2.1 and 2.2)—the pattern of cancer mortality throughout Europe, which is likely to reflect incidence, is by no means uniform.

The International Agency for Research on Cancer has recently prepared a series of maps on the geographical distribution of cancer mortality, at statistical level 3, within the EC countries (for example, at the county level in England and Wales, and the Département level in France). Unfortunately, it is not yet possible to produce comparable mortality maps for the more recently joined EC members, namely, Greece, Portugal and Spain, nor for cancer incidence. Perusal of the maps for the common sites presented shows that there are very considerable differences in cancer mortality within the nine EC countries so mapped (see Figures 2.6 to 2.13). The data are age-standardized for the European population, 1970 to 1979, and the keys represent the level of mortality (vertical axis) and the number of areas that have that mortality (horizontal axis).

Some of the more striking differences are not readily explained. For example, why do the high levels of oesophageal cancer seen in north and western France cease abruptly at the Belgian border? It is highly unlikely that differences in diagnosis would account for such large differences in mortality in this generally fatal form of cancer. The reasons are likely to lie in differences in dietary habits (including alcohol and tobacco consumption), between the two countries. Hence the need for case-control and other analytical epidemiological studies to uncover the reasons.

Why oesophageal cancer should be more common in Irish and Scottish women than elsewhere again demands solution. While the large international differences in gastric cancer are worth pursuing, we need to know why this disease is so much more common in Bavaria than elsewhere in the Federal Republic of Germany. While there are international differences in breast-cancer level, within a country there is a considerable degree of uniformity, suggesting that the risk factors are characteristic for a nation and hence should be studied internationally to provide groups of contrasting risk.

Barriers to data utilization

Although there is national cancer registration for several of the countries in Europe, in others registration is either patchy or non-existent (for a detailed review, see Coleman and Démaret, 1988). The major barriers to cancer registration and to the use of the information to be derived from death certificates seem to lie in differing concepts of confidentiality. Although there has never been an example of breach of confidentiality by a cancer registry, the collection of incidence data and their utilization to throw light on the causes of cancer is effectively blocked in several European countries, including EC member states.

The future burden

Estimates can be made of the likely future cancer burden in Europe in the year 2000, taking into account increases in population size, projected by the UN Demographic Bureau (UN, 1986), the projected rise in average age and broad estimates of changes in risk (in both directions) derived from past cross-sectional and cohort time trends (Muir, 1989). These estimates are given in Table 2.4 for the common sites listed in Tables 2.1 and 2.2. It must be stressed that these projections for the period 1975 to 2000 are rather crude, and more refined figures will doubtless become available.

The projections of cancer burden by the year 2000 given in Table 2.4, while imprecise, are not likely to be too far wrong. While demographic forecasts are frequently incorrect, the errors usually occur for births, a portion of the age span with much less impact on cancer patterns than the proportion of the population aged 60 years and over.

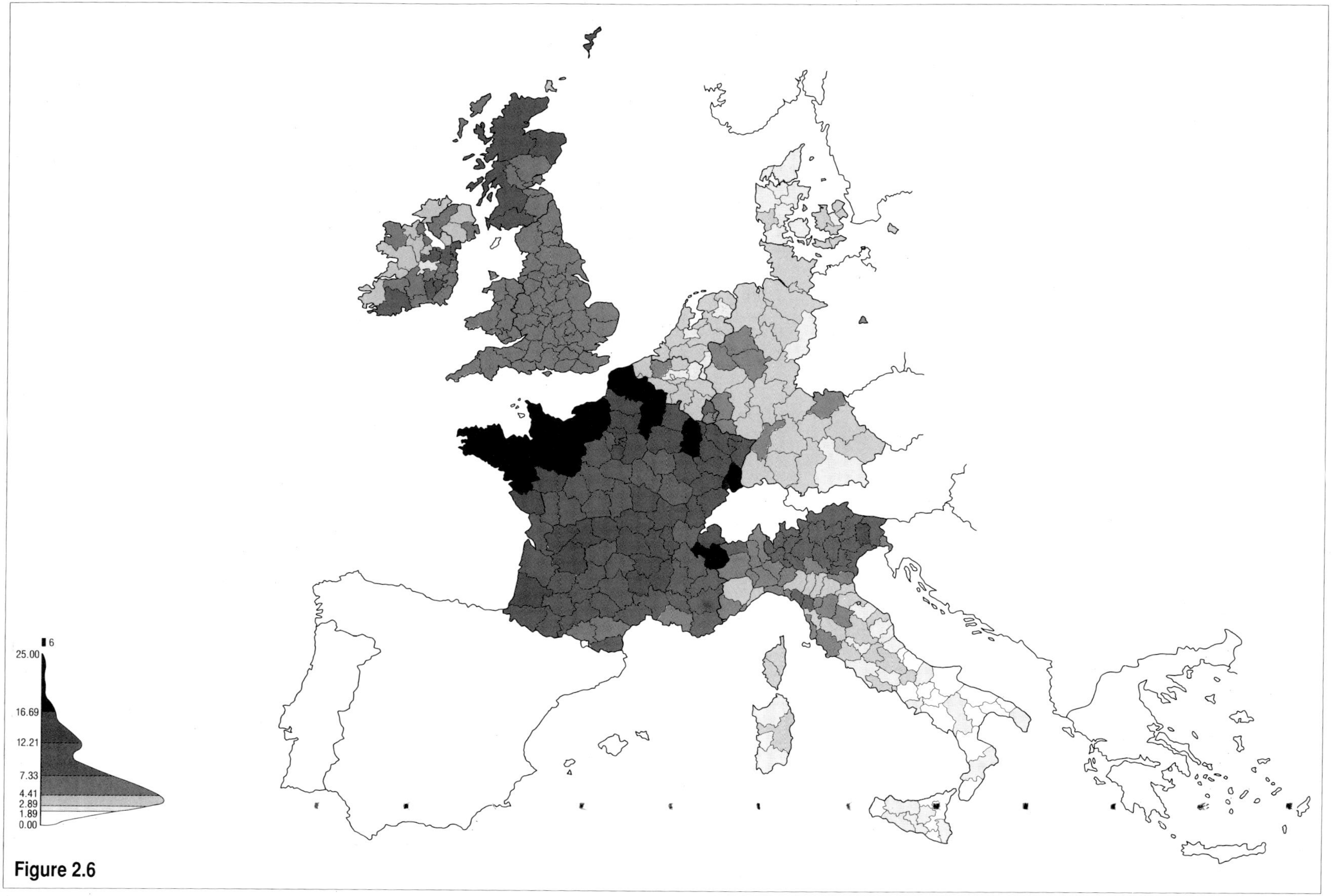

Figure 2.6

Mortality from cancer of the oesophagus in men

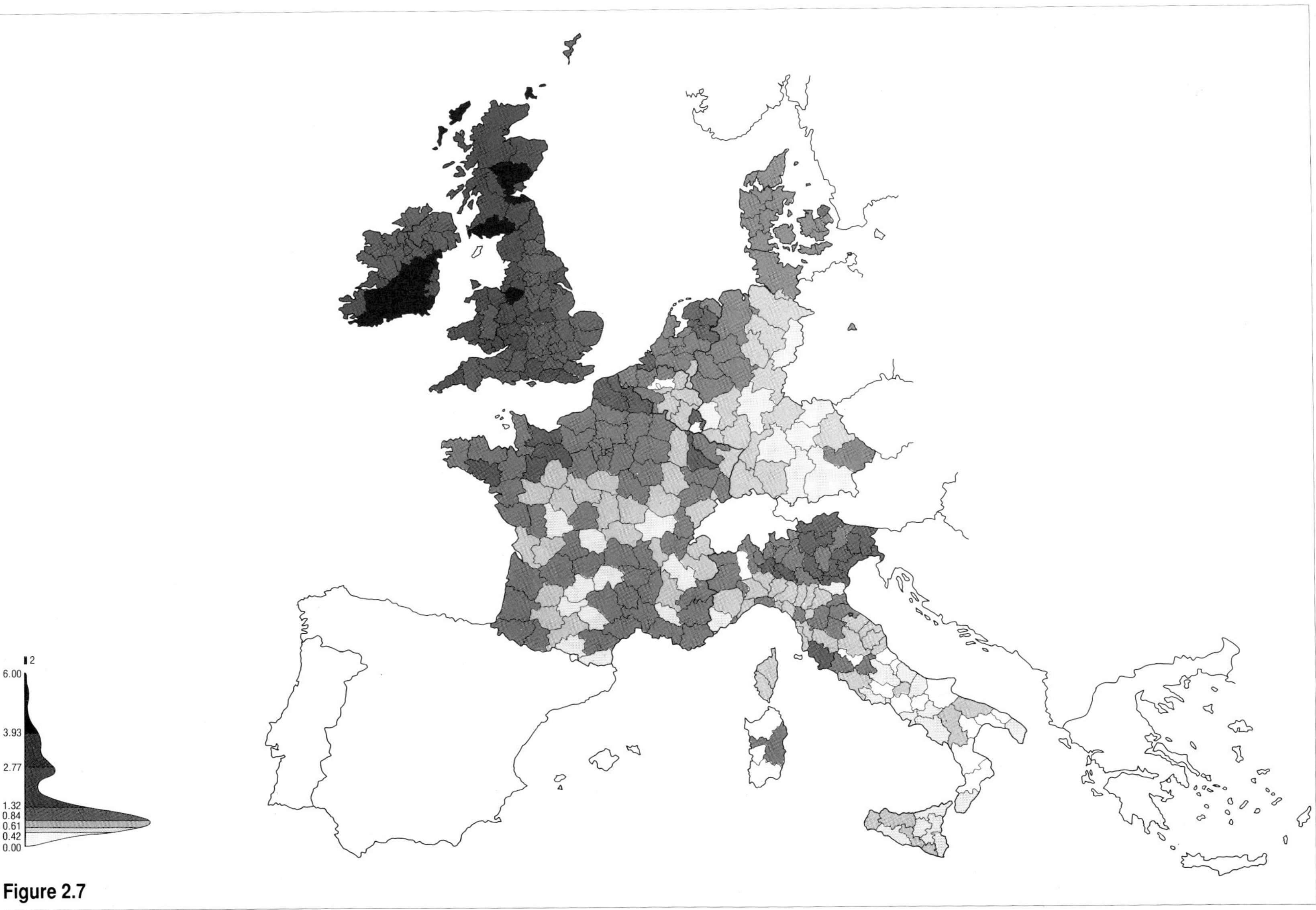

Figure 2.7

Mortality from cancer of the oesophagus in women

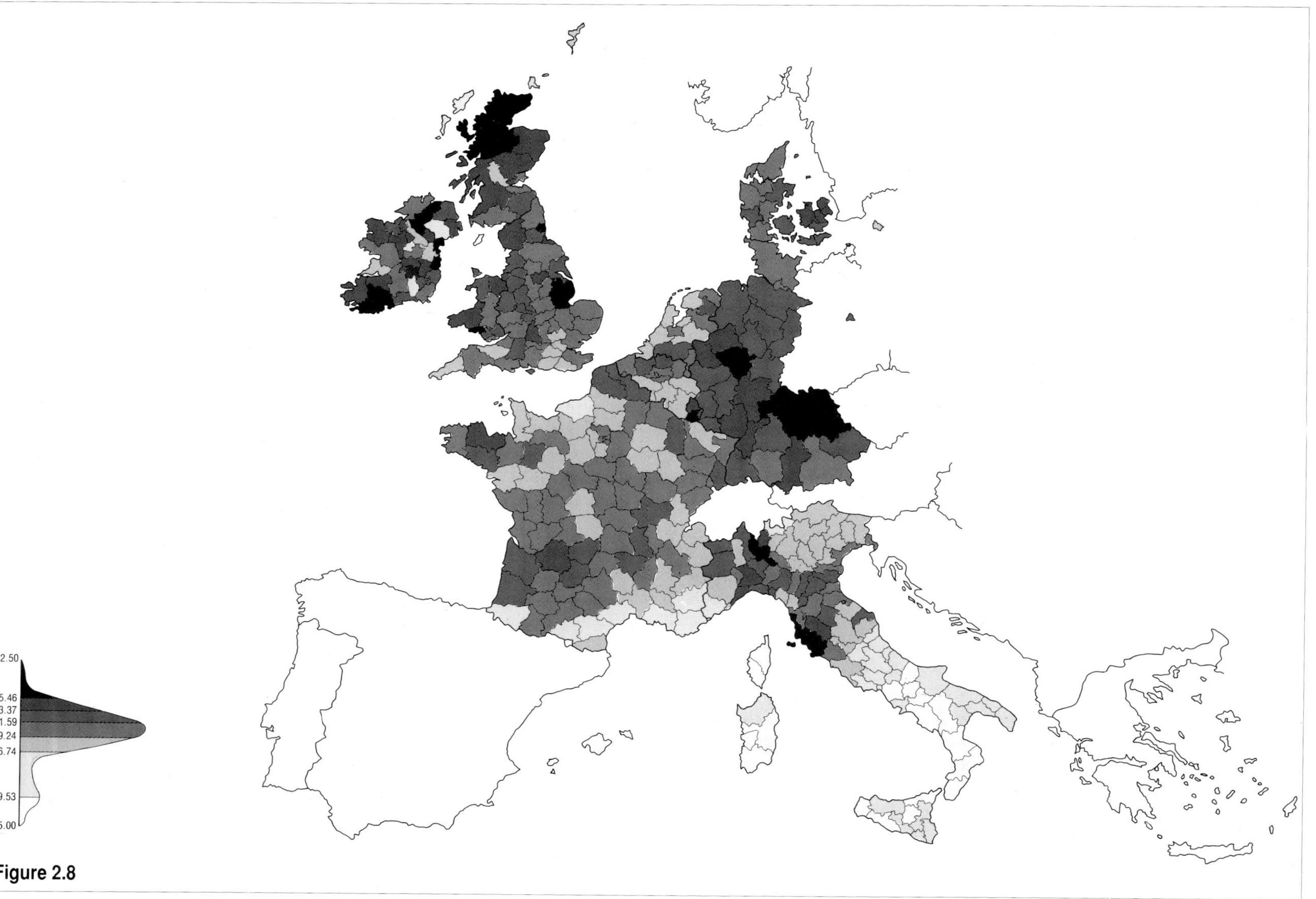

Figure 2.8

Mortality from cancer of the colon/rectum in men

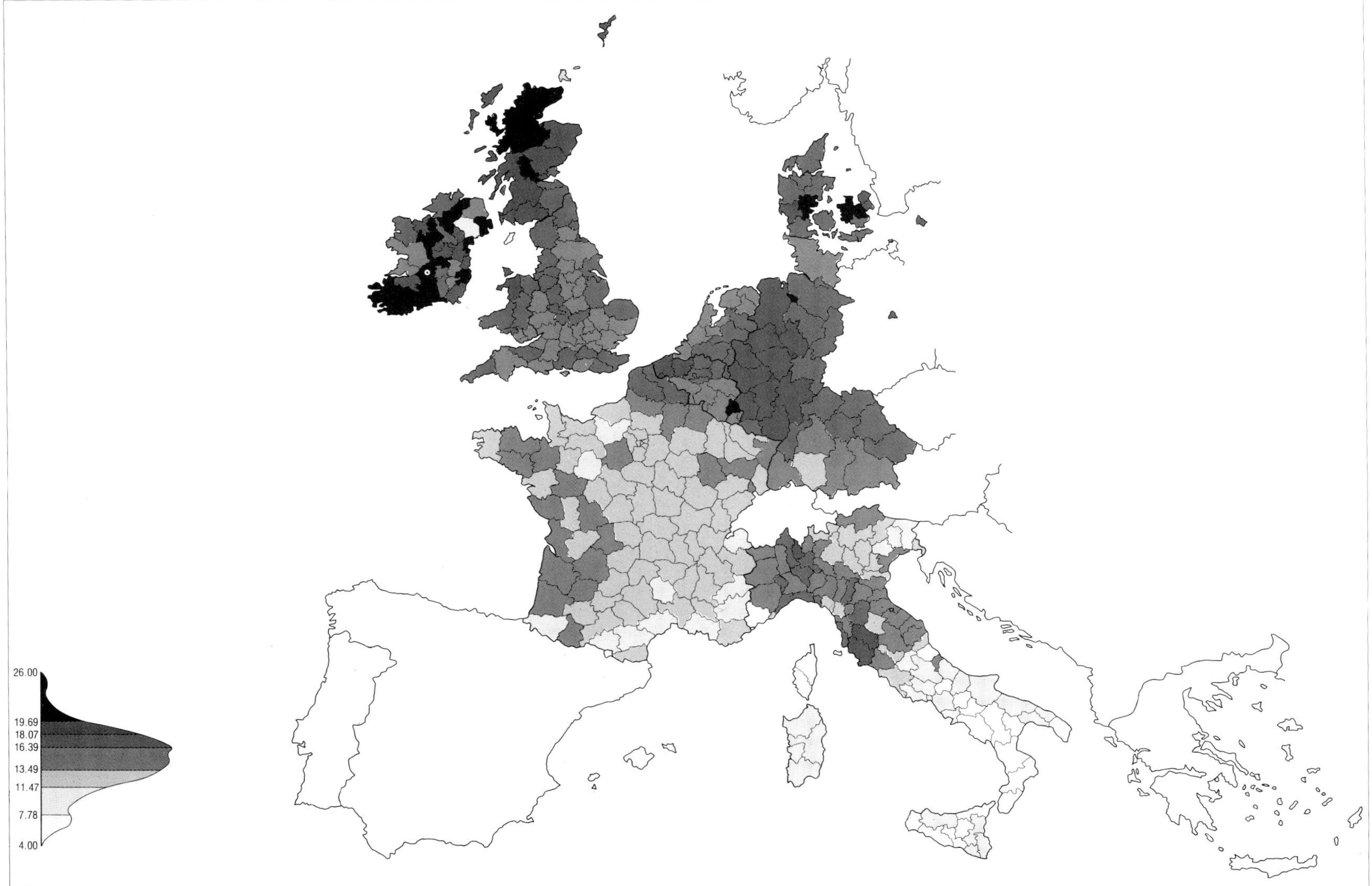

26.00
19.69
18.07
16.39
13.49
11.47
7.78
4.00

Figure 2.9

Mortality from cancer of the colon/rectum in women

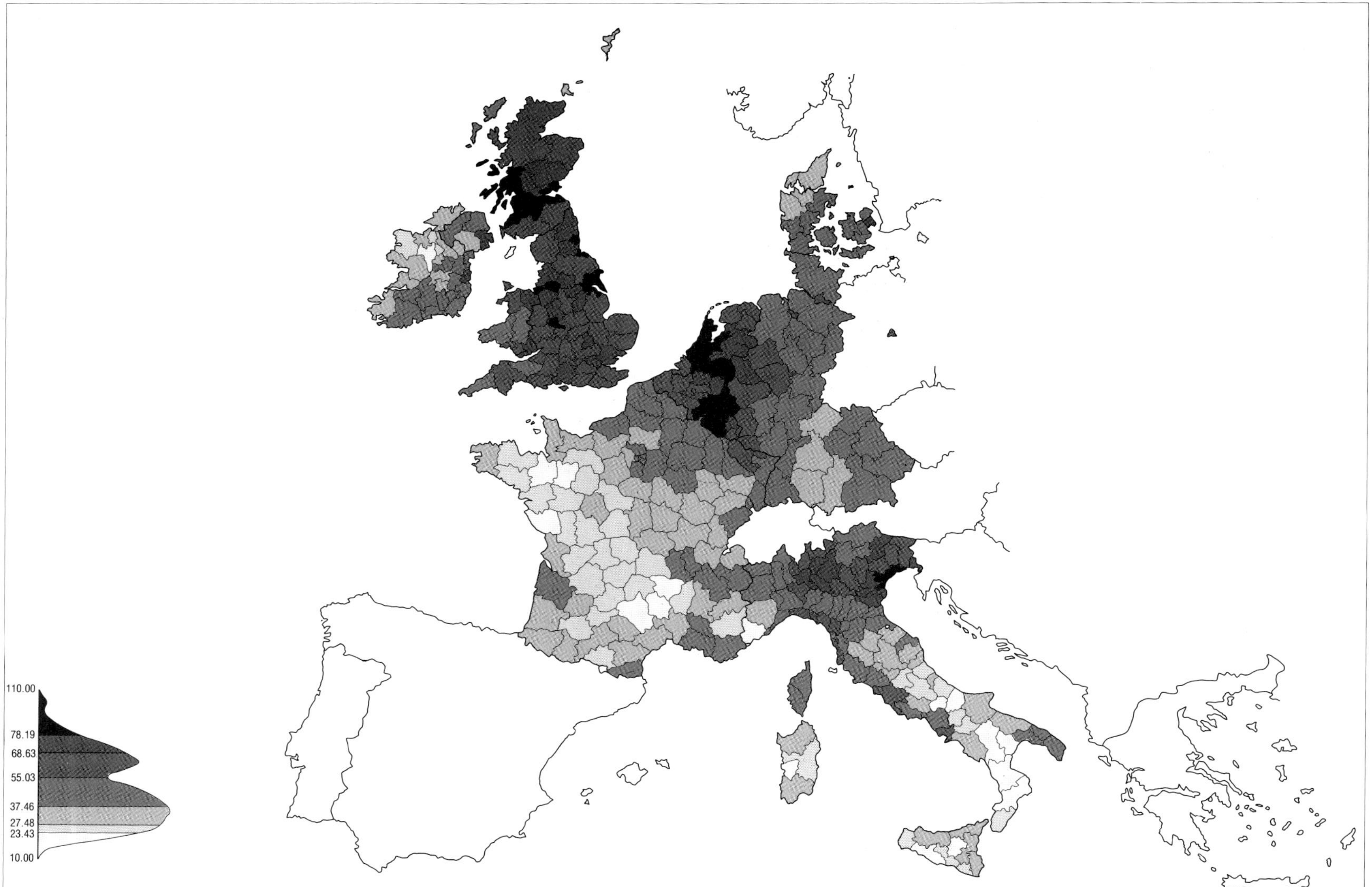

Figure 2.10

Mortality from cancer of the lung in men

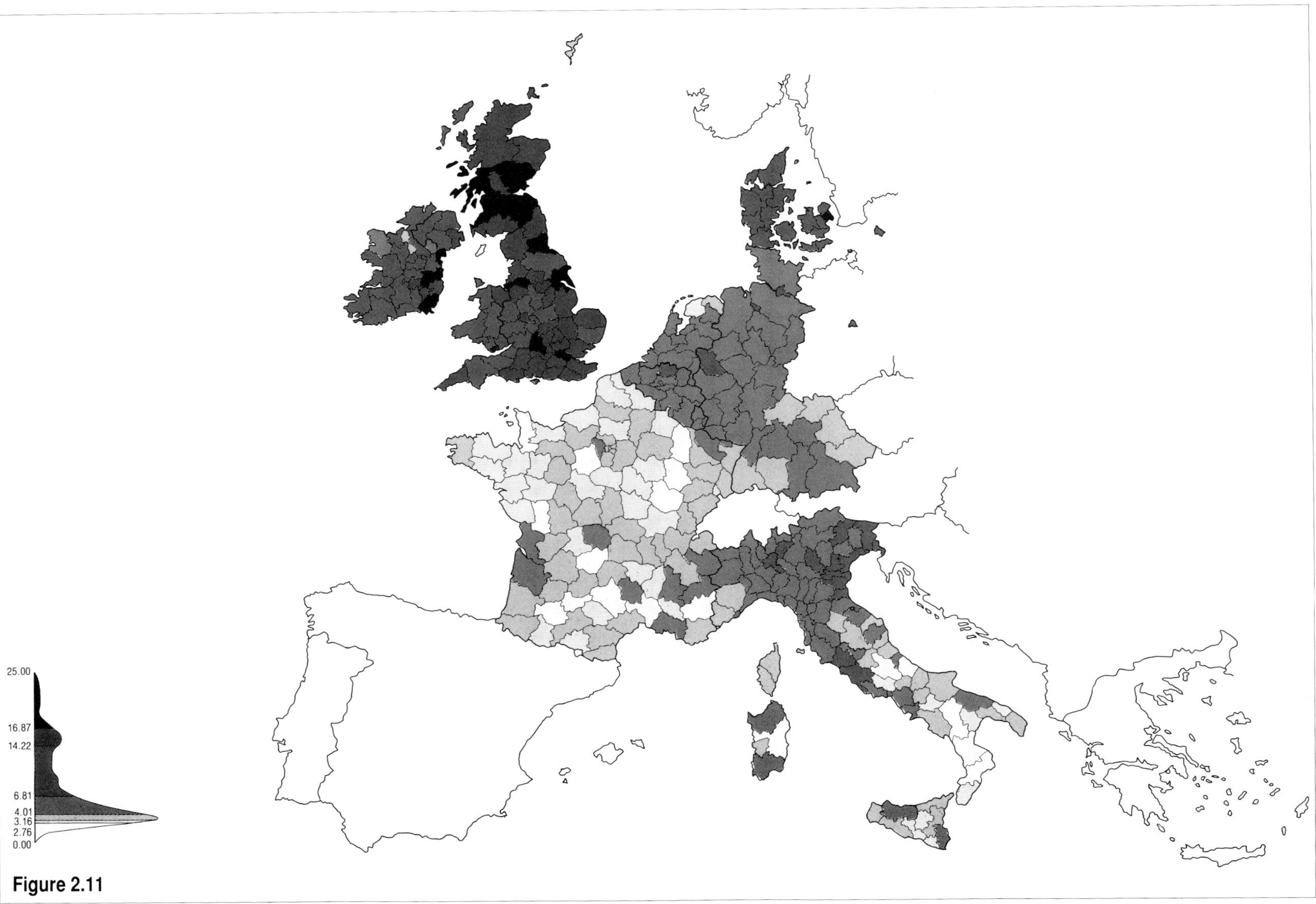

Figure 2.11

Mortality from cancer of the lung in women

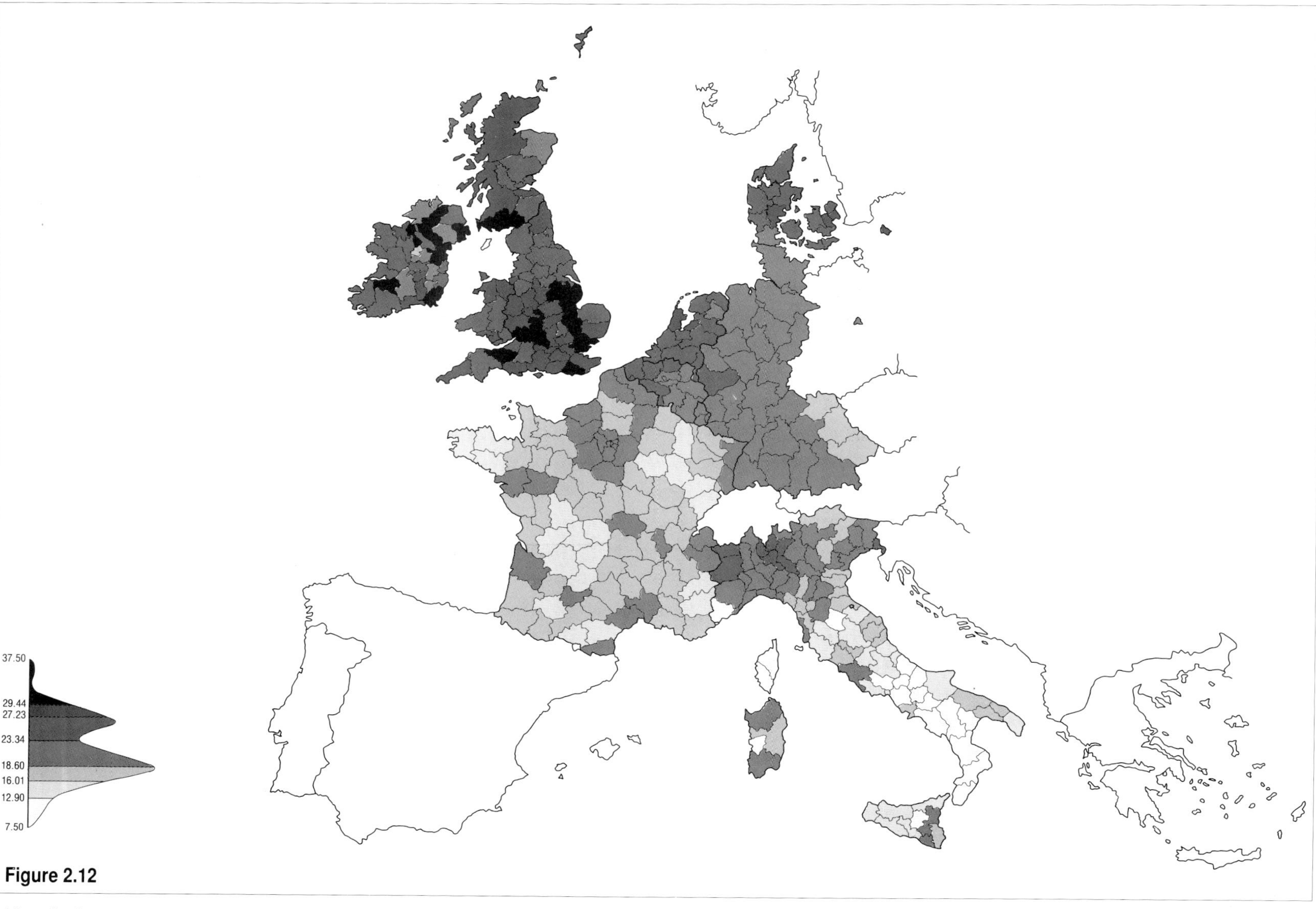

Figure 2.12

Mortality from cancer of the breast in women

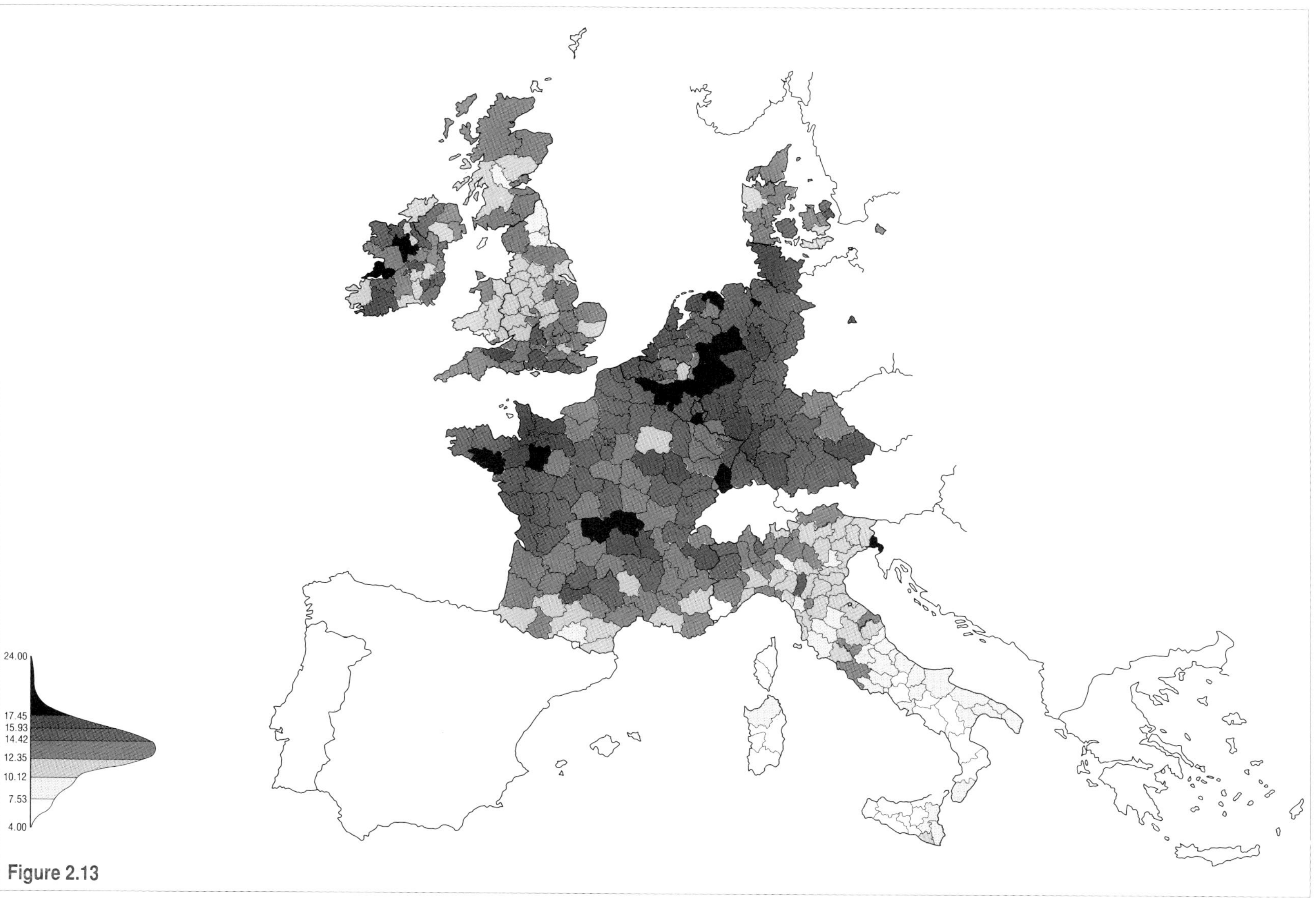

Figure 2.13

Mortality from cancer of the prostate in men

Table 2.4 Projected cancer burden (thousands) for the year 2000 assuming changes in population size and age-structure forecast by UN demographers take place, and presuming forecast changes in risk based on past time trends are valid. Ratio of 2000 to 1975 estimates in parentheses.

	Male	Female
	All sites	
North	150 (1.1)	126 (1.0)
South	361 (1.8)	288 (1.6)
West	351 (1.3)	271 (1.1)
East	195 (1.6)	186 (1.6)
	Stomach	
North	7 (0.6)	5 (0.6)
South	20 (0.7)	15 (0.7)
West	16 (0.6)	10 (0.6)
East	14 (0.7)	9 (0.6)
	Large Bowel	
North	22 (1.3)	24 (1.2)
South	42 (2.1)	45 (2.1)
West	47 (1.5)	47 (1.3)
East	18 (1.6)	18 (1.5)
	Lung	
North	44 (1.2)	15 (1.5)
South	87 (2.2)	19 (2.1)
West	88 (1.4)	15 (1.7)
East	59 (2.0)	9 (1.9)
		Breast
North		42 (1.2)
South		91 (2.2)
West		89 (1.3)
East		37 (1.9)
	Prostate	
North	19 (1.3)	
South	36 (2.1)	
West	46 (1.5)	
East	17 (1.9)	

Note: Provisional figures subject to revision
Source: Muir, 1989

Concluding comment

If primary prevention is to be successful, then a knowledge of cause—or at least of some of the causal factors operating—is essential. The cause of most lung cancer is known. Although still common in several parts of the world, gastric cancer incidence is falling everywhere, the risk being favourably influenced by diets containing adequate amounts of fresh fruit and vegetables. Large-bowel, breast and prostatic cancer also appear to be diet related, and it is here that further combined epidemiological and laboratory studies are urgently needed if these cancers are to be prevented. The current great diversity of the cancer scenery of Europe makes it all the more important that these differences be examined epidemiologically as soon as possible. The tendency towards increasing homogeneity of diet and other exposures will make it much more difficult to uncover the responsible aetiological factors.

References

Coleman, M. P. and Démaret, E. (1988) Cancer registration in the European community, *Int. J. Cancer* **42**, 339–245.

Muir, C. S. and Parkin, D. M. (1985) The world cancer burden: prevent or perish, *Brit. Med. J.* **290**, 5–6.

Muir, C. S., Waterhouse, J., Mack, T., Powell, J. and Whelan, S. (eds.) (1987) *Cancer Incidence in Five Continents*, vol. v, IARC Scient. publ. no. 88, International Agency for Research on Cancer, Lyon.

Muir, C. S. (1989) Changing international patterns of cancer incidence, in J. G. Fortner and J. E. Rhoads (eds.) *Accomplishments in Cancer Research, 1988 Prize Year*, 126-144 General Motors Cancer Research Foundation, J. B. Lippincott Company, Philadelphia.

Parkin, D. M., Läära, E., Muir, C. S. (1988) Estimates of the worldwide frequency of sixteen major cancers in 1980, *Int. J. Cancer* **41**, 184–197.

United Nations Organization (1986) *Demographic indicators of countries: estimates and projections as assessed in 1984,* UNO, New York.

World Health Organization (1977) *Manual of the International Classification of Diseases*, vol. 1, 9th revision, 1975.

Paper 2.2

RADIATION AND CANCER: OVERVIEW AND IMPLICATIONS FOR PREVENTION*

Dr. Elisabeth Cardis and Dr. John Kaldor
International Agency for Research on Cancer, Lyon, France

Ionizing radiation as a cause of cancers

Radiation is said to be ionizing when it has the capacity to accelerate electrons in matter, either directly or indirectly. Human exposure to ionizing radiation is ubiquitous. The most important source is natural, from radioactivity in the air, water, the food chain and minerals, and from cosmic rays. Exposure from human-made sources, non-existent before the 20th century, has arisen through medical diagnostic and therapeutic procedures, as well as from the nuclear industry and from nuclear weapons explosions.

The first cancers observed in association with exposure to radiation were skin carcinomas on the hands of radiologists (Upton, 1975), and several cases of what was probably leukaemia. By the 1930s, a few cases of bone cancer had been seen among young women who had ingested radium-containing paint by licking the brushes they used for painting clock and watch dials (Martland, 1931). Experimentally, the induction of tumours in laboratory animals exposed to radiation has been reported in numerous studies since 1910 (UNSCEAR, 1977).

Important epidemiological studies of radiation carcinogenesis have been carried out on the survivors of the atomic bombs in Hiroshima and Nagasaki, on a number of populations irradiated for medical reasons, and on underground miners who had been exposed to radon gas and its decay products. It is now accepted that ionizing radiation can induce cancer in any organ in which cancers occur naturally, but that organs differ substantially in their intrinsic susceptibility, in the latent period between exposure and appearance of a cancer and in the modifying effect of sex and age at the time of exposure.

Leukaemia

In the late 1940s, around the time of the establishment of the Atomic Bomb Casualty Commission in Hiroshima and Nagasaki, it had already become clear that bomb survivors were at increased risk for developing leukaemia (Ichimaru *et al.*, 1981; Kato and Schull, 1982). This increase continued as the survivors were followed up in time, and reached a peak seven to eight years after the bombing. It has been decreasing since that time, but still remains significantly higher than expected (Finch, 1984). The increased risk was observed for acute and chronic myeloid leukaemia and acute lymphocytic leukaemia, but not for chronic lymphocytic leukaemia.

An increased risk for leukaemia also exists for patients treated with X rays for ankylosing spondylitis (a chronic progressive arthritis occurring in young men) (Smith and Doll, 1982; Darby *et al.*, 1987), and for cancer of the cervix (Boice *et al.*, 1985), beginning within two years of treatment. Above a certain level of exposure, the risk for leukaemia may plateau and decrease. This is also observed among women treated with radiotherapy for cervical cancer (Boice *et al.*, 1985). This phenomenon may be due to the large number of bone marrow stem cells which are sterilized at high doses, and are thus unable to give rise to a tumour.

*Parts of this paper are drawn from the forthcoming IARC publication *Cancer: Occurrence, Causes and Prevention.*

Breast cancer

Risk for breast cancer is elevated among atomic bomb survivors (Preston *et al.*, 1986), among patients who have been treated with X rays for post-partum mastitis (Shore *et al.*, 1986), and among patients who had multiple fluoroscopies in the course of treatment for pulmonary tuberculosis (Baral *et al.*, 1977; Boice and Monson, 1977; Howe, 1984; Land *et al.*, 1980).

The risk for breast cancer appears to increase linearly with dose and at the same rate per total dose in all of the groups studied (Boice *et al.*, 1979), and to be independent of length of exposure.

Among the atomic bomb survivors, the carcinogenic effect of radiation on the breast appears to be greatest when exposure occurs around menarche, and then decreases with increasing age at exposure up to age 40 to 49, after which there may be no increase in risk (Tokunaga *et al.*, 1984).

Lung cancer

The risk for lung cancer is elevated both in populations exposed externally, such as the atomic bomb survivors (Preston *et al.*, 1986; Shimizu *et al.*, 1987) and ankylosing spondylitis (Smith and Doll, 1982), and internally, such as underground miners. Investigations on the effects of exposure to radon from natural sources in houses are being carried out in many countries, but have so far not shown clearly an increased risk due to domestic exposure.

The excess risk for radiation-induced lung cancer appears to be greater in subjects exposed later in life. Male and female survivors of the bomb have the same increase in absolute risk (Yamamoto *et al.*, 1987).

Several attempts have been made to study the interaction between exposure to radiation and cigarette smoking in causing lung cancer. The studies of atomic bomb survivors suggest that the relationship is additive (Prentice *et al.*, 1983; Kopecky *et al.*, 1986), but data on underground miners in Colorado are more consistent with a multiplicative effect (Whittemore and McMillan, 1983; Hornung and Meinhardt, 1987).

Cancer of the thyroid

The risk for cancer of the thyroid is elevated among atomic bomb survivors (Prentice *et al.*, 1982) and among people treated with radiotherapy as children, at the thymus and for tinea capitis (ringworm) (Ron and Modan, 1984; Shore *et al.*, 1980; Ron *et al.*, 1987). Iodine absorbed into the body concentrates in the thyroid gland, and its radioactive isotopes, such as ^{131}-iodine, have been used for therapeutic and diagnostic purposes without increasing the risk for cancer of the thyroid (Hoffman, 1984; Holm, 1984).

In the atomic bomb survivors, the risk for cancer of the thyroid had decreased by 30 years after exposure (Beebe *et al.*, 1977), but in other studies the increase in risk seems to persist for at least 30 years (Shore *et al.*, 1985). Children appear to be more susceptible than adults to induction of thyroid cancer by radiation.

Gastrointestinal cancers

An increased risk for stomach cancer has been observed among atomic bomb survivors (Shimizu *et al.*, 1987) and patients treated with X rays for ankylosing spondylitis (Smith and Doll, 1982), especially for people exposed under the age of 20 (Preston *et al.*, 1986). Atomic bomb survivors also had an increased risk for cancer of the colon. The incidence of rectal cancer was higher in women who had received radiation treatment for cancer of the cervix than those who had not (Day and Boice, 1983; Boice *et al.*, 1988).

Cancer of the liver

Patients who were injected with thorotrast (containing ^{232}-thorium) for diagnostic purposes, now an obsolete procedure, had a very high frequency of tumours of the liver (where thorium concentrates), specifically of cholangiocellular carcinoma and of haemangiosarcoma (von Kaick *et al.*, 1984).

Multiple myeloma

A small increase in the risk for multiple myeloma was observed in atomic bomb survivors (Shimizu *et al.*, 1987) and in patients treated with radiotherapy for cervical cancer (Boice *et al.*, 1983). Studies of workers in the nuclear industry who are exposed to relatively low doses of radiation have also showed increases in risk for myeloma (Smith and Douglas, 1986; Gilbert and Marks, 1979; Gilbert *et al.*, 1989).

Cancer of the bone

Information about radiation-induced cancers of the bone comes from studies of women who ingested a mixture of radium isotope while painting luminous dials (Rowland *et al.*, 1978) and of patients treated for various diseases by injections of ^{224}-radium (Mays and Spiess, 1984). Whatever the route of exposure, radium is mostly transferred to bone. The first sarcomas of bone appeared in less than ten years, and new cases continued to be reported among dial painters nearly 60 years after exposure; in the patients injected with shorter lived ^{224}-radium, the risk pattern is close to that of radiation-induced leukaemia.

Quantitative and qualitative aspects of radiation carcinogenesis

More quantitative information is available about radiation carcinogenesis than for any other human carcinogen. Both epidemiological and experimental studies have provided data on the shape of the dose-response curve for cancer induction following exposure to radiation, on the relative effects of different types of radiation and on the effect of exposure rate. Nevertheless, our understanding of the mechanisms underlying the process is still very incomplete. There are therefore great difficulties in predicting the life time risk attributable to exposure to radiation. Extrapolation must often be done on the basis of mathematical models built on assumptions which cannot currently be tested either experimentally or in existing epidemiologic studies. Some of the issues for which assumptions must be made are discussed below.

Threshold

Whether there is a threshold below which radiation is not carcinogenic has long been a subject of scientific debate (Upton, 1983). In fact, statistical error virtually precludes the demonstration of absence of effect in epidemiological studies where exposure assessment is difficult and biases may occur. There is, in any case, little biological plausibility that there is a threshold. Thousands of animals are required to study experimentally the carcinogenic effect of doses of radiation that cause very small increases in the risk for cancer (see, for example, Ullrich and Storer, 1979a, 1979b, 1979c; Upton *et al.*, 1969).

Dose-response function at low doses

The dose-response curve for radiation carcinogenesis appears to be well described by a linear curve at low levels of response to so-called high LET (linear energy transfer) types of radiation such as α particles and neutrons; it is probably concave upwards for low LET radiation such as γ and X rays (BEIR III, 1980; Mole, 1984). At very high levels of response, the probability of malignant transformation taking place reaches a plateau then eventually decreases, probably because of increased cell killing (UNSCEAR, 1988).

Susceptibility of tissues

It is clear that some tissues are much more susceptible to radiation carcinogenesis than others. The bone marrow is a site of particular and rapidly manifested sensitivity. The recent detection of clusters of leukaemia in children living near nuclear plants, who may have been exposed environmentally to radioactive contamination, raises the possibility that sensitivity to internally absorbed high LET emitters is much greater than was previously suspected (COMARE, 1988). The breast and thyroid are also highly radiation-sensitive.

Radiation types and pattern of exposures

It appears, based on the results of animal experiments, that, at low doses, high LET radiation is substantially more carcinogenic than low LET radiation, and that extending exposure to low LET radiation over time produces a smaller carcinogenic effect than an acute exposure to the same cumulated dose (Hall, 1978). Protraction of exposure over a long period has been the focus of recent studies (Inskip *et al.*, 1987; Smith *et al.*, 1987), but the results are difficult to compare with those of the studies of acute exposure.

The only data on human exposure to high LET radiation now comes from studies of miners exposed to α particles. The results are consistent in showing that α particles are much more efficient per unit dose (i.e. energy absorbed in the tissue) in inducing lung cancer than γ or X rays, although the relative difference has not been well quantified.

Implications for preventing cancers caused by ionizing radiation

The best available estimates of cancer risk caused by ionizing radiations indicate that the percentage of cases which can be ascribed to natural background radiation is very small indeed, even for childhood leukaemia. In any case, the ubiquity of the exposure makes any prevention strategy linked to background radiation rather impractical.

Diagnostic and therapeutic irradiation play a very important role in current medical practice. Modern techniques aim at minimization of dose levels, and optimum targeting to the tissue involved. It is likely that, within these technological limitations, the benefits of irradiation should outweigh the costs in increased cancer risk.

Workers in the nuclear industries are subject to stringent controls, and are probably working close to a level at which increased cancer risk due to occupational irradiation is negligible.

There are thus few areas where prevention strategies may substantially reduce the risk of cancer due to ionizing radiation. The one which is probably most important from the public health point of view is the lung cancer hazard posed by radon progeny. Exposure at high levels still affects a small proportion of underground miners, and a much bigger percentage of the population is exposed to low levels of radon trapped in buildings.

Extensive monitoring programmes are under way in a number of countries, with the goal of identifying areas of high radon content. Findings from these surveys should then lead to appropriate modification of buildings to prevent exposure to occupants. The number of cases of lung cancer which could be prevented in this way is very difficult to estimate, since the distribution of exposure levels before and after modification cannot be reliably estimated. Another complicating factor is the possibility that smoking and radon interact multiplicatively, so that cessation of smoking may eliminate much of the risk.

Ultraviolet radiation as a cause of cancers

Most human exposure to ultraviolet radiation is from the sun, and the most highly exposed individuals are therefore those living nearest to the equator and, at any given latitude, those whose work or recreation takes them outdoors. Much lower levels of exposure result from certain types of fluorescent lighting. The carcinogenicity of ultraviolet radiation was discussed in a detailed appendix to an IARC monograph (IARC, 1986), which is the source used for writing this section of the paper.

Data from epidemiological studies are consistent in demonstrating a causal relationship between exposure to sunlight and cancers of the lip and skin (other than melanoma). Ultraviolet radiation produces skin and other external tumours in exposed experimental animals.

Several case reports and descriptive studies also indicate that sunlight may play a role in the induction of non-melanocytic skin cancer. This is supported by observations that 80 per cent of these cancers are found on the head and neck, that incidence decreases with increasing distance from the equator, and that outdoor workers appear to have a higher risk than indoor workers. Nevertheless, the few case-control studies of non-melanocytic skin cancer have been of uneven quality and have perhaps for this reason not demonstrated a risk as clearly as one might have expected. The evidence concerning lip cancer is far clearer.

For melanoma, the epidemiological data are

more complex: the anatomical distribution is not predominantly on exposed areas of the skin, rates do not increase rapidly in old age, and in several studies indoor workers had a risk equal to or greater than that of outdoor workers. The latitude gradient does, however, appear to hold, except in Europe, where the trend may be inversed by skin pigmentation.

Theories have been advanced that individuals who maintain suntans, through extensive recreational or occupational exposure, are at lower risk for melanoma than those who tan and burn intermittently. Exposure in childhood or early adolescence may confer a greater risk than exposure in adult life.

Implications for preventing cancers due to ultraviolet radiation

There are clear links between sun exposure and skin cancer. For non-melanotic skin cancer, the relationship seems rather straightforward: the higher and longer the exposure, the greater the risk. Thus outdoor workers, such as builders, farmers and sailors, should be encouraged to minimize exposure, most simply by wearing appropriate clothing. In those parts of Europe where sun exposure is highest, the majority of the population is already protected to a certain extent by a constitutionally darker complexion.

Melanoma prevention is much more problematic. The rapid rise in risk seen over the past few decades may well be attributable to the increasing leisure possibilities brought about by affluence, and in particular the new accessibility of sunny southern European holidays to highly susceptible northern Europeans. Since one of the main goals of these leisure activities is suntanning, it is not realistic to recommend total avoidance. Furthermore, for the moment it is not known whether avoidance of *sunburn* (as opposed to suntan) through appropriate use of clothing and creams in the early parts of a summer vacation would reduce the melanoma risk. Nevertheless, this strategy is probably reasonable on general grounds, and could be a first step towards melanoma prevention.

Electromagnetic fields as a cause of cancers

Exposure to extremely low frequency (ELF, 0-300 Hz) electromagnetic fields has only recently been suspected of increasing the risk for cancer and particularly for acute myeloid leukaemia. A number of studies of men likely to have been occupationally exposed to ELF fields, carried out in different countries on different occupational groups using different designs and indirect assessment of exposure, has shown, with some consistency, greater than expected incidence of or mortality from leukaemia, and particularly the acute myeloid form (Milham, 1982; Wright *et al.*, 1982; Coleman *et al.*, 1983; McDowall, 1983; Stern *et al.*, 1986), in the order of a 20 per cent increase for all leukaemia and 45 per cent for acute myeloid leukaemia (Coleman and Beral, 1988). These results probably indicate a true increase in risk in people occupationally exposed to ELF fields, but studies in which detailed, direct assessment of exposure is undertaken are needed to confirm this.

In several studies, leukaemia and cancer risk have been examined in both adults and children in relation to residential exposure to ELF fields. The results are less consistent than those of the occupational studies. Increased risks for leukaemia were seen among children, but only a few cases were available. The major problems in estimating risks are the ubiquity of the exposure and the difficulties in measuring it (report of IARC *ad hoc* working group, 1988).

References

Baral, E., Larsson, L. E. and Mattsson, B. (1977) Breast cancer following irradiation of the breast, *Cancer* **40**, 2905–2910.

Beebe, G. W., Kato, H., Land, C. E. (1977) *Mortality experience of atomic bomb survivors, 1950–74.* Life Span Study Report 8. Radiation Effects Research Foundation Technical Report 1–77, Hiroshima.

BEIR III: Committee on the Biological Effects of Ionizing Radiation (1980) *The effects on populations of exposure to low levels of ionizing radiation*, National Academy of Sciences, Washington, D.C.

Boice, J. D. Jr., Day, N. E. *et al.* (1985) Cancer risk following radiation treatment for cervical cancer. An international collaboration among cancer registries, *J. Natn. Cancer Inst.* **74**, 995–975.

Boice, J. D., Engholm, G. *et al.* (1988) Radiation dose and second cancer risk in patients treated for cancer of the cervix, *Radiat. Res.* **116**, 3–55.

Boice, J. D., Land, C. E., Shore, R. E. *et al.* (1979) Risk of breast cancer following low-dose radiation exposure, *Radiology* **131**, 589–597.

Boice, J. D. and Monson, R. R. (1977) Breast cancer in women after repeated fluoroscopic examinations of the chest, *J. Natn. Cancer Inst.* **59**, 823–832.

Coleman, M., Bell, J., Skeet, R. (1983) Leukaemia incidence in electrical workers, *Lancet* **i**, 982–83.

Coleman, M. and Beral, V. (1988) A review of epidemiological studies of the health effects of living near or working with electricity generation and transmission equipment, *Int. J. Epidemiol.* **17**, 1–13.

COMARE (1988) (Committee on Medical Aspects of Radiation in the Environment) second report: *Investigation of the possible increased incidence of leukemia in young people near the Dounreay Nuclear Establishment, Caithness, Scotland,* HMSO, London.

Darby, S. C., Doll, R., Gill, S. K. and Smith, P. G. (1987) Long-term mortality after a single treatment course with X rays in patients treated for ankylosing spondylitis, *Br. J. Cancer* **55**, 179–90.

Day, N. E. and Boice, J. D. (eds.) (1983) *Second cancer in relation to radiation treatment for cervical cancer*, International Agency for Research on Cancer, scient. publ. no. 52, Lyon.

Finch, S. C. (1984) Leukemia and lymphoma in atomic bomb survivors, in J. D. Boice and J. F. Fraumeni (eds.) *Radiation Carcinogenesis: Epidemiology and Biological Significance*, 37–44, Raven Press, New York.

Gilbert, E. S. and Marks, S. (1979) An analysis of the mortality of workers in a nuclear facility, *Radiat. Res.* **79**, 122–148.

Gilbert, E. S., Peterson, G. R. and Buchanan, J. A. (1989) Mortality of workers at the Hanford site: 1945–1981, *Health Phys.* **56**, 11–25.

Hall, E. J. (1978) *Radiobiology for the Radiologists*, 2nd ed., Harper and Row, Philadelphia.

Hoffman, D. A. (1984) Late Effects of Iodine-^{131} Therapy in the United States, in J. D. Boice and J. F. Fraumeni (eds.) *Radiation Carcinogenesis: Epidemiology and Biological Significance*, 173–280, Raven Press, New York.

Holm, L. E. (1984) Malignant disease following Iodine-131 therapy in Sweden, in J. D. Boice and J. F. Fraumeni (eds.) Radiation Carcinogenesis: Epidemiology and Biological Significance, 263–271, Raven Press, New York.

Hornung, R. W. and Meinhardt, T. J. (1987) Quantitative risk assessment of lung cancer in US uranium miners, *Health Phys.* **52**, 417–430.

Howe, G. R. (1984) Epidemiology of Radiogenic Breast Cancer, in J. D. Boice and J. F. Fraumeni (eds.) *Radiation Carcinogenesis: Epidemiology and Biological Significance*, 119–129, Raven Press, New York.

IARC (1986) *IARC monographs on the evaluation of the carcinogenic risk of chemicals to humans,* **40**, Some naturally occurring and synthetic food components, furocoumarins and ultraviolet radiation, IARC, Lyon.

IARC (1988) *IARC monographs on the evaluation of carcinogenic risks to humans,* **43**, Man-made mineral fibres and radon, IARC, Lyon.

Ichimaru, M., Ishimaru, T., Mikami, M., Yamada, Y. and Ohkita, T. (1981) Incidence of leukemia in atomic bomb survivors and controls in a fixed cohort, Hiroshima and Nagasaki, October 1950–December 1978. Radiation Effects Research Foundation Technical Report, 13–81, Hiroshima.

Inskip, H., Beral, V., Fraser, P., Booth, M., Coleman, D. and Brown, A. (1987) Further assessment of the effects of occupational radiation exposure in the United Kingdom Atomic Energy Authority mortality study, *Br. J. Ind. Med.* **44**, 149–160.

Kato, H. and Schull, W. J. (1982) Studies of the A-bomb survivors 7 Mortality 1950–1978. part I. Cancer Mortality. *Radiat. Res.* **90**, 395–432.

Kopecky, K. J., Nakashima, E., Yamamoto, T. *et al.* (1986) *Lung cancer, radiation exposure and smoking among A-bomb survivors, Hiroshima and Nagasaki, 1950–1980.* Radiation Effects Research Foundation Technical Report 13–86, Hiroshima.

Land, C. E., Boice, J. D., Shore, R. E. *et al.* (1980) Breast cancer risk from low-dose exposures to ionizing radiation: results of parallel analysis of three exposed populations of women, *J. Natn. Cancer Inst.* **65**, 353–376.

Martland, H. S. (1931) The occurrence of malignancy in radioactive persons, *Am. J. Cancer* **15**, 2435–2516.

Mays, C. W. and Spiess, H. (1984) Bone sarcomas in patients given Radium-224, in J. D. Boice and J. F. Fraumeni (eds.) *Radiation Carcinogenesis: Epidemiology and Biological Significance*, 241–252, Raven Press, New York.

Milham, S. (1982) Mortality from leukemia in workers exposed to electrical and magnetic fields, *N. Engl. J. Med.* **307**, 249.

Mole, R. J. (1984) Dose-response relationships, in J. D. Boice and J. F. Fraumeni (eds.) *Radiation Carcinogenesis: Epidemiology and Biological Significance*, 403–420, Raven Press, New York.

McDowall, M. E. (1983) Leukemia mortality in electrical workers in England and Wales, *Lancet* 1, 246.

Prentice, R. L., Yoshimoto, Y. and Mason, M. W. (1983) Relationship of cigarette smoking and radiation exposure to cancer mortality in Hiroshima and Nagasaki, *J. Nat. Cancer Inst.* **70**, 611–622.

Preston, D. L., Kato, H., Kopecky, K. J. *et al.* (1986) Life Span Study Report 10, part 1, *Cancer Mortality among A-bomb Survivors in Hiroshima and Nagasaki, 1950–1982*, RERF TR/1-86.

Ron, E., Kleinerman, R. A., Boice, J. D. Jr., LiVolsi, V.A., Flannery, J.T., Fraumeni, J. F. Jr. (1987) A population-based case-control study of thyroid cancer, *J. Nat. Cancer Inst.* **79**, 1–12.

Ron, E. and Modan, B. (1984) Thyroid and other neoplasms following childhood scalp irradiation, in J. D. Boice and J. F. Fraumeni (eds.) *Radiation Carcinogenesis: Epidemiology and Biological Significance*, 139–151, Raven Press, New York.

Rowland, R. E., Stehney, A. F. and Lucas, H. F. Jr. (1978) Dose-response relationships for female radium dial workers, *Radiat. Res.* **76**, 368–383.

Shimizu, Y., Kato, H., Schull, W. J. *et al.* (1987) Life Span Study Report II, Part I: Comparison of risk coefficients for site-specific cancer mortality based on the DS86 and T65DR shielded kerma and organ doses, RERF TR/12-87.

Shore, R. E., Hildreth, N., Woodward, E. D. *et al.* (1986) Breast cancer among women given X-ray therapy for acute postpartum mastitis, *J. Natn. Cancer Inst.* **77**, 689–696.

Shore, R. E., Woodward, E. D. and Hempelmann, L. H. (1980) Radiation-induced thyroid cancer, in J. D. Boice and J. F. Fraumeni (eds.) *Radiation Carcinogenesis: Epidemiology and Biological Significance*, 131–138, Raven Press, New York.

Shore, R. E., Woodward, E., Hildreth, N., Dvoretsky, P., Hempelmann, L. and Pasternack, B. (1985) Thyroid tumors following thymus irradiation, 74, 1177–1184.

Smith, P. G. and Doll, R. (1982) Mortality among patients with ankylosing spondylitis after a single treatment course with X rays, *Br. Med. J.* **284**, 449–460.

Smith, P. G. and Douglas, A. J. (1986) Mortality of workers at the Sellafield plant of British Nuclear Fuels, *Br. Med. J.* **293**, 845–854.

Tokunaga, M., Land, C. E., Yamamoto, T., Asano, M. *et al.* (1984) Breast cancer among atomic bomb survivors, in J. D. Boice and J. F. Fraumeni (eds.) *Radiation Carcinogenesis: Epidemiology and Biological Significance*, 45–56, Raven Press, New York.

Ullrich, R. L. and Storer, J. B. (1979a) Influence of g irradiation on the development of neoplastic disease in mice. I. Reticular tissue tumours. *Radiat. Res.* **80**, 303–316.

Ullrich, R. L. and Storer, J. B. (1979b) Influence of g irradiation on the development of neoplastic disease in mice. II. Solid tumours. *Radiat. Res.* **80**, 317–324.

Ullrich, R. L. and Storer, J. B. (1979c) Influence of g irradiation on the development of neoplastic disease in mice. III. Dose rate effects. *Radiat. Res.* **80**, 325–342.

UNSCEAR (United Nations Scientific Committee on the Effect of Atomic Radiation) (1977) Sources, Effects and Risks of Ionizing Radiation, United Nations, New York.

UNSCEAR (United Nations Scientific Committee on the Effects of Atomic Radiation) (1988) Sources and Effects of Ionizing Radiation, United Nations, New York.

Upton, A. C. (1975) Physical carcinogenesis: radiation history and sources, in *Cancer: a comprehensive treatise*, F. F. Becker (ed.) Plenum Press.

Upton, A. C. (1983) Environmental standards for ionizing radiation: theoretical basis for dose-response curves, *Environ. Health Perspect.* **52**, 31–39.

Upton, A. C., Allen, R. C., Brown, R. C. *et al.* (1969) Quantitative experimental study of low-level radiation carcinogenesis, in *Radiation-Induced Cancer*, IAEA publication STI/PUB/228, Vienna.

Von Kaick, G., Muth, H., Kaul, A. *et al.* (1984) Results of the German Thorotrast Study, in J. D. Boice and J. F. Fraumeni (eds.) *Radiation Carcinogenesis: Epidemiology and Biological Significance*, 253–262, Raven Press, New York.

Whittemore, A. S. and McMillan, A. (1983) Lung cancer mortality among US uranium miners: a reappraisal, *J. Natn. Cancer Inst.* **71**, 489–499.

Wright, W. E., Peters, J. M., Mark, T. M. (1982) Leukemia in workers exposed to electrical and magnetic fields, *Lancet* **2**, 1160–1161.

Yamamoto, T., Kopecky, K. J., Fujikura, T., Tokuoka, S. *et al.* (1987) Lung cancer incidence among A-bomb survivors in Hiroshima and Nagasaki, 1950–1980. Radiation Effects Research Foundation Technical Report 12-86, Hiroshima.

Paper 2.3

THE ROLE OF OCCUPATION IN THE CAUSATION OF CANCER AND ITS PREVENTION

Dr. Elsebeth Lynge
Danish Cancer Registry, Institute of Cancer Epidemiology, Copenhagen, Denmark

Introduction

In the year 2000, some 28 000 cancer cases are expected in the Danish population[1] given the present sex and age-specific rates[2] shown in Table 2.5 below. If we assume that people are economically active in the age group 20 to 64 years, then about 36 per cent of the cancer patients in the year 2000 will already be pensioners today. An additional 52 per cent of these cancer patients have already been active on the labour market for at least 20 years. New preventive measures at the workplace are thus expected to have limited or no effect on the majority of cancer cases in the year 2000. A longer time perspective is therefore needed in order to assess the potential for prevention of cancers caused by occupational exposures.

The discussion in this paper will be divided into three parts: control of exposures to known occupational carcinogens; early detection of occupational cancers; and the identification of possible cancer risks that are associated with changing work conditions and new technology in the service society.

Prevention of exposure to known occupational carcinogens

Identifying carcinogens

The most comprehensive list of known carcinogens in the occupational setting comes from the International Agency for Research on Cancer (IARC) *Monographs on the Evaluation of Carcinogenic Risks to Humans*. According to the recent IARC supplement no. 7, a total of 628 agents were evaluated for evidence of their carcinogenicity before 1988[3]. A total of 246 agents were classified as carcinogenic to humans (group 1), probably carcinogenic to humans (group 2A), or possibly carcinogenic to humans (group 2B)(see Table 2.6). The majority of these carcinogenic agents occur in the occupational setting. Twelve agents are used in industries for which the specific chemical(s) has not been identified: 101 are industrial chemicals; 13 are pesticides; and 49 are laboratory chemicals. Occupational exposures might, however, also be relevant to the 58 drugs (for example, nurses administering cytostatic drugs), to the ten food ingredients (for

Table 2.5 Expected cancer cases in Denmark in the year 2000 by labour market participation in 1990

Labour market status today (year 1990)	Started working in year	Age in year 2000	Expected cancer cases in year 2000	
			Number	Per cent
children	–	0–19	17	1
entering labour market	1990–91	20–29	277	1
active, have worked <20 years	1970–89	30–49	2859	10
active, have worked ≥20 years	1945–69	50–74	14 516	52
pensioners	1900–44	75–99	10 112	36

Table 2.6 Number of agents classified by IARC in groups 1 to 4, 1987

Type of agent	IARC group Human carcinogen 1	Probable 2A	Possible 2B	Not classifiable 3	Not carcinogenic 4	Total
industry[1]	11	–	1	4	–	16
industrial chemical[2]	17	19	65	170	–	272
pesticide[3]	–	–	13	37	–	50
laboratory chemical[4]	–	8	41	67	–	116
drug[5]	18	10	30	71	1	129
food ingredient[6]	1	–	9	31	–	41
habit[7]	3	–	–	1	–	4
Total	50	37	159	381	1	628

Notes
1 Defined industrial processes involving exposure to complex mixtures of chemicals.
2 Chemicals known to be used in industrial production, either as a raw material in chemical synthesis or as a compound or additive in a product.
3 Chemicals used for pest control.
4 Chemicals known to be used for research purposes only.
5 Chemicals used as drugs for humans or animals.
6 Food additives or contaminants, often of natural origin (also additives used in cosmetics).
7 Tobacco smoking and related stimulants.

example, cooks preparing fried food), and for the three habits (for example, waiters serving in smoky rooms).

Labelling carcinogens

The most simple preventive measure is information about the potential risk. An EC directive on labelling of chemical compounds for carcinogenicity was issued in 1983[4]. According to this directive, substances known to be carcinogenic to man, and substances which should be regarded as if they are carcinogenic to man, are to be labelled with the risk phrase R45 *'May cause cancer'*. Substances which cause concern for man owing to possible carcinogenic effects are to be labelled with the risk phrase R40 *'Possible risk of irreversible effects'*. Out of the 163 industrial chemicals, pesticides and laboratory chemicals so far classified as carcinogenic by the IARC, a total of 41 has now been labelled with the risk phrase R45 *'May cause cancer'*, and 12 have been labelled with the risk phrase R40 *'Possible risk of irreversible effects'* (see Table 2.7). Ten chemicals not classified as carcinogenic by the IARC have been labelled with the risk phrase R40; two chemicals *not* evaluated by the IARC have been labelled with the risk phrase R45, and an additional two chemicals have been labelled with the risk phrase R40[5,6,7]. Separate labelling exists for asbestos[8].

Policies for preventing exposure

Production and use is prohibited for the four aromatic amines shown in Table 2.7: 2-naphthylamine, 4-aminobiphenyl, benzidine and 4-nitrodiphenyl[9]; marketing and use is prohibited with certain exceptions for crocidolite (blue asbestos)[8]. A proposal has been put forward for the protection of workers from the risks related to exposure to carcinogens at work[10].

Cancers caused by known occupational carcinogens probably represent a relatively small proportion of all cancer cases, for example, about 4 per cent of all cancer deaths estimated for the US[11]. However, the list of known carcinogens represents a fund of knowledge directly applicable to preventive measures. To maximize the benefit of this

Table 2.7 Industrial chemicals, pesticides and laboratory chemicals classified by IARC in groups 1–2B by EC label

IARC group	EC-labelling[1] R-45	R-40	No	Total
Industrial chemicals				
Group 1	9[2]	0	8	17
Group 2A	11[3]	1	7	19
Group 2B	10	6	49	65
Pesticide				
Group 1	–	–	–	–
Group 2A	–	–	–	–
Group 2B	2	5	6	13
Laboratory chemical				
Group 1	–	–	–	–
Group 2A	4	–	4	8
Group 2B	5	–	36	41
Total				
Group 1	9	0	8	17
Group 2A	15	1	11	27
Group 2B	17	11	91	119
All groups				
1–2B	41	12	110	163
Group 3	–	10	264	274
Not IARC	2	2	–	–

Notes
1 A given agent on the IARC list can have more than one EC label, eg. a given chemical and salts of this chemical.
2 Three groups of chemicals (arsenic, chromium, mineral oils) only partly labelled.
3 One group of chemicals (cadmium) only partly labelled.

knowledge, information about occupational carcinogens should be disseminated efficiently, data should be collected on their use, exposed workers should be identified and their cancer pattern monitored, and measures should be taken to eliminate future exposure.

A policy on prevention of occupational cancers should, however, also include chemicals not known to be carcinogenic and new chemicals. Statistics should be collected on all chemicals in use, so that priorities could be set for systematic testing. Some chemicals used as substitutes for carcinogens have themselves been found to have carcinogenic potential—for example, man-made mineral fibres (MMMF)[12] used in insulation instead of asbestos, and bitumen[13] used in asphalt instead of coal tars. Mutagenicity testing has been required for all new chemicals marketed in the EC since 1980[14]. When occupational groups are found to have an excess cancer risk for which the causes are not known, research efforts should be directed towards identification of the aetiological agents.

Early detection of occupational cancers

Primary prevention is expected to have limited effects on mortality from occupational cancers in the near future. Therefore, possibilities for early detection and screening should be considered as an alternative. The majority of known carcinogens occurring in the occupational setting cause either bladder or lung cancer (see Table 2.8 below).

Table 2.8 Occupational exposures causally associated with lung and bladder cancer in humans

Bladder	Lung
aluminium production	aluminium production
4-aminobiphenyl	arsenic
benzidine	asbestos
coal gasification	bis(chloromethyl)ether and chloromethyl methyl ether
coal-tar pitches	chromium compounds, (hexavalent)
manufacture of auramine	coal gasification
manufacture of magenta	coal-tar pitches
mineral oils	coal-tars
2-naphthylamine	coke production
the rubber industry	haematite mining
	iron and steel founding
	mustard gas (sulphur mustard)
	nickel and nickel compounds
	soots
	talc containing asbestiform fibres

Bladder cancer

Cytological screening of urine samples from dyestuff workers and from workers in the rubber industry has been going on for many years. These programmes have been investigated by Cartwright, who concluded that 'most screening has been done by private programmes, with little regard for the size of the screened population. These were also 'in house' exercises and were often shrouded in confidentiality. The waters are also muddied by the lack of data about the fate of patients.'[15] Cartwright also states that 'no direct assessment of the effect of bladder cancer screening on work forces has yet been published that uses mortality as an end point'[16].

Survival is better for bladder-cancer patients diagnosed and treated at an early stage of the disease than at a late stage[17]; it is therefore pertinent, if possible, to make a thorough evaluation of the effect on mortality of those bladder-cancer screening programmes that have been in operation in industrial populations for decades. Two cases of non-invasive bladder tumours were detected recently, when urine samples were examined from 370 men and cystoscopy was carried out in 67 men who had been exposed to the aromatic amine, MBOCA, known to be carcinogenic in experimental animals[18]. However, too little is known about the possible effect of bladder-cancer screening to recommend it for industrial populations.

Lung cancer

Lung-cancer screening based on combined chest X ray and sputum cytology has been evaluated in three randomized trials in the US. No significant difference in lung cancer mortality between the screened group and the control group has been found in any of these studies[19]. A case-control study has been conducted in the German Democratic Republic to evaluate the impact of chest X rays alone. No effect could be detected[20]. The data on lung-cancer screening by these methods thus do not favour recommendation of its use, not even in high-risk industrial populations.

However, lung-cancer screening based on monoclonal antibodies directed at antigens expressed by lung cancer cells is currently being developed[21], and this might turn out to be a promising screening tool for high-risk occupational groups in the future. Chemoprevention of lung cancer with vitamin A/ beta-carotene is currently being tested in a high-risk population of asbestos workers[22].

Changes in cancer patterns expected from changes in society

Limited emphasis has been put on the search for occupational risk factors that might have followed the changing work conditions and the introduction of new technology in the service society. This is of course a difficult task, due to the long latency time found for most malignant diseases in man. One possibility might be to study the cancer pattern of those occupational groups who have for a long time experienced work conditions similar to those that are now becoming common. An example of such a comparison is given in Table 2.9, where the incidence of 41 specific cancer sites is compared in male skilled workers, farmers and academics in Denmark[23]. Minor differences were found for 15 of the cancer sites between these three social groups; major differences were found for 26 cancer sites.

The skilled workers had the highest risk for 17 cancer sites. These sites include classic occupational diseases, such as cancer of the nasal cavity[24] and cancer of the pleura[25], together with cancer of the bladder and cancer of the lung related to tobacco smoking[26] and occupational exposures[3]. The high-risk cancers for skilled workers also include metastases and non-primary lung cancer, probably due to a social bias in diagnosis. Farmers have the highest risk for cancer of the lip, which is related to outdoor work[27], and for cancer of the peritoneum.

The academics who are engaged in predominantly administrative and managerial office work had the highest risk for seven cancer sites. The excess risk for melanoma is probably due to a more frequent intermittent sunlight exposure[28]. The excess risk for other skin cancers might be a diagnostic artefact. Mycosis fungoides is an extremely rare disease. Further investigations should, however, focus on reasons for the high risk of cancer of the bone, penis and scrotum, colon and kidney among academics.

The risk of cancer of the colon has been found to be greater among men in sedentary occupations compared to physically active men[29,30,31]. One hypothesis put forward to explain this finding is that physical activity appears to stimulate colon peristalsis, and this shortens the duration of contact between carcinogenic agents and the mucosa. An excess risk for colon cancer in people with low physical activity was also found in a recent study, where dietary factors were controlled for in the analysis[32]. The potential impact of these findings is illustrated by the fact that one-third of

Table 2.9 Ratio of incidence for individual cancer sites between male skilled workers, farmers, and academics in Denmark 1970 to 1980

Cancer sites with ratio < 1.50		Cancer sites with ratio ≥ 1.50, and the high risk groups being:					
		Workers		Farmers		Academics	
multiple myeloma	(1.03)	stomach	(1.66)	peritoneum	(2.40)	bone	(1.52)
non-Hodgkin's lymphoma	(1.03)	thyroid	(1.77)	lip	(3.29)	penis,scrotum	(1.66)
prostate	(1.05)	metastases	(1.82)			colon	(1.85)
testis	(1.11)	pancreas	(1.90)			other skin	(1.99)
brain	(1.13)	bladder	(2.39)			kidney	(2.12)
leukaemia	(1.13)	small intestine	(2.43)			melanoma	(2.17)
salivary glands	(1.15)	oesophagus	(2.64)			mycosis fungoides	(2.91)
connective tissue	(1.22)	lung	(3.28)				
endocrine glands	(1.24)	liver	(3.57)				
rectum	(1.28)	pharynx	(3.97)				
Hodgkin's lymphoma	(1.28)	mouth	(4.11)				
other and unspecified	(1.29)	nasal cavity	(4.28)				
gall bladder	(1.35)	larynx	(4.93)				
liver, not primary	(1.42)	tongue	(5.30)				
eye	(1.47)	breast	(5.63)				
		pleura	(5.94)				
		lung, not primary	(6.73)				

the Danish population today report having sedentary occupations[33].

The changing composition of the work force is also expected to have an indirect influence on the future cancer pattern mediated through the life style and habits adopted by various occupational groups. An example concerning women is given in Table 2.10. Academics, teachers, nurses, and related professions are high-risk groups for breast cancer[23]. This might be related to hormonal and dietary factors such as reproductive behaviour with nulliparity or late age at first birth[34]. However, as the percentage of women in these 'high-risk occupations is increasing, the future incidence of breast cancer is expected to rise if the new generations of well educated women adopt the same reproductive behaviour. Changes in industrial structure thus have an impact on cancer patterns in a broader sense than that related to specific occupational exposures.

Table 2.10 Changes in the composition of occupational groups of women in Denmark between 1960 and 1980, and the relative risk of breast cancer in these groups in 1970–1980. (Relative risk of all economically active Danish women = 1.00.)

	Percentage of women in this occupation		Relative risk of breast cancer
	1960	1980	1970–1980
self-employed, family worker	5	6	1.02
academics	–	2	1.41
teachers, etc.	4	7	1.28
nurses, bookkeepers, etc.	9	20	1.14
all other	82	65	0.95

Conclusion

Almost 90 per cent of the cancer cases in Denmark in the year 2000 will occur in people who have already left the labour market or who have already been working for at least 20 years. A long-term perspective is therefore needed to assess the potential for prevention of cancers caused by occupational exposures. Thorough regulations should be implemented to eliminate exposures at the workplace to agents that are already known to be carcinogenic. The possible impact on bladder-cancer mortality should be assessed for cytological screening of urine samples. Further efforts should be directed towards identification of the possible cancer risks associated with working conditions in the service society. An assessment should be made of the expected changes in the cancer pattern following the changing composition of the work force.

References

1 Danmarks Statistik, Statistiske efterretninger (1988) *Befolkning og Valg* **13**, 2–3.

2 Danish Cancer Society, Danish Cancer Registry (1988) *Cancer incidence in Denmark 1985*, Danish Cancer Society, Copenhagen.

3 International Agency for Research on Cancer (1987) *IARC monographs on the evaluation of carcinogenic risks to humans*. Supplement 7, *Overall evaluations of carcinogenicity: an updating of IARC Monographs vols 1 to 42*. IARC, Lyon.

4 De Europæiske Fællesskaber. 83/467/EØF. EFT 1983, L 257/1–33.

5 De Europæiske Fællesskaber. 86/431/EØF. EFT 1986, L 247/1–41.

6 De Europæiske Fællesskaber. 87/432/EØF. EFT 1987, L 239/1–20.

7 Miljøstyrelsen (1988) *Vedr. nyt direktiv om klassificering m.v. af farlige stoffer*, Miljøstyrelsen, Kemikalie-/bekæmpelsesmiddelkontoret, 29 juni.

8 De Europæiske Fællesskaber. 83/478/EØF. EFT 1983, L 263/33–36.

9 De Europæiske Fællesskaber. 88/364/EØF. EFT 1988, L 179/44–47.

10 De Europæiske Fællesskaber. 88/C 34/03. EFT 1988, C 34/9–14.

11 Doll, R. and Peto, R. (1981) The causes of cancer: quantitative estimates of avoidable risks of cancer in the United States today, *JNCI* **66**, 1193–1308.

12 International Agency for Research on Cancer (1988) *IARC monographs on the evaluation of carcinogenic risks to humans: man-made mineral fibres and radon*, 43, IARC, Lyon.

13 International Agency for Research on Cancer (1985) *IARC monographs on the evaluation of the carcinogenic*

risk of chemicals to humans: polynuclear aromatic compounds, part 4, bitumens, coal-tars and derived products, shale-oils and soots, 35, IARC, Lyon.

14 De Europæiske Fællesskaber. 79/831/EØF. EFT L 259/ 10–28.

15 Cartwright, R. A. (1985) Screening for bladder cancer, in Miller, A. B. (ed.).*Screening for Cancer*, Academic Press, London.

16 Cartwright, R. A. (1986) Screening workers exposed to suspect bladder carcinogens. *J. Occup. Med.* **28**, 1017–19.

17 Hakulinen, T., Pukkala, E., Hakama, M., Lehtonen, Saxeen, Teppo, L. (1981) Survival of cancer patients in Finland in 1953–1974, *Ann. Clin. Res.* **13**, suppl. 31.

18 Ward, E., Halperin, W., Thun, M., Grossman, H. B., Fink, B., Koss, L., Osorio, A. M., Schulte, P. (1988) Bladder tumors in two young males occupationally exposed to MBOCA. *Am. J. Ind. Med.* **14**, 267–72.

19 Fontana, R. S., Sanderson, D. R., Woolner, L. B., Taylor, W. F., Miller, W. U., Muhm, J. R. (1986) Lung cancer screening: the Mayo program. *J. Occup. Med.* **28**, 746–50.

20 Ebeling, K., Nischan, P. (1987) Screening for lung cancer—results from a case-control study, *Int. J. Cancer* **40**, 141–4.

21 Ruddon, K. (1988) New technique boosts hopes for early lung cancer detection. *JNCI* **80**, 1354–5.

22 Henderson, M. M., Kakar, F., Sarason, I., Thompson, B., Thornquist, M., Urban, N., Kristal, A., Peterson, A., White, E., Kushi, L., Chu, J., Omenn, G., Goodman, G. (1988) Cancer Control Research Unit. In IARC (ed) *Directory of ongoing research in cancer epidemiology.* IARC, Lyon, 1988, p. 395.

23 Lynge, E., Thygesen, L. (1988) Use of surveillance systems for occupational cancer: data from the Danish national system, *Int. J. Epidemiol.* **17**, 493–500.

24 International Agency for Research on Cancer (1981) *IARC monographs on the evaluation of the carcinogenic risk of chemicals to humans*, **25**, *Wood, leather and some associated industries*, IARC, Lyon.

25 International Agency for Research on Cancer (1977) *IARC monographs on the evaluation of the carcinogenic risk of chemicals to humans*, **14**, *Asbestos*, IARC, Lyon.

26 International Agency for Research on Cancer (1986) *IARC monographs on the evaluation of the carcinogenic risk of chemicals to humans*, **38**, *Tobacco smoking*, IARC, Lyon.

27 Lindqvist, C. (1979) Risk factors in lip cancer: a questionnaire survey. *Am. J. Epidemiol.* **109**, 521–30.

28 Østerlind, A., Tucker, M. A., Stone, B. J., Jensen, O. M. (1988) The Danish case-control study of cutaneous malignant melanoma. II. Importance of UV-light exposure. *Int. J. Cancer* **42**, 319–24.

29 Garabrant, D. H., Peters, J. M., Mack, T. M., Bernstein (1984) Job activity and colon cancer risk, *Am. J. Epidemiol.* **119**, 1005–14.

30 Vena, J. E., Graham, S., Zielezny, M., Swanson, M. K., Barnes, R. E., Nolan, J. (1985) Original contributions. Lifetime occupational exercise and colon cancer, *Am. J. Epidemiol.* **122**, 357–65.

31 Gerhardsson, M., Norell, S. E., Kiviranta, H., Pedersen, N. L., Ahlbom, A. (1986) Sedentary jobs and colon cancer, *Am. J. Epidemiol* **123**, 775–80.

32 Slattery, M. L., Schumacher, M. C., Smith, K. R., West, D. W., Abd-Elghany, N. (1988) Physical activity, diet, and risk of colon cancer in Utah, *Am. J. Epidemiol.* **128**, 989–99.

33 Groth, M. V. (1988) *Fysisk aktivitet og motionsvaner i dan danske voksenbefolkning 1987*, DIKE, Copenhagen.

34 Ewertz, M. (1988) Risk of breast cancer in relation to social factors in Denmark, Acta *Oncol.*, 27(6A) 733–37.

Paper 2.4

DIET AND CANCER A SOBERING LOOK

Dr. Eyvind Thorling
Danish Cancer Society, Department of Nutrition and Cancer, Århus, Denmark

Overview

The diet and cancer problem has at least two sides, which should be kept carefully separated. One is the possible influence of the diet on the induction and development of a growing tumour in an otherwise healthy person. The other is the more hypothetical effect of diets on the growth of an established tumour in the progressive phase of growth, with polyclonicity and autonomy, no longer dependent upon promoters or hormones for its growth. This overview will confine itself to the possibilities for prevention of disease. Very little indeed is known of the therapeutic side of the problem.

A great deal of information collected over the last two or three decades had led to the suggestion that the diet we eat is a (the) major modifier of our risk of cancer[1]. Much work has gone into estimating the percentage of tumours affected by our diet. This numbers game may have misled us. It is not a question of whether 90 or 95 per cent of our cancers are dependent upon our environment, or whether 30 or 70 per cent are somehow related to our diet (some more, some less). The problem is to prove that the last few per cent are completely independent of our life style. Since we all live in some kind of an environment and eat some sort of diet, the answer may elude us forever.

We know from scores of animal experiments that even for the tumours for which we 'know the aetiology' (say, a known chemical carcinogen or virus), it is still possible to influence the course of the experiment by minor changes in the 'environment'. This is best known for tumours originating in hormone-dependent tissues, perhaps best illustrated in the genesis of mammary tumours in mice and rats, or lymphomas in mice. Also, this is apparent in epidemiological studies—life-style factors are most likely to show up in tumours of hormone-dependent organs. This, of course, illustrates how intimately hormone production in our body reflects the environmental stimuli via the central nervous system and the endocrine glands. These cultural effects are often hard to quantify, but are undoubtedly involved in the modification of the risks (for example) for mammary cancer by an effect on the age of menarche and menopause and the age at first child birth.

Although the age-specific cancer mortality rate has not changed much since the establishing of reliable cancer registrations, the public has somehow got the impression that the risk of getting a cancer has increased immensely[2]. This requires an explanation, and a scapegoat is searched for. The news media bear a heavy burden in this respect, but maybe we have not exerted enough restraint ourselves in publishing our new findings. Anyhow, the request/demand from the public is one for advice concerning what diet they should eat and what life-style factors may be harmful.

In this situation we should reconsider the following argument given by Michael Hill in Århus in 1985 before the ECP conference on diet and cancer[3].

> Cancer of the large bowel is one of the most common cancers in the western world. About 5 per cent of us will get it. Consequently, 95 per cent of us will not. We do not know in advance who is who. Giving advice therefore implies giving advice to the whole population. We know of a fairly large number of risk factors for colon cancer, and fairly profound changes in the diet should be recommended. Apart from the effect on the

> society and the production of food stuff, this also has the drawback that the 95 per cent of the population make these changes completely in vain, since they are not going to get colon cancer anyhow.
>
> We should therefore be able to tell them with great confidence that this change in diet does in no way imply an increased risk of acquiring other ailments or perhaps other cancers. Since this is definitely true and obvious for colon cancer, which is a common cancer, it is of course even more so for all other cancers.

The basis for giving advice rests on a number of assumptions, some of which are indeed declarations of faith, profound convictions that, however, may be too frail and rooted in wishful thinking rather than sound skepticism. However controversial they may seem, and considering the taboos around them, they should nevertheless be discussed.

The basic concept is as follows. The Japanese, for example, have a low incidence of colon cancer, but a high incidence of stomach cancer. If they emigrate to (say) America, they may, by adopting the American diet (and life style), obtain a lower risk of acquiring stomach cancer. Providing they are able to omit from their diet the 'bad stuff' that causes an increase in colon cancer, they should ideally end up with a low incidence of both cancer types. Japanese women should likewise stick to the Japanese diet as far as the risk factors for breast cancer are concerned, and even more so for endometrial cancer, which would otherwise increase tenfold after emigration to America.

It may well be that when an increasing number of dietary risk factors become known, the permissible diet would ultimately shrink to nil. In fact, nowhere in the world does any one group eat a diet that considerably diminishes the overall risk of cancer. This basically is the 'Cramer versus Peto and Doll' case[4]. The pertinent question is 'Are we able to reduce the total incidence of cancer or are we witnessing a movement of cancers from one organ to another?' Little solid information is available to elucidate the question.

It is apparent that in Japanese migrants to America the incidence of stomach cancer decreases and that of colon cancer increases, although not to quite the same degree. A number of other cancers also change in incidence rate. There are indications suggesting that factors protective for colon cancer, such as a high-fibre/low-fat diet, are indeed risk factors for, if not stomach cancer, then at least atrofic gastritis, which appears to precede the development of stomach cancer.

In animal experiments, the same carcinogen may give tumours in different organs according to the dose given, and it is possible to move colon tumours induced by a carcinogen from the right to the left side of the colon, by giving cultures of acidophilus bacteria. Biologically speaking, it is not improbable that the target organ may be shifted by, say, dietary changes altering the metabolism of pro-carcinogens, promoter substances, the 'stress' on the organs, enzyme induction by indole derivatives, and so on. This is as yet poorly understood and the extent to which it is effective is unknown.

It is, however, striking that the total cancer incidence rate is fairly constant over extended periods of time with some cancer rates varying quite considerably. In the end, it comes down to the question of whether one should consider the individual cancer diseases as completely separate entities or whether they may somehow be connected. Although we do not at present understand how this may in fact be the case, it does not preclude the usefulness of such considerations. In human epidemiology, we must make some kind of an allowance for the effect of tobacco smoke, which is such a powerful effect superimposed upon all the other modifiers. At the same time, it is hard to conceive of any special cancer risk that could be attributed to the *stopping* of smoking.

Carcinogenesis and diet

Now, how could diet possibly be involved in the formation of tumours in man? For the sake of systematization, the following categories could be made:

Category A: diet could contain components that have an effect on the mucous membranes in the intestinal tract, making them more vulnerable to carcinogens, for example by inducing metaplasia or chronic irritation with increased proliferation, or by facilitating penetration of carcinogens.

Category B: diet could contain genotoxic carcinogens or pro-carcinogens either as a natural part of the food, as contaminants, as compounds added deliberately, or components formed during storage and preparation of food.

Category C: diet could contain modifiers in the form of promoters or anti-promoters, various forms of co- and anti-carcinogens, or factors that could be metabolized into such compounds, or factors with an effect on the bulk of the intestinal content such as water and 'fibres'.

It is inconceivable that any one of these factors works in isolation from the effects of the others. They exert their effect at all steps of the development of a cancer from initiation to promotion and progression. This is the explanation of the multifactorial origin of tumours and at the same time makes it senseless to pinpoint 'causes' in the more traditional sense of the word. All the components may, however, alter the risk for the final outcome.

In category A, the most likely compounds would be alcoholic beverages, especially the strong ones, but also high concentrations of salts, and maybe local irritants in swallowed dissolved tobacco smoke. These compounds may be responsible for the metaplasia in the stomach and the atrofic gastritis that almost inevitably precedes the development of cancer in the stomach. The effect of tobacco smoke may also be involved in the origin of cancer of the oesophagus and of course of the mouth and pharynx/larynx. The roughage in our diet may, as mentioned later, have a protective effect on the large bowel, but there are indications that a very coarse diet with low fat content may be a risk factor for the development of atrofic gastritis. The effect of alcohol has also been ascribed to the possibility that alcohol might act as a solvent for carcinogens, carrying them across the membrane barrier to the blood stream and liver.

Category B has probably attracted most attention over the last decades and maybe unjustly so. It takes little skill to explain to people that cancer-provoking agents should not be added to our diet on purpose. The definition of carcinogens and the evaluation of accepted doses has, however, given insurmountable difficulties and the 'Delaney clause' is unrealistically square and not useful for practical life. The control on food additives that followed the early discussion of these problems has led to very restrictive regulation and there is very little in today's use of additives that gives cause for anxiety.

In fact, the effect of these compounds does not show up in epidemiological investigations. The best estimate ascribes less than 2 per cent of all cancers to food additives (including lingering effects from previous, less restrictive regulations)[1]. Far more important may be compounds of natural origin, as stressed by Bruce Ames in the famous paper from 1983 in *Science*[5]. Also, carcinogens formed during storage by, for example, various moulds or during preparation in the form of pyrolysis and pyrosynthetic products, may be important. In large areas of the world, the aflatoxins certainly seem to play a major role in the occurrence of liver cancer, albeit in all probability in collaboration with the hepatitis B virus. Avoidance of mouldy food is now a general caution given in all food recommendations. The human relevance of the pyrosynthetic compounds, however, remains to be established. It is, however, probably in the category C compounds that one should look for the main effects of diet on the development of cancers in man.

In category C the main groups of compounds would be the fibres, lipids, vitamins, minerals and a large group of miscellaneous compounds. The fibre problem has attracted major interest, but is still a very complicated area. Much confusion in the past was caused by a lack of good definitions and methods of analysis. Food fibres comprise a large group of plant materials of very different chemical composition. Much confusion also stems from the fact that we do not eat pure fibres but plants, with all the hundreds of other components with unknown effect, which are difficult to separate from a fibre effect.

Several, not mutually exclusive, explanations have been given for the fibre effect in the bowel. The early explanations given by Burkitt may still hold some truth. Fibres may simply increase the volume of the bowel content giving a dilution effect on alleged carcinogens in the bowel and speeding up the passage time, thereby maybe decreasing the absorption from the bowel of harmful substances. The bulk effect is apparently not caused by water binding by the fibres, but rather by the fact that many fibres are good substrates for the microflora in the bowel and that the microflora then thrive and expand. The greater part of these bacteria is water and consequently the water content of the stools increases.

A large content of microflora also means the presence of enzymes that are not normally produced by the epithelial cells, enzymes that make digestion of fibres possible. The end products of this metabolism may alter, for example, the pH of the stools and consequently the solubility of many minerals and the binding of chemicals to fibre surfaces. These enzymes may also play a role in the metabolism of steroids, bile acids, etc.

Various fibre components will have various effects, and so far it is not possible to tell which fibre types may have the protective effect against colon cancer, although the pentosanes appear to be the most likely candidates. The lesson so far is, however, that one should not eat fibres as, for instance, tablets, but the vegetables and cereals in which they are found, as long as the effect of the concomitant plant materials is not known.

Lipids have long been considered a promoter for cancers of the mammary gland and the large bowel and, with less confidence, for the prostate gland. International correlation studies so far have been the most suggestive, whereas the person-based case-control and cohort studies have not been consistent. This may in part be due to a uniformity in fat intake of the study population and to an overload with risk factors. Most women in industrialized countries simply eat so much fat that a little more or less does not show up in the risk for breast cancer. In searching for a dose-response relation, we tacitly assume that susceptibility for the risk factor is equally distributed. This is by no means a permissible assumption since genetic differences will probably be responsible for great differences. This means that in a case-referent investigation we are likely to find, in between the cases, an over-representation of women with an increased susceptibility for the risk factor. This may completely quench the dose-response dependency that we are looking for and consequently we are left without the possibility to test our hypothesis in this setting.

There is another difficulty in interpreting the epidemiological results and the incidence trends over time. A better nutritional status at large, having improved over the century, has led to an increase in the final heights of young people by more than 10 centimetres, and also to an increase in weight, a decrease in the age of menarche, and an increase in the age of menopause. These are but a few of the significant parameters that may be of importance for the type of cancers we get. For mammary cancer, this would mean an increased incidence, which has been described over that same period. It is not fair to ascribe this solely to an isolated effect of fat intake.

Animal experiments may throw light on some of these problems, although one should be extremely careful in interpreting the results. It makes little sense to compare cats and mice when it comes to the effect of diet. Most experiments have been carried out in rodents because they are omnivorous, like man. Lipid intake has been varied usually from 5 to 20 per cent within the test groups. The studies almost uniformly show that bowel cancer and mammary cancer are enhanced in the groups receiving the high-fat diet. However, it is not at all clear whether this is due to the fat consumption *per se*, or to the high calorie intake inevitably consumed with the high-fat diet. There are good experiments to show that in animals on a high-fat diet, but with restriction of the total amount of calories given per time unit, the high-fat diet does not promote tumour formation. Consequently the *amount* of fat given, rather than the composition of the diet, is important.

It is also hard to separate the effect of a high-fat diet from the effect of the resulting obesity, since animals kept under traditional laboratory conditions will grow fat on a high-fat diet. In most experiments, only energy intake has been varied and only recently have experiments been carried out in which energy expenditure has also been varied by letting rats run in a running wheel or on a motor-driven treadmill. The experiments are so far not conclusive, although it appears that exercising the fat away does decrease the risk for mammary cancer[6]. Reddy *et al.* recently found fewer colon cancers in rats, given azoxymethane, in the groups allowed free exercise in running wheels[7]. Epidemiological evidence points to an increased risk in people with sedentary work.

Energy expenditure, however, is not only dependent upon the degree of exercise, but also on clothing and climate and more elusive factors such as temperament and the degree of 'luxury fuel' consumption. The mechanisms involved in the fat effect on mammary cancer and large-bowel cancer may, furthermore, be quite different.

Recommendations concerning diet and cancer prevention

In essence, we still have a lot to learn before we are able to give more detailed advice on diet. Up until then, recommendations in more general terms may be given, such as prudent restraint on the total calorie intake and to take a reasonable amount of exercise. Quantitation of the advice is out of the question at the moment, and so are the possibilities for differentiating between the many different types of lipids. Only theoretical considerations and a few animal experiments blame the polyunsaturated lipids for the largest effect. Even the polyunsaturated lipids consist of at least two major classes, the Omega 3 and 6 types, which might theoretically behave differently in their effect on the development of cancers.

It is extremely interesting that in the group of minerals and vitamins that have protective properties, the most conspicuous are anti-oxidants—radical scavengers such as the carotenoids, vitamin E and C and, indirectly, selenium, being part of the important glutathion peroxidase[5,8,9,10]. It is conceivable that their effect is exerted via a protection against endogenously formed, oxygen-derived radicals. This whole area appears to be very promising since it may offer a more general protection especially against the promoting effect in carcinogenesis. The effect is likely to be more unspecific and may consequently offer a more general protection against the development of tumours in the body. It is also likely that there may be a protective effect against the DNA toxicity of the oxygen-derived radicals which may be the largest single threat to the integrity of our DNA[11].

This whole area needs extensive study, and a large number of papers have appeared in recent years. Again, a more quantitative aspect is still lacking, nobody being able to tell anyone how many carrots they should eat daily. Intervention studies are under way using either carotenoids alone or combinations of carotenoids, vitamin E and selenium, vitamin C and other natural or artificial anti-oxidants. Animal studies have shown protective effects of such combinations against a variety of chemical carcinogens and ultraviolet light. Attempts at transforming this information into practical advice is, however, at present still 'skating on thin ice'.

Until the results of intervention studies more clearly show us the way to go, it is probably prudent to advise the public to consume a diet rich in the foodstuff containing these components. This, however, would be a natural consequence of efforts to avoid consuming a diet too rich in lipids. In practice, therefore, we should meet little difficulty in making the moderate changes in our diet that would meet both objectives.

In conclusion then, diet appears to be of paramount importance for the type of cancers we get and probably also for the total risk of getting a cancer. Even though a large amount of information is already at hand on the topic, we are still not ready to give specified, detailed or quantitative advice to the general public. There are, however, some more general lessons to be learned, which may have a significant impact. In 1985, these general rules were issued as recommendations by a consensus conference arranged by the ECP and IUNS in Århus in Denmark[3]. These recommendations may still serve as guidelines in the giving of advice to the public. The recommendations are given below.

- Decrease the intake of saturated and unsaturated fat in countries where, on average, fat constitutes more than 30 per cent of total food energy (calories). In other countries, people should maintain their lower fat intake. Consumption of fat can be decreased by lowering the intake of butter, margarine, cooking oil, and salad oils and dressings; by selecting fish, poultry, leaner meat products, and low-fat dairy products; and by boiling, baking and steaming foods rather than by frying.
- Eat a varied diet containing different types of vegetables and fruits, especially green leafy and root vegetables and citrus fruits; and ensure an adequate intake of vitamins and minerals through consumption of these foods rather than by using supplements.
- Consume foods that are rich in complex carbohydrates (i.e. starch and fibre) that are known to promote healthy bowel function.
- Maintain appropriate body weight. If a lower energy intake is desirable, use foods with complex carbohydrates including whole-grain cereal products, fruits and vegetables instead of the higher-energy fatty foods.
- Consume a low-salt diet. A desirable goal is less than 5g of salt per day as recommended in relation to cardiovascular diseases.
- Use fresh or minimally processed foods rather than cured, pickled, or traditionally smoked foods. Avoid eating mouldy foods.
- Drink alcohol only in moderation, if at all.

References

1 Committee on Diet, Nutrition, and Cancer. Assembly of life sciences (1982) National Research Council (ed.) *Diet, nutrition, and cancer*, National Academy Press, Washington, D. C.

2 Cohen, M. M., Diamond, J. M. (1986) Are we losing the war on cancer? *Nature* **323**, 488–89.

3 Joossens, J. V. Hill, M. J. Gebours, J. (eds.) (1986) *Diet and human carcinogenesis.* ECP Symposium/2. Excerpta Medica, Elsevier Science Publ., Amsterdam.

4 Doll, R., Peto, R. (1981) The causes of cancer: quantitative estimates of avoidable risks in the United States today, *J. natn. Cancer Inst.* **66**, 1192–1308.

5 Ames, B. N. (1983) Dietary carcinogens and anticarcinogens, *Science* **221**, 1256–64.

6 Simopoulos, A. P. (1987) Calories and energy expenditure in carcinogenesis: Conference report, *Am. J. Clin. Nutr.*, suppl. Jan.

7 Reddy, B. S., Sugie, S., Lowenfels, A. (1988) Effect of voluntary exercise on azoxymethane-induced colon carcinogenesis in male F344 rats, *Cancer Res.* **48**, 7079–81.

8 Cerutti, P. A. (1985) Prooxidant states and tumor promotion, *Science*, 375–381, Jan.

9 Cutler, R. G. (1984) Antioxidants, aging, and longevity I (1984) W. A. Pryor (ed.) *Free radicals in biology*, vol. vi, Academic Press, Orlando, 371–428.

10 Modifiers of carcinogenesis. Proceedings from the Symposium in Copenhagen, 22–23 Sept 1983. *Acta Pharmacol. Toxicol.* 1984, 55 (suppl. II).

11 Cathcart, R., Schwiers, E., Saul, R. L., Ames, B. N. (1984) Thymine glycol and thymidineglycol in human and rat urine: a possible assay for oxidative DNA damage, *Proc. Natl. Acad. Sci. USA* **81**, 5633–37.

Paper 2.5

CANCER PREVENTION AND THE NEW BIOLOGY

Dr. Graham Currie
Marie Curie Research Institute, The Chart, Oxted, Surrey, England

Cancer is a disease of genes. Cancers arise as a consequence of genetic pathology in a single cell, which passes on the malignant genotype to its cellular offspring. The characteristics of cancer cells—usually referred to collectively as the malignant phenotype—are thus inherited and such inheritance is truly genetic.

The purpose of this paper is to review some of the evidence for the above statements, to explain very briefly something of the current state of molecular oncology and to discuss how such exciting new evidence could be applied to the problem of how to prevent cancers. Before addressing the molecular basis of cancer development, it is worth giving some thought to the nature of the malignant phenotype. What distinguishes a cancer cell from a normal cell?

The malignant phenotype

Proliferation and survival of cancer cells

Although cancers are diseases of cell proliferation, they are not diseases of proliferation rate. There is a common misconception that cancer cells multiply abnormally fast. This is not necessarily so. Their multiplication is just inappropriate, in the wrong place, at the wrong time.

It is also worth bearing in mind that although the proliferation of cancer cells seems to be unrestrained, it is a very inefficient process. Comparisons of the cell cycle time of cancer cells (i.e. the time taken to complete one cell division) with the volume growth rates of tumours reveal a dramatic disproportion, which suggests that the survival rate of cells from each subsequent division cycle must be very low indeed. These rare survivors in the necrotic, avascular and disorganized mess that is characteristic of most tumours presumably represent the survival of the least unfit in an environment that is less than ideal.

Extended lifespan

Normal human cells maintained in tissue culture have a limited lifespan and, moreover, the residual number of cell doublings in a cell population declines with the age of the donor (i.e. the older the donor, the shorter the remaining lifespan of the cell). Although there is, as yet, no convincing evidence that restricted cellular lifespan is directly related to senescence of the whole organism, it remains the best *in vitro* correlate of ageing. Cellular ageing could represent a genetically determined switch to a non-proliferating, fully differentiated state. Some authors have even suggested that it may represent a vital biological clock mechanism, the function of which is to restrict the lifespan of the whole organism.

Cancer cells, as a rule, do not age. When normal human cells are grown in culture, extension of lifespan (often referred to as 'cellular immortality') is a highly significant acquired characteristic associated with malignant change. The apparently unlimited extension of the lifespan of cancer cells may represent some form of permanent arrest in an undifferentiated state. Since differentiation represents a programmed pattern of specific gene expression, cellular immortality—indeed, cancers—can be viewed as disorders of gene expression.

Other malignant characteristics

Many other characteristics are associated with malignant behaviour *in vivo*, for example, invasiveness and metastasis. *In vitro* correlates include cellular growth in the absence of contact with a substratum. These are ill-defined and complex phenomena, which are also manifested by some normal cells, and for the purposes of this article will be regarded as epiphenomena.

The probability of the malignant phenotype

The proliferation of normal cells is a very complex cascade of programmed events initiated by the binding of a chemical growth factor to a specific receptor at the cell surface. An activating signal is transmitted across the cell membrane and carried by chemical messengers through the cytoplasm to the nucleus, where complex molecular changes occur in the DNA. The DNA and subsequently the cell duplicates, and the identical offspring gradually acquire the characteristics of fully differentiated cells. The coordinated control of these events leading to the duplication of DNA, cell division and differentiation, could be subverted anywhere in the cascade. Many genes are involved and damage to any one of them could interfere with the regulation of cell division and differentiation.

A probabilistic model for cancer development would envisage damage to DNA occurring randomly throughout the genome in the cell populations most exposed to carcinogenic insult (for example, bronchial epithelium). This could result in a bewildering array of abnormalities in DNA, including deletions, point mutations, rearrangements, etc. occurring either in coding or non-coding regions. The chance must be remote of damage resulting in changes in gene function that end in a viable and autonomous cell with an extended lifespan. Deletion of regulatory genes or other controlling sequences (such as promoters or enhancers), or mutational activation or even amplification of particular genes, will only confer a selective advantage on the affected cell if there are no other harmful lesions, and if the specific lesion induced has significant effects upon some activity such as cell proliferation. This is clearly a long shot. What is more, the common lethal cancers arising in epithelial cells (for example, lung, breast, colon) seem to require multiple, and probably quite specific, combinations of genetic lesions before the cascade of events described above is subverted.

What kinds of genetic lesions cause cancers?

Dominant or recessive lesions

Normal body cells, like cancer cells, contain two versions of each gene—one inherited from each parent—arranged on pairs of chromosomes. Certain characteristics of the cell may only be expressed when both the genes at a particular location on a pair of chromosomes are described as recessive. If only one of the genes is recessive, then the characteristic that it encodes will not be expressed in the presence of its dominant counterpart on the other chromosome in the pair.

It has been known for some time from the results of cell fusion experiments (for example, Harris, 1986) that malignancy is a recessive characteristic. In other words, when a malignant cell is fused with a normal cell the resulting hybrid behaves more like a normal cell; the malignant characteristics are not expressed in the presence of normal chromosomes. (There is one major and interesting exception to this rule: the hybrids chosen for monoclonal antibody production, which retain malignant characteristics.) The re-emergence of malignant behaviour in the offspring of such hybrid cells is associated with the loss of certain chromosomes.

This has led to the notion that specific genes—known as regulatory or suppressor genes—can function to inhibit the malignant phenotype. This view is strengthened by experiments on the ageing of normal cells, which reveal that senescence is a dominant characteristic and suggest that there are regulatory genes that act to place some sort of limit on normal cell proliferation. Such regulatory genes may, of course, be important targets for carcinogenesis. Currently available evidence suggests that regulatory genes may be present on several different human chromosomes and that these are dominant to (i.e. can repress) recessive malignant characteristics, such as unrestrained proliferation and extended lifespan.

However, talk of dominant and recessive traits—more reminiscent of Mendel's wrinkled peas than of modern molecular genetics—is probably a misleading oversimplification. Many genes exert their effects indirectly, i.e. some gene products may stimulate or even inhibit the expression of other functionally important genes. Furthermore, the abnormal protein encoded by an abnormal gene could block the target sites for the normal protein that it replaces. The possible mechanisms of genetic subversion are numerous and complex.

Gene loss and cancer

The foregoing discussion points to the possible loss of regulatory genes as an initiating event in cancer cell development. What is the currently available evidence for such a view?

In the cells of childhood retinoblastoma, there is a consistent chromosome abnormality—loss of genetic material on both copies of chromosome 13 at a specific location (see Table 2.11). Knudson (1985) has therefore proposed that two mutations are necessary for the genesis of retinoblastoma, one in each chromosome of the pair. However, in the familial form of this cancer, inactivation or loss of one of the significant genes may be inherited from a parent. The normal, active gene on the other chromosome 13 has been identified and its DNA sequence has been determined. It has been named Rb. Interestingly, two well-studied DNA-tumour viruses (SV40 and adenovirus) seem to operate by interfering with the normal functioning of the Rb gene. Moreover, lesions of the Rb gene have been identified in cancers other than retinoblastoma, including osteogenic sarcoma and some cases of breast cancer. Recent studies have shown that an Rb gene clone will, when transferred into retinoblastoma cells in tissue culture, cause reversion of their malignant phenotype to the normal state.

There is mounting evidence to show that this sort of mechanism, loss of a specific gene, may operate at other chromosomal loci in other types of cancer. Sporadic cases of Wilm's tumour, hepatoblastoma and rhabdomyosarcoma seem to involve gene loss at, or close to, the locus on chromosome 11 that is associated with WAGR syndrome (Wilm's tumour, aniridia, genitourinary malformations and mental retardation). Other significant losses at specific locations are listed in Table 2.11 and the hunt is on for more.

Table 2.11 Gene losses associated with some cases of human cancer

Cancer	Chromosome number
bilateral acoustic neuroma and meningioma	22
childhood retinoblastoma	13
colorectal cancer	5, 17 and 18
ductal breast cancer	13
familial adenomatous polyposis	5
familial neurofibromatosis (von Recklinghausen's disease)	17
kidney and lung cancer	3
multiple endocrine neoplasia syndromes (MEN-1/MEN-2)	1 and 10
Wilm's tumour, hepatoblastoma and rhabdomyosarcoma	11

Experimental approaches to the identification and cloning of putative regulatory or suppressor genes are in progress throughout the world. Investigators are searching through gene 'libraries' for clones with suppressant activity, or are introducing chromosomes into malignant cells, which revert them to normal. For example, Weissman and colleagues (Weissman *et al.*, 1987) have demonstrated the presence of sequences on chromosome 11 that can suppress the malignant characteristics of human tumour cells.

Multiple genetic lesions

If one thinks of environmental carcinogens simply as genetic 'poisons', then deletion of genes seems to represent the most significant aspect of carcinogenesis. That does not mean it is true. It is just easier to imagine than other more complex genetic events! It is as yet unclear how many stages in a given cancer may be due to gene loss. The appropriate combination of types of genetic damage necessary for a cell to become malignant may require both dominant and recessive lesions.

Although many of the childhood cancers and some of those in young adults seem to develop in response to one or two genetic events in a cell, the majority of common lethal cancers of the industrialized world are the products of multistage carcinogenesis. A variety of compelling evidence from histopathology and epidemiology indicates that these cancers arise after a series of necessary, cumulative genetic events. In general, it seems that cancers with a long latent period from the initial exposure to a carcinogen pass through more stages than do the rapidly developing cancers. For example, cutaneous malignant melanoma seems to need only one or two genetic lesions, whereas cancer of the prostate may need up to ten distinct but cumulative events involving genetic damage (Cook, Doll and Fallingham, 1969).

In conclusion, it is worth emphasizing that most of the available evidence suggests that cancer is a common cellular destination that is reached by many different pathways. There is no one single cause of cancer, no single cancer gene, and there is therefore no grand unifying hypothesis or solution.

Oncogenes

The word oncogene is a misnomer, but we are stuck with it. 'A gene that causes cancer' is a concept perfectly reasonably applied to the genes carried by cancer-causing viruses, but the term has come to mean any gene that could be involved, in some way or another, in the genesis of cancer.

DNA tumour virus oncogenes

Oncogenic DNA viruses such as adenovirus or the papovaviruses (for example, papilloma or polyoma viruses and SV40) contain specific identifiable sequences responsible for their cancer-causing properties. These viruses are of considerable clinical significance in that one or more of them may be implicated in a number of human cancers, most notably cancers of the cervix and penis. The DNA tumour virus oncogenes studied so far do not show close structural similarities to any genes in the DNA of the cells that they infect. They do appear to have functional equivalents in mammalian cells, but these are not yet fully characterized or understood.

The best studied of the DNA tumour virus oncogenes have three very important properties. First, the product of a single oncogene can produce the most dramatic and diverse range of biochemical and functional changes in an infected cell—in other words, one oncogene can affect the expression of lots of other genes. Second, they extend the lifespan of a variety of cells, at least in tissue cultures. Third, cells 'immortalized' by these oncogenes are not usually fully malignant, but immortalizing oncogenes can collaborate with other oncogenes to confer all the characteristics of the malignant phenotype. For example, cells immortalized by one of the adenovirus oncogenes can be fully transformed to the malignant state by another oncogene from the same virus or by a polyoma virus oncogene.

There seems to be at least two distinct functions of these oncogenes: immortalization and malignant transformation. In the SV40 virus, a single oncogene can fulfil both functions, which may explain the ability of this virus to induce cancers in many different cell types and in several different host species. Many of these oncogenes encode proteins that interact with other proteins in the infected cell, which in their turn would normally be involved in regulating DNA replication. Studying the DNA tumour viruses and their oncogenic products has provided us with important insights into the molecular basis of normal and malignant cell biology.

RNA tumour virus oncogenes

Acutely transforming RNA viruses (or retroviruses) also contain sequences in their genetic material known as retroviral oncogenes, which are responsible for the transforming properties of these viruses. Unlike the DNA virus oncogenes, however, these retrovirus oncogenes are structurally very similar to DNA sequences present in the genetic material of normal cells. Indeed, it turns out that these DNA sequences have been 'hi-jacked' by the viruses. At some point in past evolution, these sequences have been copied from the host cell by the virus, converted into their RNA-equivalent and spliced into the viral genome, where they have since remained. About thirty of these retroviral oncogenes have been reported and they are all normal cellular genes subverted in one way or another. The discovery of retroviral oncogenes has focused attention on their counterparts in normal cells—the so-called 'cellular oncogenes'.

Cellular oncogenes

Cellular oncogenes have several properties in common with their retroviral analogues. They function as dominant genes, their structure has remained remarkably stable throughout their evolution, their products have numerous complex effects on other genes and most of those studied so far seem to play a role either in regulating cell proliferation or differentiation. Many cellular oncogenes seem to be members of large families of host cell genes with similar DNA sequences.

Some cellular oncogenes (for example, the *ras* genes) seem to be involved in the genesis of human cancers. They were originally detected by their ability to transform cells in tissue culture to a fully malignant phenotype when the gene was incorporated into the host cell DNA. Three slightly different activated *ras* genes have been identified—one in bladder-cancer cell lines, another in colon and breast cancer lines, and a third in neuroblastoma and sarcoma lines. They have subsequently been detected in a variable percentage of cases of most forms of cancer.

The *ras* genes detected in the DNA of cancer cells are usually found to be single genes activated by point mutations at specific 'hot-spots' in the DNA sequence. They are unusual in that, so far, mutation seems to be involved in the activation of only a few types of cellular oncogene. In those oncogenes in which mutation is required for activation, the oncogenic effect on the host cell is likely to be mediated by the production of an abnormal protein, which has direct or indirect effects on cell proliferation or differentiation.

It is difficult to provide an accurate assessment of the number of cellular oncogenes in the mammalian genome, since the definition of what constitutes an oncogene is so woolly. What is more, new oncogenes are being described at the rate of about one per week. At the time of writing, there are at least 100 so-called oncogenes. I suspect that there are going to be a lot more.

Oncogenes and multistage carcinogenesis

It is the prime ambition of many cancer-research workers to provide a complete explanation for the carcinogenic process in molecular terms. This is clearly going to be a massive exercise, but it is not impossible. Since the DNA sequencing of the entire human genome is an entirely practicable proposition, which is already in progress, most things are now possible in biology. They just require a lot of money and a lot of effort.

The molecular events underlying the various histopathological stages identifiable in the development of a common lethal epithelial cancer have not yet been fully characterized, but substantial progress has been made. A major international collaborative study has examined gene loss and *ras* gene activation in the history of colorectal cancers. Vogelstein and colleagues (1988) examined a large number of cases of colorectal cancer at all stages in their natural history. In adenomas under 1 cm in diameter they only rarely detected any genetic abnormality, but in larger adenomas they found a high incidence of mutant *ras* genes. Moreover, gene losses at specific locations on chromosome 17 or 18 were characteristic of either advanced adenomas or of carcinomas.

These results are consistent with a model for the multistage development of colorectal carcinoma that involves the mutational activation of the *ras* gene (a dominant lesion), coupled with the loss of several—probably at least three—genes that normally suppress the malignant phenotype (recessive lesions). It is interesting that Vogelstein's group identified four genetic lesions and that the absence of any detectable lesion in the early adenomas implies that there is a fifth. Epidemiological evidence derived mostly from age-incidence curves has suggested the presence of five discrete steps in the genesis of colorectal cancers (Cook, Doll and Fallingham, 1969).

How can molecular biology help us to prevent cancers?

How will new developments in our understanding of the molecular basis of carcinogenesis help in preventing cancers? I do not know the answer to this question, but on the basis of the results so far available, it is clear that as far as clinical application is concerned, methods may be more important than paradigms.

Perhaps the most exhilarating aspect of modern molecular genetics is its facility to do remarkable things quickly and reproducibly. Techniques have become available that make it a relatively simple task to look for a given point mutation or a deletion in the DNA obtained from a single cell. Automation of these diagnostic methods can provide large numbers of valuable results in an afternoon.

Just 25 years ago, many eminent biologists were predicting that the inner workings of the cell were far too complex ever to be comprehended—that there were impenetrable 'black boxes' at the heart of biology. The triumph of reductionism and of the New Biology is that there are no longer thought to be any black boxes. Although there is a great deal that we still do not know about how cells behave, there is every reason to believe that we will eventually know everything that we need to know. Weinberg's claim (1983) that 'the molecular mechanisms underlying cancer should be well defined by the end of this decade' would have sounded vainglorious twenty years ago. But this is no longer so. His estimate of the timescale required was a little optimistic, but his excitement and enthusiasm seem entirely justified by events.

How should our resources be deployed to maximize the impact of molecular genetics on cancer prevention? Obviously, by doing more well funded, high-quality, basic research we stand a good chance of making interesting and possibly important discoveries about how cells work and about how normal cells become cancer cells. Only then can we start talking about clinical relevance with any real confidence. But we can already review what could be done with the currently available methods of molecular genetics.

Identification of those at risk

Mutations in the DNA of ova and sperm cells play a role in the inheritance of a predisposition to some cancers. Inherited mutations are, as already mentioned, associated with a high incidence of retinoblastoma, and others have been identified in cases of familial adenomatous polyposis (FAP), the multiple endocrine neoplasia syndromes (MEN-1 and MEN-2), and in familial neurofibromatosis (von Recklinghausen's disease) (see Table 2.11).

The investigation of these relatively rare familial disorders is allowing the development of expertise, reagents and methods that will eventually be focused on familial influences in the more common cancers, for example, breast cancer. A large panel of diagnostic reagents is becoming available, which could before too long be applied in automated assays to the genetic screening of large populations to detect those at high risk of developing a cancer. There is, of course, no point in doing this unless you have some treatment to offer the patients. Clinical experience in FAP and MEN syndromes suggest that genetic screening is clinically worthwhile. While it does not necessarily prevent primary cancers, it detects tumours early enough to render the treatment effective, i.e. it prevents deaths from these cancers.

Molecular methods for early detection

The sheer sensitivity of modern molecular techniques is their main strength and enables them to be used for various types of screening assay. For example, the presence of the DNA of potentially oncogenic viruses can easily be detected in an otherwise normal cell. Cervical cytology could be revolutionized by the methods of molecular biology. Latent human papilloma virus (HPV-16) infection could be detected in cells of the cervix uteri at the same time as looking for abnormalities in cellular genes in the same sample. As mentioned earlier, the study by Vogelstein and colleagues (1988) suggests that the detection of *ras* gene mutations in early lesions of the colon and rectum may indicate the presence of pre-cancer.

Virus vaccines

Genetic manipulation techniques will be of enormous value in the production of vaccines for the prevention of some virus-induced cancers. Perhaps the most significant internationally is the introduction of genetically engineered hepatitis B vaccines, which should—if deployed in the appropriate populations at risk (for example, in the Gambia)—be of considerable value in the prevention of primary hepatoma.

Epstein–Barr virus vaccines are currently being investigated and should prove to be of value for the prevention of African lymphoma, nasopharyngeal carcinoma in the Far East and transplantation-associated lymphomas. Other virus-associated cancers, such as adult T-cell leukaemia (associated with the HTLV-1 virus), should be amenable to prevention by vaccination if directed at appropriate populations in the Caribbean and in rural Japan.

Detection of carcinogen-induced damage in cells

The detection of environmental carcinogens should be facilitated by a direct examination of the confrontation between the ultimate carcinogen and DNA. Modern biochemical techniques, such as mass spectroscopy and nuclear magnetic resonance (NMR) methods, can detect the formation of so-called adducts between carcinogens and DNA or RNA, as well as with proteins such as haemoglobin in the cell. It is therefore possible to identify individuals who have recently been exposed to carcinogens by the presence of such adducts (say) in the haemoglobin of a simple blood sample. Cigarette smokers have readily detectable adducts in their blood. The deployment of this sort of technique, for example, in factory workers, could play a valuable role in cancer prevention by providing a system for monitoring those at risk.

DNA repair

We live in a sea of carcinogens. External and internal body surfaces are regularly being exposed to physical and chemical carcinogens—in food, in air, in sunlight, in just about everything. A very long-chain replicating polymer such as DNA is clearly at risk of damage and of replication error. There is abundant evidence that we have our own in-built cancer-prevention systems, in biochemical pathways that inactivate carcinogens and in the ability to repair damaged DNA.

A range of DNA-binding proteins have been characterized with the ability to recognize damaged sequences and activate their excision and repair. Environmental carcinogens that inflict genetic damage would also have to overwhelm or subvert such an effective biochemical 'quality-control' system. This may be another clue to the multistage nature of most carcinogenesis. Inherited defects in DNA-repair capacity are well described and are associated with an increased incidence of cancer in, for example, xeroderma pigmentosum, which is characterized by an extreme sensitivity to sunlight and a high incidence of skin cancers at an early age.

In the very near future, much of the molecular enzymology of DNA repair should be comprehensively understood due to the application of molecular cloning techniques. This will generate valuable reagents that could be used for diagnostic purposes, for example, in the detection of inherited defects in DNA repair and the identification of at-risk groups. It is also tempting to speculate that a detailed knowledge of the biochemical mechanisms of DNA repair could lead to the development of pharmacological techniques for its enhancement.

Activation and detoxification of carcinogens

The activation of carcinogens by host cell enzymes and the interaction of the ultimate carcinogen with its molecular targets are two areas in which modern biochemistry has a lot to offer, and in which pharmacology could be of potential importance. For example, we now know that free radicals derived from molecular oxygen may play an important role in DNA damage and that such free radical damage has been incriminated in both the initiation and promotion stages of carcinogenesis.

Many anti-oxidant compounds have been shown to inhibit chemical carcinogenesis in experimental systems. This could lead to either a nutritional or pharmacological approach to the prevention of cancers. Dietary factors such as vitamin E, selenium and beta-carotene are currently being investigated, since they are known to play a role in anti-oxidant defence.

Molecular epidemiology

The direct application of modern molecular techniques to specific problems in cancer prevention may emerge from investigations of those cancers whose cause (or causes) is unknown, but whose incidence gives cause for concern. Examples of such cancers include testicular cancer and non-Hodgkin's lymphoma, both of which are becoming more common each year. By looking for causative genetic lesions in these cancers (for example, viral oncogene sequences), we may be able to gain insights into the main causative factors and then take appropriate action.

Gene therapy

Given the remarkable ability of modern molecular biology to engineer or tailor genes, it is easy (perhaps too easy) to speculate about the possible forms of genetic intervention that could be deployed for the prevention of cancers. Gene therapy could be envisaged for the prevention of some familial cancers. Missing genes can, in theory, be replaced and these might include missing or defective 'tumour-suppressor' genes in specific pedigrees. In tissue culture and in certain genetically-manipulated strains of laboratory animal such conjuring tricks have already been accomplished.

However, the difficulties of applying such remedies to people who are clinically well, but who are considered at high risk of developing cancer, are enormous. The major difficulty will be to target a single copy of a normal gene precisely to the correct spot in the genome and to insert it accurately without, at the same time, doing harm elsewhere. Since we cannot at present do this, gene therapy for cancer prevention remains science fiction.

New drug development

The main hope of modern molecular genetics and cancer prevention must lie in its ability to identify specific targets for pharmacological intervention. Most of the significant events involved in cancer cell behaviour involve specific protein-protein or protein-DNA interactions. The mechanisms of these interactions can be modelled by computer graphics and drug development can then, in theory, take place. New discoveries about 'zinc fingers' or 'leucine zippers' suggest that drug design for the specific regulation of gene expression may be feasible and highly effective.

Conclusion

The New Biology has revolutionized our understanding of what cancer is and how it develops. Molecular genetics will undoubtedly have a major impact on our knowledge of, and ability to manipulate, carcinogenesis. Such optimism should, however, be seen in context. It can, and no doubt will, be argued that even the most complete understanding of the molecular basis of malignant change will not necessarily provide optimal approaches to cancer prevention. Up to 400 000 Europeans die each year from smoking-related cancers. You do not need molecular genetics to deal with that problem.

One of the most significant effects of modern clinical oncology is seen in the improved survival of cancer patients under 40 years of age. Cancers occurring in patients over 40 are still largely unresponsive to systemic therapies and death rates are largely unaffected by new treatment methods. However, epidemiological evidence leading to programmes of carcinogen avoidance (smoking, dietary factors, etc.), are likely to have their major impact on the incidence of cancers in elderly people. Cancers in the young—due presumably to inherited and/or viral causes—will not, by and large, be preventable by life-style modification. The application of molecular biology and future research efforts should, I believe, be targetted on the study of cancers that occur in people under 40 years of age.

References

Cook, P. J., Doll, R. and Fallingham, S. A. (1969) A mathematical model for the age distribution of cancer in man, *Int. J. Cancer* **4**, 93–112.

Harris, H. (1986) The genetic analysis of malignancy, *J. Cell Sci.* suppl. 4, 431–444.

Knudson, A. G. (1985) Hereditary cancer, oncogenes and anti-oncogenes, *Cancer Res.* **45**, 1437–45.

Vogelstein, B. and nine others (1988) Genetic alterations during colorectal-tumour development, *New Engl. J. Med.* **319**, 525–532.

Weinberg, R. (1983) A molecular basis of cancer, *Scientific American* **249**, 102–116.

Weissman, B. E., Saxton, P. J. and four others (1987) Introduction of a normal human chronosome 11 into a Wilm's tumour cell line controls its tumorigenic expression, *Science* **236**, 175–180.

Chapter 3

CANCER EDUCATION AND THE GENERAL PUBLIC

Summary

The background papers and subsequent wide-ranging discussions of the working group on 'Cancer education and the general public' at the Lisbon Colloquium emphasized the need for action in four main areas:

1 The need to integrate cancer education, from the early stages of planning, into general health-education programmes. However, it must be recognized that the acceptability of health education is reduced if social norms and government legislation do not encourage the adoption of healthier behaviour. Health-education programmes must be balanced by health-promotion activities that make it easier for people to maintain their health and minimize their risks of developing disease.

2 Cancer-education programmes for the general public should be:

- built on proven models of health education; continued research on this is necessary.
- based on a community development approach that involves truly interactive consultation at all levels.
- aimed at enhancing the competency of individuals and groups to take action to protect their health.

3 The need for education and training of those involved in cancer education so that, within a multidisciplinary team approach, a broad range of health educators' skills can be drawn upon.

4 The approach should emphasize keeping risk factors low—'Stay low', rather than lowering risk factors; this requires cancer-prevention education to 'Start Young'. Research is needed to establish the most effective interventions with young people, as is education and training for those who work with them. Priority should be given to preventing young people becoming regular smokers.

Paper 3.1: *Health Education in the Community* Dr. Emer Shelley

Paper 3.2: *Primary Prevention of Cancers: the need for health education and intersectoral health promotion* Professor Gerjo Kok and Dr. H. de Vries

Paper 3.3: *Educating Early about the Prevention of Cancers* Dr. Anne Charlton.

The working group concentrated on reaching the general public through the community groups to which individuals belong. The main theme was primary prevention. The background papers covered a wide range of specific projects and most of these projects had transferable elements that could be used in planning other projects. The working group emphasized, however, the importance of making local projects culturally specific to the target community group.

The group recognized the importance of delivering cancer education within whole health-education programmes. These health-education programmes must, in turn, be supported by the health-enabling social, economic and political changes that health promotion seeks to bring about. However, many of the projects described in the background papers were not planned as part of integrated health-promotion programmes. Such integrated plans can meet opposition, as Kok (Paper 3.2) admits when describing work in the Netherlands:

> An integrated health-promotion programme is not realizable at this time in our country. There is a change in the right direction, but the resistance against an effective anti-smoking health-promotion policy is still very strong.

This form of opposition was exemplified immediately after the Colloquium, whilst this book was being written, by the opposition of a single member of the European Community, the UK (although supporting the Europe Against Cancer project) to the introduction of compulsory *Smoking kills* warnings on the fronts of cigarette packets.

PM attacked over stance on tobacco

Aileen Ballantyne
Medical Correspondent

THE Prime Minister came under mounting attack from European cancer experts yesterday for her opposition to compulsory "smoking kills" warnings on the front of cigarette packets.

Experts running the Europe Against Cancer campaign want to go further than the European Economic Community Council of Ministers' agreement, unsuccessfully opposed by the British Government. They want to ban tobacco sponsorship of the arts and sport, and all tobacco advertising by the end of the year.

Mr Michael Wood, honorary secretary of the Cancer Education Co-ordinating Group for the UK and Ireland, called for the bans at the European Parliament in Strasbourg on Wednesday and strongly attacked the British-supported voluntary agreements with the tobacco industry.

Speaking after a meeting with Mrs Thatcher and Mr Kenneth Clarke, the Health Secretary, in London yesterday, Professor Maurice Tubiana, chairman of the committee of experts for Europe Against Cancer, stressed that their priority was the fight against tobacco – which caused a third of all cancers in Europe.

Dr Michel Richonnier, co-ordinator of the Europe Against Cancer programme, said that without a common policy on tobacco advertising and cigarette health warnings there would be nothing to stop the tobacco industry concentrating on the country with the weakest regulations.

Newspapers and magazines, printed in any language, carrying the strongest advertisements and weakest health warnings permitted, could be distributed freely by the tobacco industry in the EEC after 1992, he said.

Mrs Thatcher, who launched Europe Against Cancer Information Year in Britain in January as part of the Europe Against Cancer programme, is likely to go to the European Court of Justice over Britain's right to veto health directives.

● Dr Martin Raw, adviser to the British Medical Association on tobacco and Europe, accused Mrs Thatcher of "breathtaking hypocrisy" in personally supporting the Europe Against Cancer programme, yet opposing proposals aimed at putting it into action.

In yesterday's British Medical Journal, Dr Raw writes: "The European Commission expected a rough ride for the tobacco directives from the tobacco industry. It had not expected the British Government to do the industry's job for it."

Figure 3.1 Although the UK supported the Europe Against Cancer campaign, it was the only EC member to vote against the introduction of compulsory 'Smoking kills' warnings on the front of cigarette packets.

Other chapters in this book cover the discussions, relevant to this chapter, by the groups on health policy (Chapter 4) and business interests and cancer (Chapter 5). Chapter 7 attempts to draw together the wide range of discussions to throw light on the planning and delivery of integrated programmes.

For this chapter, the introduction to the three accompanying papers examines:

- **the nature and practice of health education** Helping people to change; using a community development model of health promotion; and taking action to improve health—educating the health consumer.
- **ethical issues** Keeping risk factors low; priority target groups; the importance of role models; the potential to cause harm; evaluation must be done; and the need for further research and development.
- **cancer education: plans and priorities** Is the community ready for a cancer-education programme? Clarifying the message; planning the intervention; avoiding a premature launch; and planning, implementation and evaluation: balancing the use of resources.
- **competency-based training for health educators** Health educators' competencies and cancer education.

A The nature and practice of health education

The fundamental need of those whose work involves them in cancer education for the general public is for education about the nature of health education and training for its practice.

The temptation for cancer 'experts', who are inexperienced in the practice of health education, is to leap from what is known about the causes of cancers into exhorting the individual to change his or her ways. Such prescriptive advice to the general public assumes that if only people knew what they were doing wrong they would change their ways. A conclusion that is easily drawn from this approach is that those who, despite being warned, do not change, can be blamed as foolish or as lacking in will power.

Health education aims to maintain and improve individual and community health through the process of education. Individuals and communities can be helped to learn about their possible health choices and the constraints that operate on these choices. They can be helped to build up their skills so that they can make, for themselves, informed decisions as to what action to take to improve their health.

However, many health workers who are required to move into this field may not be familiar, or at ease, with educational approaches that seek to empower the learner. They may be more accustomed to the approach that assumes that, as health experts, they know best what decisions other people should make.

Many people will need support to build up confidence in their ability to change. If, at heart, they don't believe they *can* change their ways, they are more likely to discard the evidence that they *should* make the change. Once they are committed to making a change, they may then need help to build up adequate skills to make and maintain the desired change. Of course, nothing succeeds like success—a person's confidence in his or her ability to make changes is immensely reinforced by succeeding in making a change! Conversely, failure can be demoralizing and can make someone less likely to want to try again. Fortunately, it is often quite easy to show just how much can be learned from a previous failed attempt; it can be seen as making a subsequent attempt much more likely to succeed.

When planning how to make changes, most people will identify constraints that make it difficult for them to make the desired change. Some of these constraints may be overcome by the individual or by community action. Other constraints will need action at a higher level, perhaps even by means of government legislation, if the barriers to change are to be removed.

These constraints that make it difficult to adopt a healthier life style must be minimized as far as is possible. In Paper 3.1, Shelley concentrates on health education within the community but makes it quite clear that such an approach, if it is to be effective and indeed ethically acceptable, must be embedded in a wider health-promotion programme in which the economic constraints and social problems that hinder change are tackled.

Helping people to change

Cancer education requires far more than passing on information about the causes of cancer. It is equally important to help people to change their way of life. These two needs can result in conflicting approaches. Health-education messages often deliver information in an authoritarian way that assumes the 'learner' is a passive recipient who will obey the advice without questioning it. This authoritarian style can conflict with the approach needed to help people to change their ways.

The aim of messages that increase competency must be to encourage people to feel confident in their ability to reach informed decisions and to change their behaviour. This latter approach draws upon theories of the determinants of self-esteem and on how to build up a sense of self-efficacy and actual competency (Paper 3.2). Such an approach puts a high value on the ability of an individual to make up his or her own mind. (Ironically, the professional training of some health workers may have emphasized the importance of their expert knowledge and may have thereby encouraged them to believe that they know what is best for other people!)

Education within groups Educational interventions that are tailor made for specific community groups are a particularly effective way in which to build up both individual and group competency in order to take action to improve health.

Since the social norms of groups frequently affect the acceptability of the information, the basic messages of cancer education can often be best delivered through these community groups. Kok and de Vries (Paper 3.2) remind us that the use of paraprofessionals, i.e. specially trained influential members of target groups, can be particularly effective with these groups.

The group approach is particularly effective with those people whom traditional health-education approaches have failed to influence. Such people often belong to a group that is culturally distinct, for example minority language groups, immigrant communities, travelling people (gypsies); or to a group that has rejected the cultural norms of their society, for example school drop-outs, drug users and many teenagers involved in the normal process of establishing a separate adult identity! Health education with these 'difficult to reach' groups may have failed because the message is unacceptable or because the people feel unable to change.

Community groups may be work, social-network, or neighbourhood based. (Table 3.1 identifies key components of health-education projects with work-based groups.) These groups need to be understood, consulted and worked with collaboratively; but health workers may require additional education and training in order to be able to use this approach. Of course, community groups may not be used to being consulted! They may need help with 'how to be consulted', i.e. how to speak up as health consumers.

Table 3.1 Workplace programmes

These can be very effective if they:

- are part of a general health programme rather than deal with specific issues of health and work
- have been developed in consultation with management and with unions
- can employ work-based health-and-safety workers whose traditional role is now reduced
- use existing networks in the workplace
- discover what the workers' expressed health needs are, i.e. what worries them most
- enter via a popular programme, for example weight loss or fitness
- tailor make the programme to the company's style

Using a community-development model of health promotion

The community development model of health promotion has to be understood by those involved in planning and delivering health-promotion programmes. In essence, such an approach seeks to build up both individual and group competency to take action to improve health. The approach requires :

Working with the community, at local level

- in small steps, carefully and with the right people
- considering, at each step, the consultation and education that will be needed
- using an intersectoral approach, so that all health workers and other professionals work together from the start in the planning and delivery of the programme
- with key representatives from community groups
- establishing a clear benefit for this cooperation
- involving, in particular,
  - teachers, pupils and school resources
  - opinion leaders in the community
  - community nurses and doctors (Involvement of local doctors is essential, but they often need encouragement and training in this community approach.)
  - local employers and retailers, who, with education, will become involved provided they do not lose money.

Taking action to improve health: educating the health consumer

Health education aims to increase the ability of individuals and groups to tackle health problems. This involves two elements: improving their sense of efficacy (their perception of their ability to do things) and their actual competency (the skills needed to do things)(see Paper 3.3).

This empowerment should go beyond enabling individuals to take action to improve *personal* health by life-style changes. Education about the determinants of health, and the issues and strategies involved in health promotion, can lead to action by individuals and groups to protect the health of their *community*—thus complementing the actions of health-promotion workers and policy makers.

Informed community action Community groups can, for example, become involved in:

- action to improve access to local cancer-screening facilities
- supporting the work of community health councils, which provide a consultative link with local health authorities
- exerting consumer pressure on local food stores—including the use of publicity for good practice—to provide a wider choice of healthier foods
- encouraging local schools to provide appropriate health education for all pupils
- lending weight to national consumer representative bodies seeking changes such as better food labelling
- convincing local employers of the community's concern about health risks associated with manufacturing processes or products, or conditions of employment
- bringing home to the politicians, who depend on their votes, the strength of community feelings about environmental health risks and government policies that 'promote ill-health'
- urging legislation and policies that make it easier for people to take care of their health.

The importance of cancer registries There is a need to educate people about how they can contribute to a better understanding of cancers and cancer risks. The release of personal data on causes of death and previous medical history for confidential use by cancer registries is needed if baseline data and correlation of cancer-associated factors is to be established. If health educators do not know how much cancer there is in their communities, and in which segments of the population cancers are more prevalent, it is almost impossible to target health education to high-risk groups effectively. It is also much more difficult to evaluate the process and outcomes of intervention programmes. As yet, not all members of the European Community agree to the release of such information. However, if the vital work of national cancer registries is explained to the general public, then resistance to the release of personal health data—which can be used to benefit future generations—can be overcome.

B Ethical issues

The ethical requirement only to offer health education for the individual as part of a health-promotion programme has already been considered.

Health-education programmes represent a major financial investment and should be proved to be cost effective. But financial considerations, on either side of the cost/benefit equation, are not the only factors to be taken into account. These programmes can raise fear and anxiety; can be invidious if they appear to single out a particular target audience; and are unprofessional if they are not based on what has been learned from earlier health-education programmes or if they do not allow for formative and summative evaluation.

Keeping risk factors low

Shelley reminds us in Paper 3.1 that even though a causal effect is established, it does not necessarily follow that reversal of the risk behaviour will lead to a reduction in the disease. The important thrust of prevention education should be towards avoiding the risk behaviour in the first place—'keeping risk factors low'—rather than giving up risk-related behaviour—'reducing risk factors'.

The emphasis should be 'Start Young'—the focus should be on the new generation that has not, as yet, adopted a life style that may damage their health. For dietary advice in particular this may entail educating parents-to-be or new parents about starting the child on a healthy pattern of eating. With smoking, priority should be given to reducing the number of young people who become regular smokers.

Priority target groups

The Colloquium recommended that, where resources are limited, cancer education should give top priority to preventing young people becoming regular smokers. At the Colloquium, much of the discussion within the working group looking at 'Educating the general public' was based on the work described by Kok and de Vries (Paper 3.2) and Charlton (Paper 3.3).

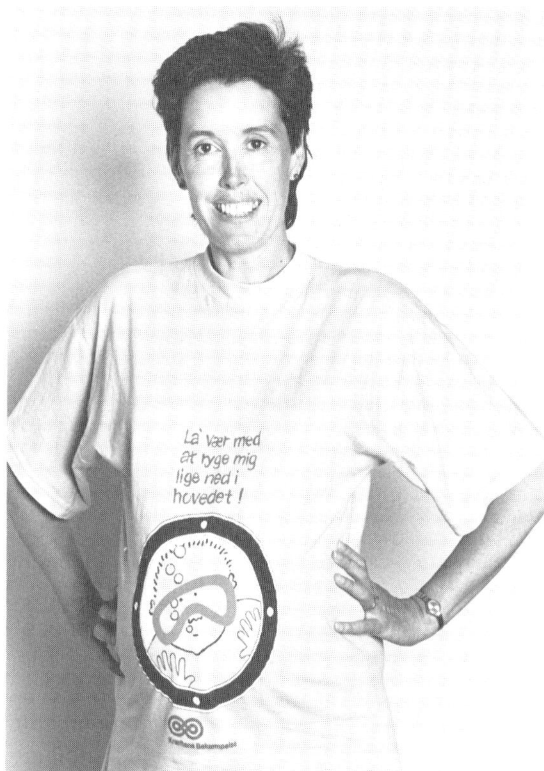

Figure 3.2 Start very young—and let the unborn generation spread the message. This Danish message says something like: 'Don't let the smoke get into my system.'

Charlton emphasizes that 'In order to plan prevention strategies, it is vital to know not only what the current prevalence is, but what underlies it', i.e. what determines young people's health beliefs and behaviours. Her analysis of this throws light on girls' positive beliefs about smoking. Her approach to health education and young teenagers could be summed up by her conference comment advocating 'Health by Stealth'. At adolescence, when an adult identity is being established, health education should concentrate particularly on building self-esteem and autonomy. In anti-smoking programmes with teenagers, it can be counterproductive to emphasize health risks. These young people are at a time of their life when they want to take risks and also the 'punishment' seems a lifetime away!

The Dutch Smoking Project described by Kok and de Vries in Paper 3.2 also focuses on young people and, interestingly, decided that:

> Preventing initial and experimental smoking is probably hard to realize, and may be unwise and counteractive. The goal of the Dutch programme is, therefore, to prevent the transition from initial and experimental smoking to regular smoking.

The dangers of singling out a target group

Singling out a target group for special attention can sometimes be undesirable and actually ineffective. Drawing attention to one group can make others feel that it is not so important for them to change; it can also encourage 'victim blaming', particularly if the target group ('them') is seen as not like 'us'. The targeted group's sense of victimization is increased if the rest of society is seen as uncaring. This highlights the difficulty of planning under-resourced programmes where some priorities must be established.

The working group, although recommending that priority should be given to preventing young people becoming regular smokers, emphasized repeatedly that young people may well reject an isolated project targeted only at them:

> Smoking prevention is only credible if it takes place within a society that takes a clear stand on health and health promotion. Smoking prevention is not credible in a society stimulating health but at the same time also actively promoting health-damaging advertisements. ... Adolescents will have a difficult question to solve: Why are we advised not to smoke? If smoking is really that bad, why aren't cigarettes, and certainly cigarette advertisements, forbidden? (Paper 3.2).

On ethical grounds, the working group urged that a European commitment is needed to the principle that 'People have a right to be free of the hazards of tobacco.'

The importance of role models

We know that people are more likely to accept the advice of those people who they admire, respect or identify with and, more importantly, they are more likely to copy their behaviour. Obviously, not all role models provide good examples of healthy behaviour. Some role models are highly culturally specific—but parents, teachers and health workers are important to almost all groups.

In health education materials Using stereotypically 'healthy people', for example famous sportspeople, as good role models in health programmes can be counterproductive if the gap between their image and ordinary people's self-images is too wide. 'Supermen' and 'superwomen' turn many people off; they seem impossibly healthy, beautiful and attractive. Since the 'beholder' despairs of reaching any of these standards, none of the proposed role model's healthy habits, such as not smoking or eating plenty of fresh fruit and vegetables, will be copied. Role models should be a little better (and older for teenagers) so that they can be more easily identified with and their behaviour copied.

Parents as models Parents are the first, and often remain the most potent, role models for their children. Fortunately, some parents can be persuaded to change their habits so as not to set a poor example to their children. Other parents are at least prepared to admit to their children that they, the parents, should change their ways.

Health educators as role models All those involved in health education also act as role models: they may, therefore, face the same dilemma as do parents. In most, but not all, member countries of the European Community, doctors do appear to practise what they preach. But there is general concern about the example set by teachers and nurses. The knowledge and attitudes of teachers and nurses concerning cancers and the possibility of reducing the risk of developing cancers will influence their own behaviour and possibly also their willingness to become involved in cancer education. If they are forced into becoming involved without adequate education and training, their own anxieties and doubts are highly likely to be passed on with the health education.

Charlton (Paper 3.3) looked at the reasons given by teachers who oppose cancer education in schools and concluded that:

> ... the message is clear. Teachers often reject cancer education for two groups of reasons: (1) practical reasons such as lack of time, finance or materials; (2) their own personal reactions to cancers or in some cases, the former reasons because of the latter ones. It is important before planning any cancer education that is to involve schools to consult, involve and educate the teachers.

The potential to cause harm

Health-education programmes can, potentially, do much more harm than merely providing counterproductive, discouraging role models.

Anxiety and fear The more people fear a disease, the less likely they are to believe in their ability to prevent it. Those people with good self-esteem (efficacy and competency) can be spurred on by moderate fear to find out what they have to change, how to make the change and who can help them. However, in those people with feelings of low self-esteem, fear generates further feelings of helplessness and dependency and can make matters worse.

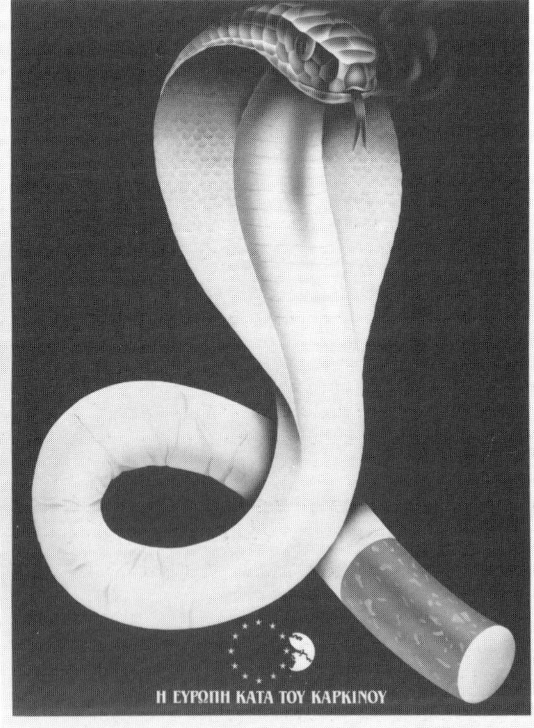

Figure 3.3 A potent symbol, but think carefully before deciding to use messages that raise anxiety.

Emphasizing the risks of a disease that provokes high anxiety to people with low self-esteem and also many constraints on their choices can only lead to an increased sense of helplessness and frustration, i.e. it increases the stress in their lives. To distance themselves from such stress, some people who believe that they cannot do anything to reduce their risks may totally deny the validity of the message and discard all advice from 'health experts'.

'Denying the message' is particularly likely to occur where exhortations to attend for cancer screening (secondary prevention) has not been preceded by an effective campaign to get across the message that some cancers can be cured. People are afraid of what might be discovered when they go for screening: they need the reassurance, which increases their sense of competency, of knowing that good treatment that offers a better chance of survival is available when cancers are discovered early.

Feelings of guilt The ethical imperative to avoid doing harm is even weightier in health programmes for young people. Charlton points out:

> Education about cancer prevention can be carried too far. If someone, be it child or adult, is given to believe that they hold the responsibility as to whether they personally get cancer or not, terrible guilt and destruction of faith can result if they or their relatives get cancer in spite of their efforts. A child is often not in a position to take or encourage the recommended action, thus unresolvable fear can result. People will probably always get cancer. It cannot always be prevented. (Paper 3.3)

It is much better to talk of reducing the risks of developing cancers rather than of avoiding cancers. Many people do wish to feel that at least they are doing all that they reasonably can to minimize their risks of developing cancer or to detect it at an early stage when the chances of a cure are higher.

However, the dilemma cannot be avoided. When emphasizing primary prevention, it must be recognized that this can generate fear related to 'Have I put myself—or others—at risk?'; and also guilt in those who already have cancer or who feel responsible for anyone who has cancer. But this is a general problem in health education and it is not morally justifiable to withhold the information that can protect future generations. Such education should also, of course, generate anger and a determination to see matters set right about those aspects of risk reduction that the individual can not control.

Evaluation must be done

Because of the potential to cause harm to healthy individuals, health-education programmes should not be undertaken lightly. Shelley (Paper 3.1) points out that:

> ... even with modest education activities, the possibility of inflicting harm, for example by induction of anxiety, on relatively healthy people, increases the ethical requirements to measure the effectiveness and the outcomes of the programmes as well as possible.

It is imperative that appropriate evaluation be funded, carried out and published. Health programmes are costly, and health educators must be accountable for their programmes. In addition, if programmes are not evaluated, other health educators can not learn from the successes and failures of earlier programmes. There is already much to be learned from the published accounts of other cancer-prevention programmes and from coronary-heart-disease reduction programmes.

The need for further research and development

Since information alone often just produces 'informed worriers', the working group made several suggestions as to specific areas of research that relate to helping people to change their ways.

- How are our messages understood by the target audience?
- What do health educators mean by health? What do lay people mean by health?—and what do they think health workers mean by it?
- What motivates community groups?
- What is the best way to approach 'difficult to reach' groups? This research would have to be culturally specific.

- How can we reach groups that have rejected cultural norms, particularly school drop-outs? Where do they meet? What is known about them as a group? Who are acceptable to them as health educators?
- Why is it easier to reach women with health education and how can men best be reached?
- What should go into a core national curriculum for health education in schools?
- How can social skills, and other determinants of self-esteem and competency, be enhanced?
- In additional to epidemiological data, baseline information is needed on the knowledge, attitudes and health beliefs of specific target groups.
- There is a need to apply the dietary advice in the European Code to all countries and cultures in the European Community.
- There is a need for further research into the determinants of dietary choice.
- How useful is food labelling? A European standard for labelling is needed.

C Cancer education: plans and priorities

An unbalanced approach to health education can easily degenerate into victim blaming; the polarizing of what should be complementary approaches; and spending much money and energy on an ineffective effort or one that cannot be evaluated.

'Thought before action' can avoid these potential pitfalls. Careful attention should be given to these questions:

- Is the community ready?
- Is the 'message' clear?
- Does the programme make a balanced use of resources?

Is the community ready for a cancer-education programme?

Health-education programmes have to be designed to match the needs of the target community. Shelley (Paper 3.1) suggests that a key step in planning is to ask: 'Has preliminary assessment of the community suggested that the programme will be well received?'

The Europe Against Cancer survey, Europeans and the Prevention of Cancer (1987) showed that people wish to have information on health matters. Eight out of ten said they were often or sometimes interested in information on health. But further work is needed to establish their health beliefs that will determine whether or not they:

- see the information as relevant to their own situation
- believe that changing their ways really will reduce the risk of cancer. The survey showed that nearly four out of ten Europeans are ill-informed or underestimate the potential for cancer prevention and cure. The survey concludes that there is still 'a major role (for campaigns) in proving that 'cancer is avoidable', and in combating the traditional erroneous image of the inexorable nature of cancer'.
- believe that factors other than those covered by the Cancer Code play a part in causing cancer. The survey revealed that many people overestimate the relative importance of cancer risks from radioactivity and the environment. However, people need their worries and misapprehensions to be recognized and responded to by cancer-education projects in order to set in perspective the risks that they fear.

Clarifying the message

Agreeing on the message—in itself a huge task—is the domain of cancer specialists; transforming the message into 'working knowledge' that is of use to people in their everyday lives is the domain of health educators. Many of the discussion groups at the Colloquium wrestled with the transformation of such messages as 'No more than 35% of total dietary calorie intake should come from saturated fats' at one extreme and 'Eat more fresh fruit and vegetables' at the other. Converting these statements into culturally specific advice that enables an individual to chose what food to eat is a challenge for health educators throughout the member countries of the European Community.

The general message should:

- be clear, agreed by all EC countries, and not conflict with other health messages;
- explain that cancers have many causes;
- emphasize that the risks can be reduced and that some cancers, especially those detected early, can be cured;
- be delivered within a healthy life-style approach;
- be for everyone, but culturally specific for the target group.

'Why' and 'How' Kok and de Vries (Paper 3.2) emphasize that 'planned health education is a form of planned behavioural change'. The advice of cancer experts must be stated in terms of specific behavioural changes that will reduce the risks of cancer. As Chapter 2 makes clear, this is not always easy to do. *Why* to change and *how* to change are completely different messages and need separate consideration. People may know their current life style is unhealthy but not know exactly what to change to make it healthier.

Getting information across is only a small part of what is involved in health education and is relatively easy to do. There now exists a large body of 'informed worriers' who know why they should change and would like to change ... but who have so far been unsuccessful. Some changes are perceived as particularly hard to make. The advice to stop smoking was the best known item of the European Code Against Cancer but it was also seen as the most difficult to comply with. And yet, 48 million Europeans have succeeded—one in three people who have ever smoked have given up.

On ethical grounds, 'informed worriers' deserve special attention; their plight is often due to earlier cancer-education campaigns that raised their fears but did not offer help with how to make the changes, nor support while the change is being made.

Planning, implementation and evaluation: balancing the use of resources

Some of the projects described in the background papers for the Colloquium can be criticized on the grounds of insufficient planning, hasty implementation and lack of planned—or in some cases any—evaluation. Budgeting for health interventions should include the costs of the long period of planning, including pretesting, together with the cost of evaluation. The temptation is to rush into action—'Why waste time when the problem is pressing?'. Kok and de Vries' response to this is that 'the

Figure 3.4 'Things you can do instead of smoking ...' This Danish poster suggests positive actions within a healthy life-style approach.

Danse med den du elsker

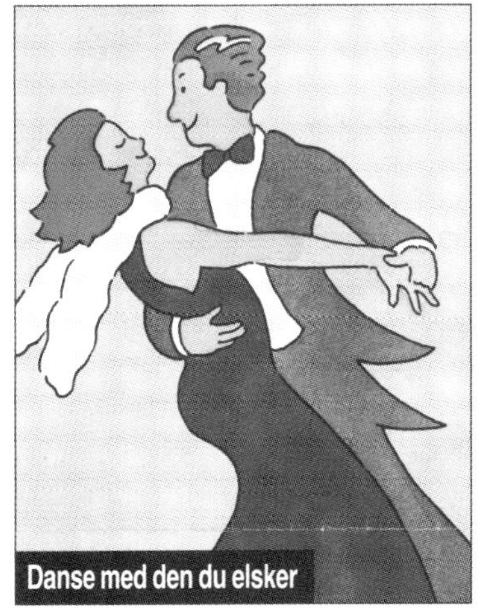

Dance with the one you love

Synge en sang

Sing a song

Kigge på fugle

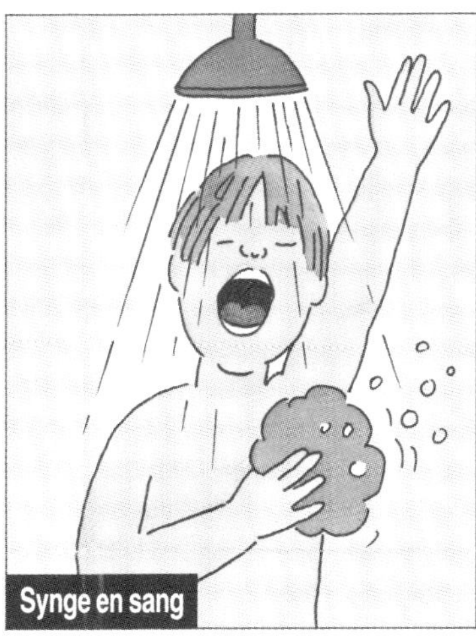

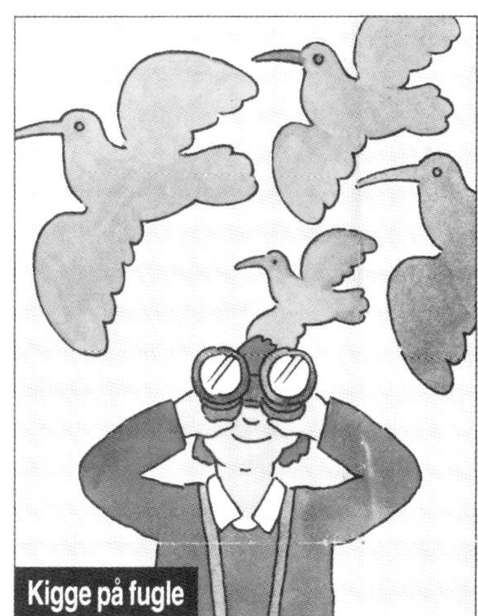

Watch birds

effectiveness of an intervention has been shown to be determined by the quality of the planning.' Their paper provides a detailed model of health-education planning, and also clearly analyzes the components of a health-education (planning) matrix.

Avoiding a premature launch To achieve commitment to a multisectoral collaborative effort, all those who are to be involved in a programme need consultation and, if need be, education, before the main programme starts. For all but the simplest projects, a pilot stage to pretest and validate the process, and if possible the outcomes, is an ethical requirement. As Shelley points out in Paper 3.1:

> Premature introduction of community education increases the likelihood of controversy surrounding the programme, thereby diluting, if not entirely negating, the desired effect. In addition, a negative outcome from one programme may place future proposals for funding in jeopardy and affect the credibility of future education initiatives.

Since controversy makes for good news stories, the media may work against the programme if they have not been well briefed about its aims and the rationale behind the chosen approach. Health educators themselves may need educating about how to work effectively with journalists who they often perceive as liable to distort their message.

D Competency-based training for health educators

All those involved in policy making and planning for cancer education should know about what health educators do. And, of course, health educators must have education and training so that they know how to do it, i.e. have the skills to be effective health educators. Health education work can be understood more clearly if the curriculum for education and training is described in terms of the skills or competencies that the worker will build up.

Health educators' competencies and cancer education

The working group's discussion generated many items that relate to the competencies of those involved in health education. These can be drawn together into the following guidelines to key competencies:

1 Allocate sufficient time and money at the planning stage of the programme The eventual success or failure of the project depends on this (see above).

2 Be clear about what the 'message' of cancer prevention is What may cause cancers? Which of the known risk factors can be avoided or at least reduced? (Chapter 2, *Current Knowledge about Cancer Prevention,*

Figure 3.4 'Things you can do instead of smoking ...' Danish Health Promotion Poster

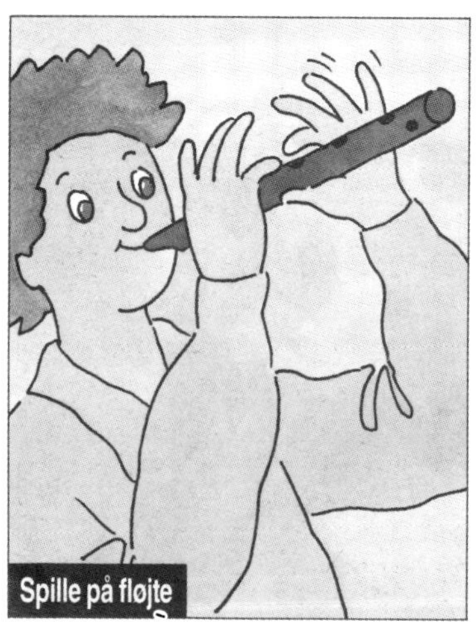

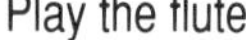
Play the flute

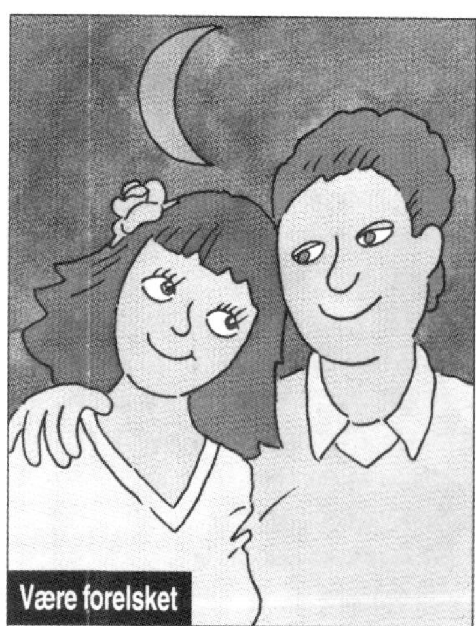

Fall in love

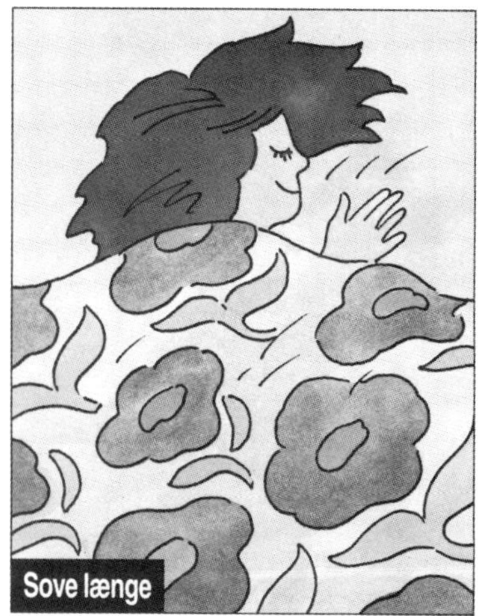

Sleep late

presents the working groups' discussions as a commentary on the Ten Points of the European Code Against Cancer.)

3 Restate this 'message' in terms of behavioural change It is generally more effective to state positively the behaviour that should be adopted rather than to proscribe the negative behaviour that should be eliminated.

- What changes should be made in order to minimize the risks?
- Who has to change? Remember, it is not only the individual's own behaviour that needs to be changed. The behaviour of politicians, policy makers and those whose business affects the health of the people also needs to be changed!

4 Know the target audiences' way of life and the constraints that operate on their choices What are the determinants of the behaviour?

- How acceptable is the advice? Do people want to give top priority to health? What would make it difficult for them to change? Would the social norms of the target group make it difficult for individuals to change? Interventions that involve changes in life style have to be culturally specific.
- Can the advice be acted upon? i.e. does it specify desirable behavioural changes that can be made bearing in mind the target groups' levels of competency and the barriers to change. Do people believe that they could make the change?

5 Survey the target audiences' existing level of knowledge and health beliefs about cancer Asking people what they already know or believe about the causes of cancer can highlight the health beliefs that may hamper them in accepting cancer education.

- How ready are they to pay attention to health advice about reducing the risks of cancer?
- How well informed are they already?
- What beliefs or attitudes do they have that might make it unlikely that they will:
  - accept the message?
  - see it as relevant to their circumstances?
  - feel able to act on it?

6 Apply the theory of what is known about the steps involved in making changes in life style to the needs of their specific target audiences The process of making a life-style change can be broken down into smaller steps, i.e. intermediate goals. These intermediate goals, for which people need advice and support from health educators, include:

- exploring the health beliefs and attitudes that may affect their commitment to change or their confidence in their ability to change

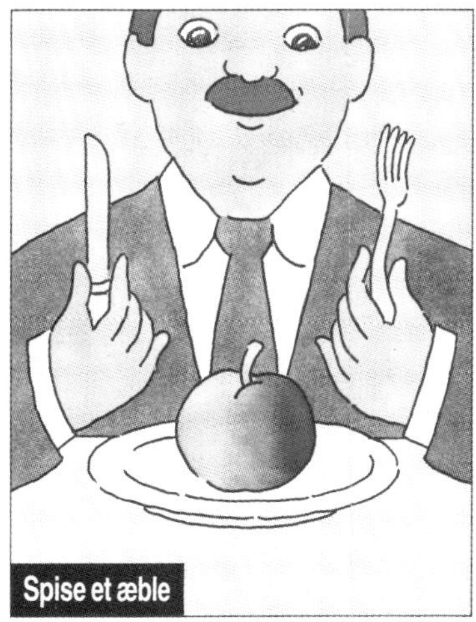

Eat an apple

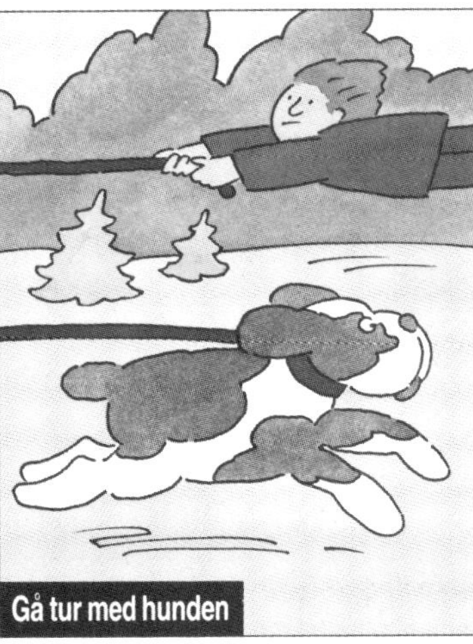

Walk the dog

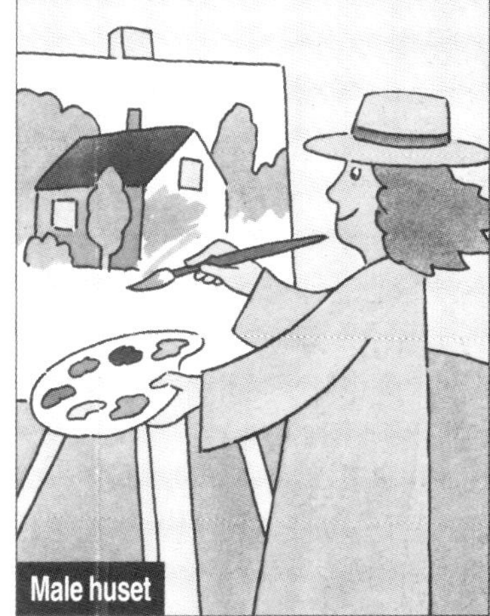

Paint the house

- making a personal commitment to change—a 'contract with yourself'
- reviewing the resources which help them to change and the constraints that make it difficult to change
- making and implementing plans for change
- learning from apparent 'failure' so that the next attempt can build on what has been recognized as potential difficulties
- monitoring and maintaining these changes, which must become part of their everyday life.

7 Analyze the social and economic structure of the target communities Help and support are generally best provided via existing community groups (neighbourhood, work or leisure interest groups). Which existing community groups must be consulted and involved in a supportive programme? What individual and community action is needed to make it easier for people to change?

8 Review—and where possible pursue—alternative strategies What action is needed and by whom to:

- reduce the risks over which the individual has no control?
- make it easier for people to change?

What part can health workers play in bringing this about? Is it unethical to proceed with the proposed intervention if these constraints are not tackled within a larger health-promotion programme?

In conclusion

The education and training of those whose work requires them to participate in cancer-prevention education should include building up the eight competencies described here. At the very least, it should be ensured that health workers realize the importance of working within a multidisciplinary team, which encompasses these competencies. 'Cancer experts' have an influential voice in educating health policy makers and politicians but these cancer specialists may also need educating so that they *understand the nature and value the contribution* of health education and promotion. They can then add the weight of their opinion to advocate the approaches described in this introduction and the following papers.

Paper 3.1

HEALTH EDUCATION IN THE COMMUNITY

Dr. Emer Shelley
Kilkenny Health Project, Kilkenny, Republic of Ireland

Health-education programmes aimed at 'individual environmental factors', such as tobacco, alcohol, diet and sexual habits, are considered an essential element of a community-based cancer-control programme[1].

Health education has been described as 'educational activity involving some form of communication, designed to improve knowledge, and develop understanding and skills, which are conducive to health'[2]. Health education aims not just to increase knowledge but to promote positive health behaviour and appropriate coping strategies.

Modern theory recognizes that information and education are necessary and core components of health promotion[3]. While this paper focuses on the topic of health education in the community in order to prevent cancer, it must be remembered that such education can only achieve its aims when it is carried out in a physical, social and cultural environment which is conducive to the health-promoting behaviours. Programmes will be successful only if economic and social problems are being tackled simultaneously.

Preliminary questions

Before embarking on a health-education programme in the community, it is necessary to consider a number of issues. Screening programmes can be justified only if the disease is an important contributor to morbidity or mortality, and if there is a satisfactory treatment available for those found to be at high risk or to have early disease. Similarly, health-education programmes in the community must address important health problems, and must be able to suggest actions that carry a reasonably high probability of reducing the problem[4]. There should be adequate grounds for expecting that the probability of inducing good will be greater than the probability of bringing about unwanted effects.

There is ample evidence that avoidance of smoking would reduce the total mortality from all cancers by about one third[5]. There is also broad agreement on the type of diet which would be likely to lead to the avoidance of coronary heart disease, hypertension, diabetes, obesity, diverticular disease and some forms of cancer. However, even when the association between a risk factor and a disease is well established, it does not follow that reversal of the risk factor will lead to a reduction in disease. This has been shown to be the case for drug treatment of hypertension which does not bring about a reduction in myocardial infarction. Further research is required to establish the protective effect of a prudent diet in relation to cancer.

Premature introduction of community education increases the likelihood of controversy surrounding the programme, thereby diluting, if not entirely negating, the desired effect. In addition, a negative outcome from one programme may place future proposals for funding in jeopardy and affect the credibility of future health-education initiatives.

Some of these problems may be overcome by directing public education towards, for example, coronary heart disease or accident prevention, where the associations with life-style factors have been more clearly delineated, and measurable benefits can be expected within a shorter time span. There are logistic benefits also from the integration of cancer and other chronic disease prevention programmes[6].

Other preliminary questions relate to whether or not the time is right to start an education programme. Are there other programmes in progress which are likely to be in competition with the proposed programme? Has preliminary assessment of the community suggested that the programme will be well received? Will the health services reinforce messages and be able to cope with those who present for counselling or screening as a result of the programme? Would funds be better spent in further preparation for a prevention programme, perhaps gathering more information on the problem in the community, training professionals, purchasing equipment and improving services, assessing community attitudes or preparing and evaluating education materials?

In summary, it is wise to consider carefully the overall aims of the undertaking and to modify them until the aims are consistent with current knowledge, the available resources and the prevailing social and cultural climate.

Evaluation: how much?

It is desirable, particularly when implementing programmes which have not previously been evaluated, to measure the effect of the health-education programme. Ideally there would be information on the epidemiology of the disease or behaviour in the population, preferably with knowledge of trends over time. In addition, it is desirable to be able to separate the effects of the programme from the effect of other forces for change within the community, though this presents complex problems for programme design[7]. Strategies for evaluating a community intervention programme for cancer prevention through dietary change have been discussed recently in the context of the Stockholm Cancer Prevention Programme[8].

The extent to which it will be appropriate or necessary to evaluate the outcome will depend on a number of factors, including the scope of the programme and the available resources. All programmes are likely to benefit from formative evaluation as part of the planning and development process[9]. An intensive community-based cancer-prevention programme would require evaluation at all stages of the undertaking and a major proportion of programme funds should be allocated to this. In contrast, for a local smoking-prevention programme, a short post-programme evaluation with participants might suffice to assess the outcome of the programme and to consider how future programmes might be improved. However, even with modest education activities, the possibility of inflicting harm, for example by the induction of anxiety, on relatively healthy people increases the ethical requirements to measure the effectiveness and the outcomes of the programmes as accurately as possible.

There may be occasions when, despite there being an important and potentially preventable health problem, it may be unethical to undertake an education programme due to inadequate resources being available for satisfactory implementation and evaluation.

Learning from other projects

Those planning health-education programmes in the community for cancer prevention can learn from the experiences of cardiovascular-disease-prevention programmes[10]. The major projects have reported their designs and methods[11,12] and those which started during the 1970s have reported on the changes in morbidity, mortality and risk factors which occurred during the projects[13,14]. In addition, these projects have formulated and evaluated the effectiveness of education programmes aimed at specific behaviours and at different target groups, using a variety of communication channels[15,16]. These programmes aimed at reducing the risk factors for cardiovascular disease have facilitated the testing and further development of theories for communication and community organization[17].

The North Karelia project was expanded to address the problem of cardiovascular disease within the whole of Finland. Subsequently, programmes were developed within Finland to address other chronic diseases, including cancer, diabetes mellitus and road accidents. The World Health Organization CINDI (Countrywide Integrated Non-communicable Disease Intervention) programme coordinates the development and evaluation of such comprehensive community programmes in a number of European countries[18].

Even where it is not possible to mount such extensive programmes, the lessons of these and other community interventions should be applied when new programmes are being planned. Just as the ethical undertaking of clinical research requires that proposals be scientifically sound, community education programmes must use the knowledge base available to plan a programme with the greatest likelihood of achieving the desired behaviour change, while minimizing harmful effects. This is particularly so in the case of a disease such as cancer which can engender harmful emotional reactions.

Planning

Early planning involves consideration of the overall aims of the programme and the statement of more specific objectives which it is desired to achieve. For example, the aim of a regional cancer-prevention programme may be to reduce the incidence of cancer by 15 per cent by the year 2000. The objectives of such a programme might include the implementation of a cancer-prevention programme, the alteration of knowledge, attitudes and behaviour in relation to cancer-promoting and health-promoting behaviours, and the evaluation of the programme which is being developed.

It may be necessary to carry out base-line measurements before deciding on sub-programme goals and outcome targets. In addition to knowledge of the base-line prevalence of any particular health-related behaviour, an assessment of resources, including those available within the community, is required. Consideration of the current attitudes of the community will permit the development of goals and targets which, while challenging, are perceived as attainable by the educators, the professionals in the area and the community itself.

Education programmes may be divided into two main areas, dealing with education and the environment. The latter seeks to make the healthy choice the easier choice. By changing the physical environment, the social and cultural environment also becomes more supportive of healthy choices, thereby making it easier for individuals to adopt and maintain health-promoting behaviours. The environmental changes may have a direct educative effect, as in the provision of specially designated areas for smoking within buildings which are otherwise non-smoking. The education programme in its turn may make it easier to introduce the necessary environmental changes.

The education programme may include mass-media programmes, training of health professionals, training of teachers and supporting health-education programmes in schools and in workplaces, working with voluntary organizations and community groups, and special events or campaigns. All aspects of the education programme require attention to the process of communication and its impact on behaviour.

Communication

Health education in the community for cancer prevention aims to communicate with groups or individuals in order to reduce health-destructive behaviours and to increase health-promoting behaviours. The process of health communication and behaviour change relies on theories of human behaviour and learning[19]. In addition to the provision of information, health-education programmes seek to alter attitudes, to raise awareness of the importance and personal relevance of the particular problem. It is also necessary to generate motivation to change, to teach the skills necessary to adopt the behaviour, to provide opportunities to do so and to facilitate the maintenance of the new behaviour.

There is not an ordered axis from awareness to maintenance along which the educator can move in the development of messages for the community. For example, people can have good knowledge of the factors which are associated with a disease but may not be aware of the disease as being important in their community or for themselves or their families. It is necessary to consider not just people's awareness of the problem, but their awareness of other health problems, their perception of the feasibility of change and their ability to successfully make such changes. Attitudes to proposed alternative behaviours must also be considered.

The public perceptions of those advocating healthy life styles may not always be attractive and flattering. One description refers to 'killjoys who go around putting up posters to tell people not to do things. Health educators are hearty people who jog around city centres in track suits wearing badges saying "I've given up" (they probably mean smoking)'[20].

The base-line survey of the Kilkenny Health Project found that knowledge of factors associated with coronary heart disease was high. Over 90 per cent of those surveyed knew that cigarette smoking was associated with coronary heart disease and with lung cancer. It was necessary to carry out an attitude study to gain some understanding of why knowledge had not been translated into more healthy behaviours[21]. It transpired that people in rural Kilkenny did not perceive coronary heart disease to be a major health problem for the community. Higher priority was given to diseases which were more visible within the community, such as cancer or arthritis. Furthermore, coronary heart disease was perceived as something which appeared suddenly, in contrast to the medical view of the process of atherosclerosis building up over many years. Coronary artery disease was considered an inevitable part of growing older. This contrasted with the view of people who had migrated into the area, who were already living a relatively healthy lifestyle which they believed would improve the quality of their lives. People in rural Kilkenny also had difficulty in reconciling health messages with the existence within their community of apparently healthy octogenarians who had smoked for many decades.

When embarking on a programme for cancer prevention, it would be necessary to study the very complex concepts and attitudes which exist towards cancer and its prevention. It is difficult even for experts to formulate a unifying concept of the development of cancer, which in reality is a group of diseases with differing aetiologies. While public perceptions of cancer are that it is an important disease, it is likely that fears and taboos surrounding the disease are such that people may deny their personal susceptibility even more than in the case of coronary heart disease. It is also likely that the greater the fear of the disease, the less likely people are to believe in their ability to prevent its occurrence.

It is now generally recognized that the mass media play a useful role in raising awareness of specific health issues, in reducing taboos and stigmas, and in providing information. Behaviour change is most likely when media programmes are reinforced by face-to-face discussion with a respected individual, preferably using reference to the individual's own behaviours and physical characteristics. Health professionals can play a key role in motivating people to change their behaviour. In addition, the omission of advice in relation to behaviour change may be interpreted by the individual as meaning that such change is not relevant to him or her.

The role of the mass media in engendering behaviour change may however be important because of the large numbers of people who may be reached by such channels. While only a small proportion may change their behaviour, the absolute numbers of people who do so may be large[22].

Social marketing

The objectives of the education programme, the base-line knowledge, attitudes and behaviours, and the available resources will determine the target groups, the communication channels and the intended function of the specific programmes. The content and format should be influenced by the principles of social marketing, to maximize the acceptability of the programme to the target audience, to increase participation and ultimately behaviour change[23]. The key elements have been summarized as the 'four Ps': the right **product**, backed by the right

promotion, put in the right **place** and at the right **price**. Elements of the marketing process are analogous to the base-line surveys, community assessment and formative evaluation.

Successful marketing of the education programme requires an intimate knowledge of the community and its subgroups and an instinct for what is likely to prove acceptable and attractive, requiring a mixture of common sense and creativity. The involvement of staff from the locality can help in the development and implementation of programmes which are appropriate to the particular social and cultural setting. Feedback from friends and community contacts can be an important, though informal, part of the formative evaluation of programmes. Popular appeal has to be balanced with adequate expertise to maintain credibility with professionals and with lay leaders.

Community organization

The practical application of diffusion theory and that of community self-development has been termed 'community organization for health'[19]. The essence of diffusion theory is that communication flows through natural social networks and that opinion leaders are required as allies in order to achieve widespread adoption of health innovations. For community self-development, community residents and organizations must collaborate with the education programme in order to achieve maintenance of the new behaviours.

One implication of diffusion research is that the use of professionals from within the community increases the likelihood of collaboration of other community members. Another is that the education programme should seek, where possible, to generate interpersonal communication, for example by encouraging representatives at a seminar to report back to their organizations.

Implicit in the need for successful diffusion and community organization is that key individuals and organizations in the community do not oppose the initiative. Supportive attitudes and a willingness to cooperate can be translated into collaborative programmes when the opportunities arise. Community self-development can be facilitated by the provision of training and materials to key individuals within organizations, following consultation as to the type of support desired.

The education programme should seek, where possible, to work through existing organizations and structures. For example, by supporting health and education professionals in the incorporation of preventive and educational activities into their day-to-day work, the programme can have more lasting effects than would be the case for education undertaken directly with the community. Such professionals have a more intimate knowledge of their clients and so can ensure that the advice is appropriate. They may undertake follow-up, thereby providing an incentive to the maintenance of new behaviours. Professionals working in a community are also likely to have greater access to those who are less well educated and those who have been difficult to reach in traditional education programmes.

Conclusion

Health education in the community for cancer prevention is a complex undertaking. The aims of the programme require careful consideration. An assessment of the resources available within the community, together with base-line information on relevant knowledge, attitudes and behaviour, will facilitate the planning of the education programme. Provision should be made in programme design for formative evaluation, to develop the most effective programmes, and for summative evaluation to measure the overall impact of the undertaking. An intimate knowledge of the community, together with formal and informal feedback, will create a programme suitable for the community. Mass media programmes can provide information and skills training. Face-to-face discussion is most likely to lead to lasting behaviour change. The incorporation of aspects of the education programme into the activities of organizations and professionals within the community will maximize the long-term benefits of the education programme.

Because of the potential to cause harm to healthy individuals, health-education programmes should not be undertaken lightly. They should be carried out in a professional manner, taking account of modern theories and the lessons of successful community programmes in disease prevention and health promotion.

References

1 WHO Working Group (1982) *Development of cancer centres and community cancer control programme*, Euro Reports and Students 70, World Health Organization, Copenhagen.

2 Nutbeam, D (1986) Health promotion glossary, *Health Promotion* **1**, 113–27.

3 WHO Working Group (1984) *Health Promotion. A discussion document on the concept and principles*, ICP/HSR 602 (MOI) World Health Organization, Copenhagen.

4 Kemm, J. R. (1985) The ethics of food policy, *Community Medicine* **7**, 289–94.

5 Doll, R. (1983) Prospects for prevention, *Br. Med. J.* **286**, 445–53.

6 Epstein, F. H. and Holland, W. W. (1983) Prevention of chronic diseases in the community-one-disease versus multiple-disease strategies, *Int. J. Epidemiol.* **12**, 135–7.

7 Farquhar, J. W. (1978) The community-based model of life style intervention trials, *Am. J. Epidemiol.* **108**, 103–11.

8 Sanderson, C., Svanstrom, L., Eriksson, C. (1988) Development of strategies for evaluating a community programme for cancer prevention through dietary change, *Community Medicine* **10**, 289–97.

9 Farquhar, J. W., Fortmann, S. P., Flora, J. A., Tilov, C. B. (1987) Stanford projects on health promotion and non-communicable disease prevention: an overview, in E. Leparski (ed.) *The prevention of non-communicable diseases: experiences and prospects*, 387–97, ICP/NCD 028/6, World Health Organization, Copenhagen.

10 Puska, P. Nissinen, A. Tuomilehto, J. *et al.* (1985) The community-based strategy to prevent coronary heart disease: conclusions from the ten years of the North Karelia Project, Ann. Rev. Public Health 6, 147–93.

11 Farquhar, J. W. Fortmann, S. P., Maccoby, N., *et al.* (1985) The Stanford Five-City Project: design and methods, *Am. J. Epidemiol.* **122**, 323–34.

12 Blackburn, H. (1983) Research and demonstration projects in community cardiovascular disease prevention, *J. Public Health Policy* **4**, 398–421.

13 Puska, P., Salonen, J. T., Nissinen, A., Tuomilehto, J., et al. (1983) Change in risk factors for coronary heart disease during 10 years of a community intervention programme (North Karelia Project) *Br. Med. J.* **287**, 1840–4.

14 Farquhar, J. W. Maccoby, N., Wood, P. D., et al. (1977) Community education for cardiovascular health, *Lancet* i, 1192–5.

15 Fortmann, S. P. Williams, P. T., Hulley, S. B., Haskell, W. L. Farquhar, J. W. (1981) Effect of health education on dietary behaviour: the Stanford Three Community Study, *Am. J. Clin. Nutr.* **34**, 2030–8.

16 Perry, C. L., Mullis, R. M., Maile, M. C. (1985) Modifying the eating behaviour of young children, *J. of School Health* **55**, 399–402.

17 Rasanen, L. Ahlstrom, A., Rimpela, M. (1974) Pretesting the channels of distribution for a nutrition education leaflet, *Scand. J. Soc. Med.* **2**, 135–40.

18 Nussel, E., Saarelma, D. (1987) The CINDI programme in Europe: joint approaches and experiences, in E. Leparski (ed) *The prevention of non-communicable diseases: experiences and prospects*, 249–61, ICP/NCD 028/6, World Health Organization, Copenhagen.

19 Farquhar, J. W., Maccoby, N., Wood, P. D. (1985) Education and communication studies, in W. W. Holland, R. Detels and G. Knox (eds.) *Oxford textbook of public health*, vol. 3, 207–221, Oxford University Press, Oxford.

20 Perkins, E. (1982) Health education—a new field for adult educators? *Adult Education* **55**, 21–6.

21 Conroy, R. M. and Shelley, E. Culture, health beliefs and attitudes in a rural Irish community, *Health Promotion* (in press).

22 Puska, P. Wiio, J., McAlister, A., *et al.* (1984) Mass media in national health promotion: development and evaluation of a theory-based method (the 'Keys to Health' television programme in 1982 in Finland, Terveyskasvatustutkimuksen vuosikirja 1984), 161–76.

23 Catford, J. Nutbeam, D. Social marketing and health: the experience of 'Heartbeat Wales' see ref. no. 18 above.

Paper 3.2

PRIMARY PREVENTION OF CANCERS: THE NEED FOR HEALTH EDUCATION AND INTERSECTORAL HEALTH PROMOTION

Professor Gerjo Kok and Dr. Hein de Vries
Department of Health Education, University of Limburg, The Netherlands

During the last years, the focus of health research has shifted from curative to preventive activities. The prevention of cancers seems to have many potentialities. However, most cancer-related activities still have a curative nature. We do not contest the need for and the importance of finding a cure. We do, however, stress that both primary and secondary prevention needs to be encouraged much more because:

- it can prevent and reduce the incidence of cancers;
- it will improve quality of life, as cancers lead to much physical, psychological, and social discomfort;
- it may reduce costs due to hospitalization and absenteeism.

Preventive health research, as a relatively new research tradition, is confronted with many different issues that need attention. These issues pertain for example to the relation of health problems with several specific behaviours, programme development, and programme diffusion. Hence, there is a great need for a model or framework which can place these issues in a single context. The advantage of such a model is that many relevant aspects are dealt with in a systematic way. For instance, primary cancer prevention will probably have hardly any impact if we initiate preventive programmes without knowing why individuals have an unhealthy life style. Therefore, prevention of cancer needs a systematic approach in which all kinds of problems are analyzed, and actions are carefully planned.

We first describe a general planning model of health education (Green and Lewis, 1986; Kok, 1988). Then we specify this model for primary prevention of cancers and describe a primary cancer-prevention strategy, called the ABC framework, that has been developed in the Netherlands (de Vries, 1989).

Planned health education

Planned health education is a form of planned behavioural change. Planned behavioural change consists of two phases: a planning phase and an evaluation phase. Figure 3.5 presents the model of planned behavioural change (based on Green and Lewis, 1986).

In the planning phase we attempt to answer five questions:

1 How serious is the problem?
2 Which behaviour is involved?
3 What are the determinants of that behaviour?
4 What options are there for change (intervention)?

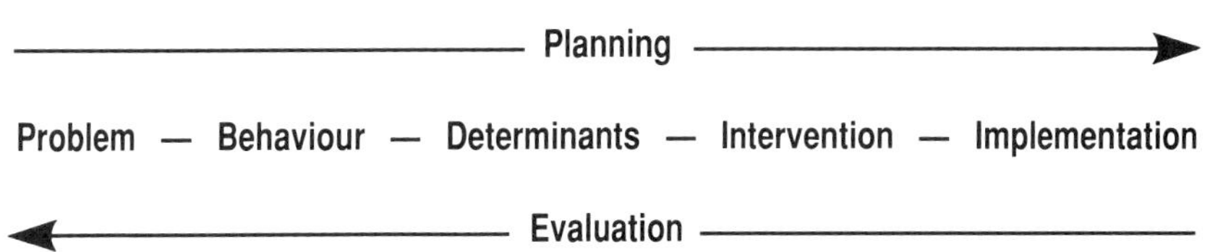

Figure 3.5 Planning and evaluation

5 How can these options be implemented?

In the evaluation phase we attempt to answer the same kind of questions in the reverse order:

6 Has the implementation been carried out as planned?

7 Has the intervention been realized as planned?

8 Have the determinants of behaviour changed?

9 Has the behaviour changed?

10 Has the problem been lessened?

When the problem is a health problem and when the intervention is educational, this model is a model of planned health education. It can be argued that this general model can be applied to all kinds of social problems, environmental pollution, discrimination, etc. Moreover, there are other types of intervention than educational intervention. Further on wel describe an intersectoral health-promotion model that integrates different possibilities for intervention.

We can illustrate the model of planned behavioural change with an example concerning the prevention of smoking (de Vries *et al.*, 1988).

The planning phase

1 Problem: cancer, cardiovascular diseases

2 Behaviour: smoking

3 Determinants: social pressure from peers, parents, mass media

4 Intervention: a social resistance programme

5 Implementation: in schools for students, aged 13 and 14 (as the increase of smoking is more rapid)

The evaluation phase

6 Implementation: Did the schools implement the programme?

7 Intervention: Did the students understand the message and did they appreciate the programme?

8 Determinants: Has social resistance against smoking increased?

9 Behaviour: Did fewer students start smoking?

10 Problem: Has the prevalence of cancer decreased?

The last question with respect to this health problem is not a realistic evaluation question as this concerns a longitudinal approach. With some other health problems, the question may be easier to answer, for instance the number of accidents with fireworks. This example of the application of the model is not very specific or thorough, and other or more complete answers are possible. The illustration is only meant to show the usefulness of the planning model in asking and answering the questions.

Why this somewhat exaggerated planning model? Why lose time considering theoretical questions while the problem is pressing? These are common questions asked by people from the field of health education and cancer prevention. The answer is simple and clear—because research has shown that only planned health education can be effective in reducing the health problems we are dealing with (Green and Lewis, 1986; Jonkers *et al.*, 1988). Intervention strategies are not in themselves more or less effective. *The effectiveness of an intervention has been shown to be determined by the quality of the planning.* An implication therefore is to carefully analyze each of the ten questions and answers. The most common mistake is that policy makers or health educators jump from the problem to the intervention without answering the questions in between. The ineffectiveness of such badly planned interventions remains unnoticed as they rarely evaluate their interventions. Evaluation is necessary to check previous decisions and for making corrections to improve the interventions. Careful planning can prevent a number of possible pitfalls that we will describe and illustrate with examples from different fields.

Possible pitfalls

Pitfall 1 the development of an intervention for a problem that does not exist. An example was an intended development of a programme against alcohol drinking by pregnant women in the Netherlands. A short literature review showed that negative health consequences were only found as a result of drinking more than one glass of alcohol a day. A short survey study showed that only 2 per cent of the pregnant women in our country said they sometimes drank more than one glass a day. Clearly there was no reason for a large educational campaign (Tholen *et al.*, 1988).

Pitfall 2 the development of an intervention addressing behaviour that has no clear relationship with the health problem involved. An example is the prevention of ski injuries. Bouter (1988) showed that participating in ski gymnastics does not prevent ski injuries. Bouter also showed that taking ski lessons and having ski bindings correctly adjusted do in fact prevent ski injuries. So an intervention to promote ski gymnastics can be successful, in that it has a high participation rate, without being effective, because no injuries will be prevented.

Pitfall 3 the development of an intervention that is based on a misconceived idea about behaviour determinants. An example is the proposal to produce a brochure encouraging parents of young children to use child safety seats while driving to improve children's safety. A short survey study showed that almost all parents did possess safety seats and were convinced of their safety-improving effects. However, half the parents stopped using safety seats because of problems with the child complaining. An intervention to increase the use of safety seats should address ways to handle bothersome children instead of only the safety aspects (Pieterse *et al.*, 1987).

Pitfall 4 the wrong intervention, for instance an intervention for the wrong target group. For example, drug education is mostly targeted at younger people, but we know that drug education can only be effective when problems at home, at school or at work are addressed (Jonkers *et al.*, 1988). Therefore it is also necessary to target drug education at parents, teachers and headteachers, and provide them with the means to relate to the younger person's problems and hence their potential drug use.

Pitfall 5 the development of a potentially effective intervention with the wrong implementation. An example is the development of an intervention programme for schools that in itself could be very effective, but which does not have adequate implementation. For example, where the material is good but schools do not know about the existence of the programme, about the ways to order the programme, or about the ways to use it.

Pitfall 6 unjustified satisfaction about the intervention. Sometimes evaluators choose the wrong or insufficient goals for evaluating their effects. For instance, satisfaction about the large number of brochures that has been handed out, without noticing that actual prevention of the health problem has not occurred.

Planned health education or planned behaviour change is a way to handle these possible threats to effective prevention. The first two steps, analyzing the problem and analyzing the behaviour, are often most efficiently dealt with by epidemiologists. The task for health educators is to carefully plan and evaluate the interventions. This implies that epidemiological findings have to be translated into behavioural goals (no smoking, less fat consumption). Then our next question concerns the determinants of those unhealthy behaviours.

Determinants of behaviour

For an answer to the question of behaviour determinants we lean upon social-psychological theories and models. Figure 3.6 on the next page presents a recent model of behaviour determinants (de Vries *et al.*, 1988).

There are three kinds of determinants:

- attitude
- social influence
- efficacy/barriers.

Attitude An attitude to behaviour is the weighing of all the advantages and disadvantages of performing that behaviour. Health is only one of the possible considerations and is often a relatively unimportant one. When health is

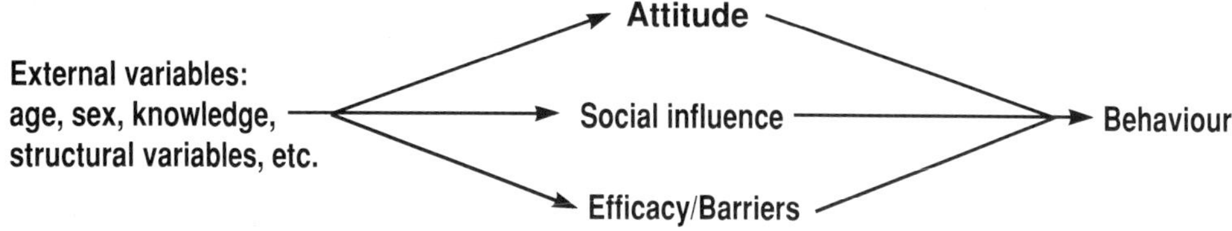

Figure 3.6 Determinants of behaviour

considered to be a part of the attitude, we suppose that the motivation to act in a manner conducive to good health is a combination of the perceived severity of the health risk, the perceived susceptibility to the health risk and the effectiveness of the preventive behaviour. But, again, health considerations are mostly not dominant and other considerations such as costs, (dis)like, status, etc. are more important. Knowledge about health risks is for most people not enough. A painful example is the unhealthy life style of many doctors.

Social influence This refers to the influence of others, directly, by what others expect; indirectly, by what others do (modelling). Social influence is often underestimated as a determinant of behaviour. Social-psychological studies show that social influence can lead to behaviour that conflicts with one's own previous attitudes. The bases for social influence are two principles: (a) people like to have the right information, and the ideas and behaviour of other people are sources of information; and (b) people like to receive social rewards, such as getting compliments from others and belonging to a group. People are themselves often quite unaware of the strong influence of others on their own behaviour.

Efficacy/barriers This stands for the determinant: is the person able to perform the (desired) behaviour? Self-efficacy is an estimation of ability to cope with possible barriers inside or outside the person. Examples of inside barriers are: not enough knowledge, not enough abilities, and not enough endurance; and outside the person: resistance from others, time and money not available, and conflicting life style. Self-efficacy is the perception of the ability to perform the behaviour; barriers are the real problems people face, sometimes unexpectingly, in actually behaving. Self-efficacy is shaped by experiences with barriers, experiences with successes, vicarious learning, verbal persuasion and physiological information (de Vries *et al.*, 1988).

There is a logical relation between perceived efficacy and real barriers, but there is also an important relation between efficacy and success in performing the behaviour. People with a higher efficacy have a higher chance of succeeding, independently of real barriers. But the discrepancy between perceived efficacy and real barriers should not become too large. Health educators can try to increase perceived self-efficacy in order to motivate people to perform the preventive behaviour. At the same time they should help people to overcome real barriers to performing that behaviour.

Other possible factors (external variables) are supposed to influence behaviour through these three determinants. If there is a relation between sex and the behaviour, for instance, there will be a difference between boys and girls with respect to attitude, social influence and/or efficacy/barriers towards that behaviour.

We have described the three kinds of behaviour determinants. Later we will specify these determinants for smoking prevention. Now we proceed with a general description of behavioural change interventions, assuming that the determinants of behaviour are known.

Health promotion

As we indicated before, health education is only one possible intervention. Other possible interventions are facilities or regulation, and probably a combination of the three is the most effective. Health promotion is the integral combination of all possible interventions to achieve the health goals: primary prevention, early detection and patient care (de Leeuw, 1989). Figure 3.7 presents the health-promotion matrix.

Health promotion	Primary prevention	Early detection	Patient care
Education			
Facilities			
Regulation			

Figure 3.7 The health-promotion matrix

Goals The health-promotion matrix provides a framework for health-promotion decisions. With respect to health-promoting goals, non-smoking interventions fall primarily under the category of primary prevention. Other health problems fall primarily under other categories, for instance breast cancer falls under early detection, asthma falls under patient care. The latter two problems cannot at present be dealt with in primary prevention.

Strategies With respect to health-promoting strategies to prevent cancer, all three options for interventions are available. We can educate, we can provide facilities and we can regulate. The distinction between those three is not very sharp, but on the one hand, there is education based on the assumption that people change their behaviour when they become motivated, and on the other hand there is regulation based on the assumption that people change their behaviour because they are forced to do so. With the second assumption, control and sanctions are necessary. But a combination of both strategies is possible and even very effective in certain circumstances, for instance education about the sanctions for drunken driving. Facilities are provided, but can be used voluntarily. Education can give information to people about facilities, for instance about possibilities for a medical check-up with advice about changes in life style. Governments could regulate the provision of such facilities.

Health promotion is integral, intersectoral, and makes use of an intervention mix.

- Integral means that health promotion is concerned with health, but also with for instance, economics.
- Intersectoral means that health-promotion activities involve several and different governmental agencies (Departments of Health, Economics, Education) and non-governmental agencies (industry, consumer organizations).
- An intervention mix involves some combination of regulation, long-term planning, health education facilities, financial stimulation, and an ongoing evaluation of the effectiveness of that combination.

Historically, health education has moved from isolated educational activities to health education as an essential part of health promotion. In the next paragraph we will describe recent views about health education as one intervention to promote health.

Health education as a behavioural change intervention

Health education starts with a clear behavioural goal: we have an undesired and a desired (preventive) behaviour, and we want people to change from behaving in the undesired way to behaving in the desired way; for instance, the cessation of smoking. Having a clear behavioural goal, we try to change the behaviour determinants: attitudes, social influence, efficacy/barriers. Changing by health education means changing by communication. Therefore the first goal is to get attention for the intervention and comprehension of the message. The second goal is changing the determinants of behaviour. The third and last goal is the maintenance of the behavioural change. A one-time-only change is not enough. We want the desired behaviour to become a habit.

One major problem in getting maintenance of behaviour change is the possible negative experiences people have with performing the desired behaviour. Messages should always be realistic regarding the experiences or consequences that follow after the change to a new healthy behaviour. Mostly those experiences are in the short run not very positive. These three health-education goals are combined with four communication variables in the health-education matrix (McGuire, 1985), as shown in Figure 3.8 below.

Decisions have to be made for each of the cells of this matrix; for example:

- Which source attracts the most attention?
- Which channel is able to change social norms?
- Which group of receivers should be especially prepared for negative experiences?

In the literature (see McGuire, 1985) a rich amount of empirical data can be found with respect to every possible decision. We will specifically elaborate on two issues here: the need for pretesting and the community approach as the most promising health-education/promotion intervention.

Pretesting of educational materials This is meant to check, for example, if the materials have the intended effect, with respect to attention, comprehension, credibility of the source and feasibility of the implementation. It is not enough that all kinds of specialists on the health problem agree (the first step) that the information in the materials is correct. A next step is to have communication specialists judge the materials and a final step is to try out the materials on a sample out of the target group. Only then is it possible to prevent all kinds of possible unwanted side-effects that have not been recognized by the health educators themselves. Pretesting is therefore very much needed and should be integrated in the materials development process.

A community approach The most promising approach at the moment seems to be the integration of health education in a community approach, especially with 'difficult' issues and with 'difficult' target groups. Community approaches are characterized by five more or less essential elements.

1 Community approaches are directed at the existing social networks, for example, neighbourhood, city, region, school and workplace. The social network is crucial in achieving the educational goals: attention and comprehension, change of determinants, maintenance of behaviour change.

2 Community approaches are multi-sectoral. They can involve many different groups, for example, health educators, national and local governments, industry and school educators. In this respect, community approaches link directly with the health-promotion approach.

3 Community approaches are multi-media activities. They use mass media as general facilitators, interpersonal communication and local mass communication, intermediates (from the network; and paraprofessional).

4 Community approaches see health as a part of life style. Programmes on cancer prevention

Health education	Source	Message	Channel	Receiver
Attention and comprehension				
Change in attitudes, social influence, efficacy/barriers				
Maintenance of behaviour change				

Figure 3.8 The health-education matrix

should not deal with, for instance, smoking, as an isolated issue, but as a part of a healthy life style. A healthy life style involves such issues as group membership, risk-taking behaviour, nutrition and exercise.

5 Community approaches can be very effective by using paraprofessionals as a source. The basic idea of paraprofessionals is the training of some relatively influential members of the target group itself to become educators. Especially with 'difficult' groups, such as people with low income and low education, this approach has proven to be the *only* effective approach, but fortunately, a *very* effective one.

Health education can be an effective way to change unhealthy behaviour to healthy behaviour. We have shown that the effectiveness of health education and health promotion depends on the quality of planning. That means, a careful analysis of the problem, the behaviour, the determinants, the intervention, the implementation, and of the strength of the relationship between those five aspects. So far, the theory and data have been related to general health education and health promotion. We will now specify our application with respect to primary cancer prevention: the Dutch ABC framework.

The Dutch ABC framework for primary cancer prevention

Following the general model of planned behaviour change (Figure 3.5), we distinguished three phases: A: analysis of the problem; B: behavioural change interventions; and C: continued health promotion.

A Analysis of cancer-related behaviours and their preventability Relevant issues for this phase are: the severity of the health problem, the relationship between different behaviours and cancer, the preventability of cancer-related behaviours, and the relevant target groups. Contributions will mostly come from epidemiological research.

B Behavioural change interventions: development and evaluation Programmes focusing on changing unhealthy behaviours have to be developed and evaluated on a small scale. Firstly, one needs to know why people behave in an unhealthy way: for example, the determinants of unhealthy behaviour such as the advantages and disadvantages of a particular behaviour, perceived social pressure. The second step is to change behaviour. Hence we need to know which methods will be most effective for cancer prevention, and how we can evaluate the effects of cancer-prevention programmes. In this phase findings from health-education research in combination with other disciplines (for example, social psychology and sociology) will be highly relevant.

C Continued large-scale health promotion Prevention will probably not be effective if prevention programmes are not used on a large scale, and if they are used only once. Therefore, implementation of successful programmes on a large scale (for example, regional or national programmes) is a prerequisite for effective cancer prevention. For successful implementation, successful programmes are not enough. We also need implementation strategies, health-promotion policies, and we need to use health projects in different health sectors. In this phase, health education will be enlarged to health promotion, including important disciplines focusing on policy development, organization psychology and management.

Analysis of the problem

Severity of the problem: the analysis phase indicates that cancers are the second largest cause of death in the Netherlands, causing 30 000 deaths yearly, which is 26 per cent of all deaths (Nota 2000). At the moment, the percentage of cancer cases that are related to behavioural and environmental factors is estimated to be around 80 per cent (Doll and Peto, 1981). Therefore, more priority should be given to primary prevention, both in practice as well as in research.

Behaviours related to cancers Cancers seem to be related to a variety of behaviours, as shown in Table 3.2 (Doll and Peto, 1981).

Table 3.2 Cancer-related behaviours and preventability

Behaviour	Best estimate %	Range	Prevention
nutrition	35	10–70	Y,A,W
tobacco	30	25–40	Y,A,W
sexual behaviour	7	1–13	Wo
occupation	4	2–8	?W
alcohol	3	2–4	Y,A
pollution	2	1–5	?
industrial products	1	1–2	?
medicines and procedures	1	0.5–3	?
sunlight	1	1–2	Y,A

Y=Youngster, A=Adult, W=Workplace, Wo=Women

Doll and Peto assume that 35% of cancer mortality can be ascribed to nutrition habits, although these estimates are not very precise. Compared to the impact of nutrition, the estimates of the impact of smoking on cancer mortality, 30%, are more precise. Reproductive and sexual behaviour is estimated to account for 7% of cancer mortality. Behaviours related to occupation account for 4%, alcohol for 3%, pollution for 2%. Industrial products, and medicines and medical procedures are each estimated to account for 1%. It is estimated that ultraviolet radiation accounts for 1% to 2% of all cancer deaths.

The next step is to consider whether these cancer-related behaviours can be prevented and whether these behaviours are relevant for the population in general, or for specific at risk groups. If the risk is spread over a large general population, mass media oriented prevention is a useful method. If a risky behaviour is limited to easily identifiable groups within the population, specific programmes for these groups may have more effect. A second factor for considering preventive activities is that we should know in which direction behaviours should change to decrease the chances of developing cancer.

Nutrition Some general goals can be formulated which can have an impact on the whole population, such as:

- a reduction of average fat content from 40% to 30%.
- well balanced diets that contain sufficient vitamins, minerals, trace elements and dietary fibre to supply the recommended amounts. Vegetables, fruits and whole grain product should be included as well.
- avoiding the consumption of badly burned parts of food.

Preventive activities for the population focusing on nutrition are feasible. However, we need more information on the factors underlying people's motives for eating an unhealthy diet. More research is also necessary to analyze whether specific population groups are at risk, in order to develop specific prevention programmes.

Smoking The most effective approach is probably smoking prevention focusing on adolescents. Smoking cessation programmes in general, and smoking cessation programmes at workplaces are other feasible methods of cancer prevention. We elaborate on smoking prevention and cessation in the next sections.

Sexual behaviour The most obvious relationship between sexual behaviour and cancer is that observed between sexual intercourse and cancer of the cervix uteri, which accounts for 1.5% of all deaths from cancer in the USA. Preventive activities for cancer of the cervix can be formulated for specific groups, such as better personal hygiene, especially the use of barrier contraceptives, for women having sexual intercourse with several partners; and cervical screening.

Doll and Peto conclude that it is not clear how far it will be possible to reduce the incidence rates of cancers of the breast, ovary, and endometrium. Fortunately, secondary prevention by breast self-examination and mammography can reduce the risk of cancer mortality.

Workplace hazards Preventive activities focusing on reduction of exposure to chemicals is relevant for small groups in the working population. Moreover, situations will differ from workplace to workplace. Although necessary, it may be difficult to formulate general prevention programmes for these risk groups.

Alcohol Excessive alcohol use increases the risk of developing cancer of the mouth, pharynx and oesophagus. Preventive activities can be formulated in terms of enhancing moderate drinking instead of excessive drinking. However, studies do not yet agree on a definition of moderate drinking. Preventive activities focusing on alcohol abuse should also incorporate other health and social effects, in order to enhance impact. Target groups can be young people, adults in general, and adults in the workplace.

Sunlight The carcinogenic effect of sunlight is ascribed to ultraviolet radiation. Preventive recommendations can be formulated which focus on reduced exposure to ultraviolet radiation. However, as individuals will always be exposed to radiation, there is a need for more precise information on the critical amount of radiation, correcting for the type of skin.

The role of smoking in primary cancer prevention is the most clear. We describe in the next section the efforts that have been made in the fields of prevention and cessation of smoking.

Cessation of smoking: the Dutch smoking cessation project

Strategies for the cessation of smoking are only partly effective, but with recent applications of theoretical insights they seem to have become more effective. In the USA, the health educator's interest in smoking has a long tradition, and review studies are regularly published on smoking, prevention of smoking and cessation of smoking. A recent and elaborated review on cessation of smoking strategies is Schwartz' (1987) report, *Review and Evaluation of Smoking Cessation Methods: the United States and Canada, 1978–1985*. We will summarize Schwartz' findings.

1 Most people stop smoking without an organized method (group, therapy, etc.) We do not know very much about this group except that the successful try has normally been preceded by some failures. A large number of these have been stimulated by a warning or advice from a health professional. Some of them use self-help manuals. Others get help from television or radio, public campaigns, articles in papers, journals and books.

2 Research programmes on the effectiveness of smoking cessation methods still have limitations. The programme descriptions are often unclear, research designs not adequate, and the comparison between the different methods is hindered by the great variation in programme implementation, participants, definitions, length of follow-up periods, etc. Most of the behavioural measurements are self reports. In recent years, we have seen a lot of improvements. Abstinence is now the goal and the follow-up period is at least one year. The self reports are checked with physiological measurements.

3 Most smokers want to stop on their own or with a minimum of help; a number of self-help manuals are available, but many of these have not been evaluated systematically. Where they are, it seems that 16 to 20 per cent of the people who try to stop individually are successful in their attempt.

4 A number of stop smoking aids are not effective: special filters, medication, hypnosis, and acupuncture do not help. Nicotine gum in itself is not very effective, but it is more useful in combination with other methods.

5 Health professionals can be very stimulating. Many doctors think they should help their patients to stop smoking. The number of people stopping after being warned by a doctor is small. With a more intensive approach, by using self-help manuals and nicotine gum, doctors can give their patients a higher chance of success. Patients who have lung or heart problems react more strongly to warnings and advice than healthy smokers do.

6 Public campaigns have very limited effects. In combination with individual or group interventions, the effect is stronger. Help by telephone seems to be effective. Community programmes are on the whole quite successful.

7 Behavioural and therapeutic methods show great variability in effect. Aversive methods are not successful. Self-control strategies are somewhat successful, especially in combination with relapse prevention strategies (see 9).

8 Many workplaces organize cessation of smoking programmes. The participation rate is low, but the success rate is relatively high.

9 Relapse prevention is essential for long-term success. Social support is very important, as is the ability to cope with difficult situations. The most common reasons for relapse are negative emotional situations (stress, frustration) and positive social situations (being offered a cigarette after dinner). Stop smoking programmes must focus on increasing their success by helping people to learn better coping skills. A lapse need not be a permanent relapse; it can be a learning experience for future coping (Marlatt and Gordon, 1985).

The most effective programmes are community interventions, health professionals' advice, and relapse prevention methods. At this moment, we are developing a Dutch Smoking Cessation Programme using these three elements. The main component of the project is the Dutch version of the recently developed smoking cessation manual, *Freedom from Smoking for You and Your Family*, by the American Lung Association. This manual is based on the recent models of behaviour suggesting three types of determinants of smoking or quitting: outcome expectations (attitude), social norms and self-efficacy. Interventions for smoking cessation traditionally focused mostly on outcome expectations. In this intervention, the roles of social support and self-efficacy in smoking cessation and maintenance are acknowledged. Special attention is given to relapse prevention: thinking about reasons for former failure and finding (and practising) ways to cope with these temptations.

In the Dutch Smoking Cessation project, existing community resources will be utilized and strengthened. Messages to local and regional mass media and general practitioners refer the smoker wanting to quit to a telephone 'Quit line' which will serve as a central reference point in the intervention. Quit line, general practitioners and local mass media refer the smoker to one of three quitting methods:

- Individual: a manual is sent by mail after a request on the Quit line or can be handed out by the general practitioner.
- Individual prompted by the general practitioner. Through minimal contact, general practitioners encourage the patient to quit with the help of the manual.
- Group interventions with counsellor. Integrating the manual into an existing or developed group method for smoking cessation.

For all smokers enrolled in these interventions, the telephone Quit line provides additional counselling.

In the Dutch programme, the intervention is made on a small scale in one city in the Netherlands with another carefully matched city serving as a control group.

Prevention of smoking: the Dutch smoking prevention project

Before developing a prevention programme, the Dutch Smoking Prevention Project started with a study on determinants of initial and regular smoking in 10 to 15-year-old students (de Vries and Kok, 1986). It appeared that non-smoking students connected smoking solely with disadvantages, while smokers mentioned several advantages. This discrepancy may create a challenge for non-smokers to initiate smoking in order to discover which side is right. Smokers may influence non-smokers, because the former group is minimizing the significance of the disadvantages. Smokers experienced more peer group pressure on smoking from their peers than non-smokers. Both groups experienced pressure to smoke from cigarette advertisements and companies.

Regular smoking was associated with long-term hazards, whereas initial smoking was associated more with short-term disadvantages, and with advantages (satisfying curiosity). However, initial smoking was not strongly connected with continued smoking. This latter finding is important as studies indicate the opposite (Hirschman *et al.*, 1984). Furthermore, non-smokers were at risk in several situations where they had less negative intentions towards non-smoking. As well as situations in which they want to experiment with smoking, other situations also seem to exert a social pressure (at parties, in cafes and discos, being outside, in the street, and when they are with friends).

Based on these results and its implications, a peer-led video programme has been developed for adolescents aged 13 and 14 (8th grade) during the second year. Although many try smoking (90%), this does not necessarily lead to regular smoking (Hirschman *et al.*, 1984). Many adolescents experiment with smoking. Preventing initial and regular smoking is probably very difficult and indeed may be unwise and counterproductive. The goal of the Dutch programme is, therefore, to prevent the transition from initial and experimental smoking to regular smoking. Regular smoking is defined as smoking at least one cigarette a week.

In structuring programme development, a programme matrix has been developed, an adapted version of McGuire's health-education matrix (see Figure 3.8). In discussing the development of the programme, we will follow the programme matrix as a guideline.

The programme

It is important that the message is attractive to adolescents as their attention is selective and motivation to participate in a prevention programme may be low. Using the school as a place of intervention will increase the chance of exposure to the message. To prevent implementation failure (a bad or non-use of the programme), we contacted teachers and school directors to analyze the factors that might cause a bad or non-use of the programme. They indicated that a programme had to be easy to apply and should have a clear structure without requiring special time-consuming training sessions. In order to realize these wishes and the above-mentioned theoretical notions, we developed a peer-led video programme.

The structure and content of the lessons were explained on video by youngsters. This method contains several advantages. First, the teacher only needed to follow a short special introductory training, as his main task consisted of coordinating the lessons, assisting the students, and stimulating them to participate. As the programme's didactic structure was simple, the teacher didn't have to spend much time in discovering how to use and prepare the lessons. The teacher did not have to follow a special course on the content as it was clearly explained on video. A special teachers' manual goes with the programme. Second, using adolescents who introduced the video lessons made the programme more attractive to students and improved comprehension.

The structure of the lessons can be summarized as follows: (a) introduction of the theme on video, presented by two adolescents (7 minutes); (b) activities in small groups, peer-led (15 minutes); (c) continuation of the lesson on video; presentation of real-life situations by adolescents (8 minutes); (d) activities in small groups, peer-led (15 minutes); (e) home activities.

The programme was implemented in November 1986 in four vocational and five high schools. The pre-test was conducted in September 1986 and three post-tests in May and September 1987, and June 1988. The programme has been evaluated by questionnaires and by group discussions, and evaluative questions were asked on the video programme, the activities, the manual, the peer-led structure, and the assistance by peer leader and teacher.

Results

Fewer young people started smoking The programme had a preventive impact on regular smoking. One year after the pre-test, regular smoking increased with 4.8% in the experimental group, compared to 7.4% in the control group ($p<.05$). Furthermore, the programme was very successful for vocational school students. Regular smoking increased with 6.7% in the control group, while it increased with 15.9% in the control group ($p<.005$). The results of the effects of the programme are discussed elsewhere in more detail (de Vries *et al.*, 1987).

Students and teachers liked the programme The prevention programme appeared to be attractive to both students and teachers. Use of videos and activities prevented boredom and inattention. The video-led nature of the programme increased chances of implementation, because teachers did not have to follow time-consuming training sessions. This made it also possible to use the programme during various different lessons, for example, mathematics, biology and history. Using the activities helped adolescents to integrate the information into their life style. Active learning in this way will make students aware of their own lack of knowledge, which will make them more open to new information.

The teacher's role was more important than predicted The most predictive factor in students' evaluation of the programme was their evaluation of the teacher's assistance. This finding was unexpected, because the programme was constructed in such a way as to make it independent of the teacher. Although we stressed that teachers needed to be encouraging and stimulating, we did not expect such a great impact of the teacher's role. Apart from stimulating students, the teacher is probably also an important source for students to assess the significance and importance of a programme. If teachers do participate in the programme, but also show (perhaps unintended) signs of skepticism, this is likely to influence students' perception of the programme.

The determinants of students' responses were clarified It appeared that students with a positive evaluation of their teacher liked the programme much more than students who had neutral or negative evaluations of the teacher. Similar results were found if students were divided by their score on the evaluation of their peer leader. The target group for the programme was vocational school students as they are at higher risk of becoming smokers. We therefore expected that they would be more positive towards the programme than high-school students, who have a different educational level. The results of the programme evaluations supported this expectation, and they also supported our assumption that smokers would be less positive towards the programme, although smokers did not differ in their evaluations of the programme and the lessons on video. Girls liked working in groups more than boys. No differences were found between 13 and 14-year-old students. Most importantly, the programme resulted in a significant preventive impact in general, in particular among vocational school students.

Continuation of prevention

An attractive and effective programme, however, does not guarantee successful prevention of smoking. Schools often have different and conflicting priorities. Health education should therefore become a major subject within the curriculum—which is presently neither the case in the Netherlands nor in Europe. Even if it were integrated into the curriculum, one might still wonder whether smoking prevention can be really effective.

Smoking prevention is only credible if it takes place within a society that takes a clear stand on health and health promotion. It is not credible in a society promoting health but at the same time also actively promoting health-damaging advertisements. In this context, smoking prevention and health education can not be optimally effective. Adolescents will have a difficult question to solve: why are we advised not to smoke? If smoking is really that bad, why aren't cigarettes and certainly cigarette advertisements, forbidden? One implication should be a promotional view on health, in which health activities are part of a larger project, which also incorporates consistent health policies and legislation.

Conclusions

We started with an overview of planned health education and we have presented an illustration of primary cancer prevention. Not all of the variables that have been mentioned in the first part were applied in the second part. For instance, an integrated health-promotion programme is not attainable at this time in our country. There is a change in the right direction, but resistance against an effective anti-smoking health-promotion policy is still very strong.

The ABC approach with regard to prevention of smoking has been specifically applied in the school situation. That programme has only some of the characteristics of the ideal community approach. In planning smoking cessation programmes or nutrition education programmes, a community approach can be developed within small cities, neighbourhoods or regions as communities. Also the workplace can be a very effective entrance for community approaches (Jonkers *et al.*, 1988).

Cancer prevention has many potentialities. Planned health education can be shown to be an extremely effective way to prevent and reduce the incidence of cancer.

References

Bouter, L.M. (1988) *Injury risk in downhill skiing*, De Vrieseborg, Haarlem, Netherlands.

Doll, R. and Peto, R. (1981). The causes of cancer: quantitative estimate of avoidable risks of cancer in the United States today, *J. natl. Cancer Inst* **66**, 1191–1308.

Dutch Nutrition Council (1986) *Factoren in de voeding en het ontstaaan van kanker* (Factors in nutrition and the development of cancer), Den Haag, Netherlands.

Green, L.W. and Lewis, F.M. (1986) *Measurement and evaluation in health education and health promotion*, Mayfield, Palo Alto, California.

Hirschman, R.S., Leventhal, H. and Glynn, K. (1984) The development of smoking behaviour: conceptualization and supportive cross-sectional survey data, *J. Appl. Soc. Psy.* **14**, 184–206.

Jonkers, R., Liedekerken P.C., Haes, W.F.M. de, Kok, G.J. and Saen, J.A.M. (1988) *Effektiviteit van GVO* (Effectiveness of Health Education), Gezondheidsbevordering, Rijswijk, Netherlands.

Kok, G.J. (1988) Health motivation: health education from a social psychological point of view, in S. Maes, C.D. Spielberger, P.B. Defares and I.G. Sarasen (eds.), *Topics in Health Psychology*, 295–300, Wiley, New York.

Leeuw, E. de (1989) *The sane revolution: health promotion*, Van Gorkum, Assen, Netherlands.

Marlatt, G.A. and Gordon, J.R. (1985) *Relapse prevention: maintenance strategies in the treatment of addictive behaviors,* Guilfort, New York.

McGuire, W.J. (1985) Attitudes and attitude change, in G. Lindsay and E. Aronson (eds.) *Handbook of Social Psychology*, vol. II, Guilfort, New York.

Pieterse, M., Kok, G.J. and Verbeek, J. (1987) Kinderbeveiligingsmiddelen in de auto: een onderzoek naar de determinanten van aanschaf en gebruik (Acquisition and usage of automobile child restraint devices: a study of determinants) Rijksuniversiteit Limburg, Maastricht, Netherlands.

Schwartz, J.L. (1987) *Review and evaluation of smoking cessation methods: the United States and Canada 1978–1985*, U.S. Department of Health and Social Services, Public Health Service, National Institute of Health, Bethesda, Maryland.

Tholen, J., Siero, S. and Kok, G.J. (1988) Alcoholgebruik tijdens de zwangerschap; een empirisch onderzoek in Drenthe (Alcohol and pregnancy) *Tijdschrift voor Sociale Gezondheidszorg* (J. Soc. Health Care) accepted for publication.

Vries, H.de (1989) Towards primary cancer prevention: the Dutch ABC framework. *European J. for Cancer and Clin. Oncol.*, accepted for publication.

Vries, H. de and Kok, G.J. (1986) From determinants of smoking behaviour to the implications for a prevention programme, *Hlth. Ed. Res.* **1**, 85–94.

Vries, H. de, Dijkstra, M. and Kok, G.J. (1987) *A Dutch smoking prevention program: development, implementation and results,* paper presented at the 6th World Conference of Smoking and Health, Tokio, 6–9 November.

Vries, H. de, Dijkstra, M. and Kuhlman, P.(1988) Self-efficacy: the third factor besides attitude and subjective norm as a predictor of behavioral intentions, *Hlth. Ed. Res.* **3**, 273–282.

Paper 3.3

EDUCATING EARLY ABOUT THE PREVENTION OF CANCERS

Dr. Anne Charlton
Cancer Research Campaign Education and Child Studies Research Group, Department of Epidemiology and Social Oncology, University of Manchester, England

The overall aims of cancer education for young people are threefold:[1]

- to present a realistic picture of the cancers, in order to prevent the excessive fear that can cause delay in seeking treatment or reluctance to accept screening
- to encourage prevention wherever possible
- to provide an atmosphere in which all cancer patients, young or old, ill or cured, will be enabled to live a happy, normal life.

It is the second of these aims which is the topic of this paper, although there is of necessity some overlap, especially where young people are concerned[2,3].

Cancers rarely occur in young people. For example, in the United Kingdom about 1200 children will be diagnosed with some form of cancer each year, which means in effect that one child in about 350 will suffer from cancer during childhood. This figure is very different from the overall statistic, when people of all ages are included. In this case, about 1 in 3 people will suffer from some form of cancer at some time in their lives. It is not surprising, therefore, that children can fail to see the relevance of cancer prevention, particularly as childhood cancers have as yet no known preventive measures.

Younger children tend to see cancers as 'just another illness'. Just as you are likely to get mumps, measles, chicken-pox and so on, you are possibly going to get cancer, they think. Unless there is an immunization to prevent a disease, many children find the idea of prevention by any other means a very difficult concept to grasp.

In addition to this mental barrier, children often find the idea of preventing adult disease too distant to concern them. At the age of nine or ten, a disease at 40 not only seems too far away to be concerned about, but also, to children's eyes, quite inevitable. The idea of being 20, let alone 40, is just untenable to a young child. 'Of course old people get ill and die; everyone dies; everyone dies of something.' 'When I am as old as 40, I would expect to be dead. What is all the fuss about?' say the youngsters.

Related to this, children's thinking is usually very logical. If, by preventive action, 15 per cent fewer people will die of cancers, then that 15 per cent will die of something else. All that will happen will be an increase in deaths from some other disease, they reason, not entirely incorrectly, and children are extremely likely to spot this apparent flaw in the logic. So, in encouraging prevention of cancers, children often need a completely different message and approach from those which are effective and meaningful to adults.

This short paper considers four aspects of starting cancer-prevention education early in life. It focuses on the European situation, but it is important to bear in mind that in other parts of the world the problem and the preventive measures and education needed are quite different. The four aspects considered here are:

1 the current state of knowledge:

the evidence of the need to start cancer prevention in childhood

2 what should be told:

the format this preventive education should take in order to be relevant to children

3 who needs to know:

the problems of finding a place for cancer-prevention education for young people in the school, home and community situations

4 getting the message across:

possible ways of solving these problems and what is already being done.

1 The current state of knowledge

There is no need here to go into details of carcinogenesis. Suffice it to say that there may be several factors in the initiation of a cancer and its subsequent development, and that a considerable time can elapse between the initiation and the appearance of an observable cancer[4]. Thus it is that the initiation and the early promotion stages of a cancer, if not the appearance of the cancer itself, can occur in childhood or adolescence. Evidence for this is stronger for some cancers than for others, and two are especially important: lung cancer and cancer of the uterine cervix.

Smoking

Doll and Peto[5] and others[6] have clearly shown that the earlier in life regular cigarette smoking begins, the greater is the risk of lung cancer. In Britain, and in some other European countries, there is considerable evidence that the age of nine or ten years is the most popular age for trying a first cigarette[7]. Most of these young experimenters try one cigarette to satisfy their curiosity, dislike it and never try another one. Unfortunately, there are those who persist and by the age of 12 or 13 years, a small but well established band of regular smokers exists[7,8].

A national survey in England and Wales in 1986[9] showed how this group of regular smokers increases in size until in the last year at school (aged 15 and 16 years), 19 per cent of the boys and 30 per cent of the girls were smoking regularly at least one cigarette per week, and some of them were already smoking quite heavily. These figures are also reflected in some other European countries. Whilst smoking amongst boys has decreased considerably in recent years, smoking among girls has fallen by a much smaller percentage and in some countries has even increased.

In order to plan prevention strategies, it is vital to know not only what the current prevalence is, but what underlies it. Why is the smoking rate so high, especially amongst girls? Many recent studies on young people's smoking have addressed this issue and a picture is emerging. First, the parents provide a medium in which smoking is, or is not, the norm. In the process of primary socialization, a very young child can associate mother's smoking with security, and with intrinsic acceptance of the habit.

Research in several European countries has shown that children whose parents smoke are twice as likely to be smokers as are those with non-smoking parents[10,11]. This is not surprising; not only does the parental example create a norm for smoking, but also cigarettes are more likely to be easily available in those households. However, if children perceive strong disapproval of their smoking by their parents, they are less likely to become smokers, even if their parents themselves smoke. A Cancer Research Campaign-funded study in England showed that children who thought their parents approved of their smoking were seven times more likely to be smokers than those who perceived parental disapproval.

Much has been said about peer pressure to smoke[12]. It is not completely clear whether young smokers tend to choose each other as friends, or whether one smoking child within a group of friends acts as the catalyst which converts the rest into smokers. Nevertheless, there is considerable evidence to show that young people smoke because their friends smoke and because they wish to conform with the group norm.

School ethos and school policy[13], together with the teachers' example[14] with respect to smoking, and health education about smoking given by teachers[15], could all play a significant part in the child's decision whether or not to smoke. It is, however, important to remember that, whatever is done in school with respect to smoking, if a child returns to an environment outside school in which smoking is not merely acceptable, but is an integral part of family and community life, then any efforts on the part of the school to discourage smoking are likely to be overridden[16].

Not only are home, friends and school factors in a child's decision whether or not to smoke, there are many macro-influences too. Cigarette advertising[17,18], portrayal of smoking in films and television programmes[19], sale of tobacco to under 16s[20], and cigarette prices[21] are all to some degree involved in the uptake and maintenance of smoking by children, as they are also with adults.

Probably related to the portrayal of cigarette smoking in films and to the messages of advertising, many young people hold positive beliefs about what smoking will do for them. The beliefs that smoking calms the nerves, gives confidence, controls weight and looks grown up are widespread among young people, especially among young smokers. Beliefs about cigarette smoking change as young people get older[22]. Under the age of 11 years, the appearance of smoking is all important; after that age, psychological and physical 'benefits' take priority and the importance of the appearance of smoking diminishes.

Knowledge about the health risks of smoking, at least as lip service, apparently increases with increasing age in the eight to 19 years age group. In a recent study in England[23], a sample of 12 and 13-year-olds was given a questionnaire on their smoking habits and the opinions and background factors mentioned above. Four months later they were surveyed again and the opinions and background factors that were reported in the pre-test were considered in the light of whether or not those who were non-smokers at the pre-test stage had subsequently taken up smoking. A logistic regression was carried out. For girls, parental smoking, positive beliefs about smoking, awareness of a cigarette brand name and best-friend's smoking were all significant. For boys, although best friend's smoking was the most strongly related factor, none was significant. The most crucial factor was that boys expressed very few positive beliefs about smoking, while for the girls these beliefs were extremely significant in their uptake of smoking.

It is vital, therefore, to begin the prevention of lung cancer at a very early stage. Teaching health-risk information is not enough. The environmental and psychological factors must all be tackled in some way during childhood.

Cervical cancer

The second type of cancer for which it is very necessary to begin the prevention message early is cancer of the uterine cervix. This cancer has always been frequent in countries where early marriage is usual[24]. In most European countries, marriages under the age of 16, and sometimes under the age of 18 years, have been relatively uncommon, if not actually prohibited. Recently, however, whilst marriage is rapidly falling out of favour amongst young people, the age when young people become sexually active has decreased and many young people have numerous sexual partners[25].

Concurrent with this change in habits, there has been a sharp and alarming rise in cervical cancer in young women[26]. The two factors may or may not be directly related, but there is no doubt that at this age, the cells in the developing tissues of the teenage uterine cervix are at their most sensitive[27]. It appears that whatever content of the sperm or semen triggers cervical cancer, these young cervical cells are at their most vulnerable to it.

There is clear evidence that sexual intercourse started at early or mid to late teens is related to an increased risk of cervical cancer, as is having multiple sexual partners. If either the girl or the boy has several sexual partners, the girl's risk of cervical cancer is increased[28]. Cervical cancer is also most frequent in specific occupational groups. These groups are mainly, but not entirely, in the skilled, semi-skilled and unskilled manual working groups[29]. Boys as well as girls need education about cervical cancer while still at school. It is too late by the time they have left school. Either the damage is already done by then, or else the women at the highest risk have become largely unreachable by any educational messages. Primary and secondary prevention by the cervical smear test need to be presented at school, even if the girls are too young to have the test done at that stage.

Other cancers

Other cancer prevention messages relevant to young people which need to be started early are those related to protecting the skin from strong sunlight, eating a balanced diet, not drinking excesses of alcohol, and observing safety precautions at work. The sunlight problem is an important one in Britain, where suntanned skin is considered fashionable. Sunbeds are also popular and their risk, though known, is largely unpublicized as yet. There is evidence that excessive exposure to sun in young childhood increases the risks most, again indicating the need for early education.

Most children are not able to choose their everyday diet, which is governed by what the family can afford and their established life style. Moreover, the evidence for specific dietary factors increasing or decreasing cancer risks is, as yet, rather indefinite[30]. Nevertheless, defining and encouraging a balanced diet when we are teaching children can have wider spin-offs in initiating changes in family diets and, of course, has wider health benefits than merely helping to prevent cancers.

At present alcohol consumption among adolescents in Britain seems to be an even more frequent habit than smoking[31]. Education about this topic should start in school.

Preventive action for breast cancer is still a debatable subject. Breast self-examination, itself far from being of proven effectiveness for adults, is even more suspect for young people. There are four main reasons for this, but there are other underlying problems too. The main reasons against teaching breast self-examination in schools are:

- if it is not learned correctly, it is not effective and creates a false sense of security;
- young girls' breasts are often lumpy, so to go to a doctor at that stage would probably bring a negative reply and perhaps deter another visit for a suspicious lump later in life;
- the prognosis for breast cancer in someone so young is poor;
- it could create excess anxiety.

2 What should be told

It is clear from the foregoing review that merely teaching about the health risks is a non-starter[32]. To children the facts are boring, the distant future is not relevant and some children like to take risks anyway. In many ways, the type of education needed hits right at the foundations of what many present-day European children accept as desirable. Imagine how many children at present hold most or even all of the following beliefs: it is part of life to smoke; all my family do; so do my friends and teachers; cigarettes are sold in ordinary shops, so they cannot be that bad; it is attractive to be as thin as possible, if not even thinner; fat people are ugly and laughable; it is good to be calm, cool, confident and sophisticated—cigarettes do this for you, films and advertising tell you so; it is old-fashioned not to have at least one boyfriend or girlfriend and quite unmentionable not to have sexual relations with them; it is beautiful to be tanned; not to eat meat every day is a sign of poverty; it is friendly and sociable to drink alcohol.

When anyone, including a child, makes a decision concerning their health, they weigh up whether or not the health risk threat is serious enough and personal enough to merit making a choice. They then balance what they will gain with what they will lose[33]. A young person may stand to lose a lot because many of the health messages undermine their established normative beliefs. What health educators must do is to decide how positive health behaviour can be incorporated into a young person's chosen life style.

It is often difficult for a health-oriented adult to be aware of just how threatened a young person can feel when presented with so many healthy life-style messages. Equally, it is difficult, but necessary, for the health-educating adults to distinguish just how far they can expect young people to change at their request, and it is just as difficult to separate elements of the young person's behaviour that are hazardous to health from those that are not. It is neither feasible, nor desirable, that all young people should be turned into athletic, conformist 'ideal' youngsters whose one main concern is their health. There is nothing intrinsically wrong with not liking sports, with going to rock concerts, wearing leather jackets and having pink hair. Health education must meet young people where they are, and not try to negate their culture.

How can health-education messages be integrated into young people's life styles?

- by involving parents, whole families, communities, and legislation, if need be. Parents are especially important in the education of younger people.
- by making clear which aspects of a person's life style would best be changed and providing young people with the determination and methods for making these changes; for example, the practicalities of how to resist peer pressure, and the processes needed to make decisions.
- by helping build up self esteem among young people. It is important that they should know and accept their own value. In the words of a well known saying, 'Grant us serenity to accept the things we cannot change, courage to change the things we can, and wisdom to know the difference.' Young people often lack confidence in themselves. If anything in them fails to conform to the current ideal, they often feel a failure. Cancer-prevention education can help a person to see that it is not necessary to be skinny and anorexic (and hence often a smoker) to be beautiful; that being suntanned is not vital to being attractive; that being a virgin at 16 is certainly not a matter for shame and despondency. In this way a foundation can be created on which health negotiations between educator and young people can begin.
- by making health risks relevant, for example by showing that some risks are immediate, such as the increased carbon monoxide in smokers' expired air.
- by making all health messages realistic, logical and above all *relevant* to young people.
- by solving some of the real practical problems that underlie some of the unhealthy choices, for example finding out what is causing the stresses which appear to necessitate smoking as a means of calming nerves. How do non-smokers cope with the equivalent stresses?
- by taking care that our messages do not have the opposite effect to the one intended; for example, being sure that looking at advertisements for cigarettes as part of a lesson or competition is not, in fact, encouraging children to smoke rather than discouraging them; that there is no stigma attached to the cervical smear message; that the diet messages do not lead to the belief that fat is bad, sugar is bad, meat is bad, starch is bad, only fibre is good, which has led to malnutrition in some wealthier areas.

3 Who needs to know

Unfortunately, achieving successful cancer-prevention education is not as easy as the theory suggests. The problems are many and varied. Below is a list of those problems often raised by teachers[34]:

- We do not know enough about cancer.
- We have no time available in the curriculum or syllabus.
- Cancer-prevention messages could frighten the children.
- Children are too young to be bothered by such things.
- We have no money for materials.
- I (the teacher) am frightened of cancer.

The list could extend indefinitely, but the message is clear. Teachers often reject cancer education for two groups of reasons. Firstly, for practical reasons, such as lack of time, finance or materials; and secondly, their own personal reactions to cancers, or, in some cases for the former reasons because of the latter ones. Before planning any cancer-prevention education that is to involve schools, it is important to consult, involve and, if necessary, educate the teachers. This would be best achieved by including it as an element in the basic training course and failing this, in-service training, and certainly participation in planning of materials.

4 Getting the message across

One means of solving both problems is to involve teachers at all stages, thereby educating them about cancer and cancer education and thus enabling them to face and sort out their own fears and supposed lack of knowledge. This process also ensures that materials are planned to fit in with their courses and examination syllabi. Many schools do not have health education courses. In fact, this lack need not present too many problems. Cancer prevention has many aspects and fits well into a range of academic and practical subjects[35].

Teachers who might balk at teaching about cancer may be very happy to teach an aspect related to their own specialist subject. For example, teachers of Home Economics will happily plan balanced diets and look at meals worldwide. Chemistry teachers will include carcinogenic chemicals and safety in handling them. Physics teachers will carry out experiments on protection against the ultraviolet radiation from the sun, and so on. It is unnecessary and could be counterproductive to teach about cancer in the form of a 'cancer week', because the children may become bored and may even develop a resistance to the messages presented in this way.

There are now some excellent teaching packages available from a number of organizations in Europe; *Karin en 50 000 anderen*[36] by the Queen Wilhelmina Fund in Amsterdam is a particularly good example of a general package. There are numerous smoking education packages. The Cancer Research Campaign Education and Child Studies Research Group, Manchester, England, has a general cancer-education package entitled *Cells, Cancers and Communities*[37], which takes into account the cross-curricular approach mentioned above. In controlled trial evaluation, various parts of it were shown to be effective in increasing knowledge, fostering a less emotive attitude, and encouraging 16-year-old girls to take the cervical smear test. The International Union Against Cancer has a general package of seven modules on cancer education[39]. These materials are guidelines and are intended to be adaptable to the needs of teachers and other educators in every country.

It would be impossible to list all the excellent cancer-prevention packages available. Suffice it to say that many steps have been made. Smoking rates amongst boys are falling in several countries, which might be the first indicator of success. It is too soon as yet to make this assertion. New methods are constantly being developed. Although materials often cannot be transferred from one country to another, ideas can and should be.

In conclusion, a word of warning and a word of hope. Education about cancer prevention can be carried too far. If someone, child or adult, is given to believe that they hold the responsibility for whether or not they personally get cancer, terrible guilt and destruction of faith can result if they or their relatives do get cancer in spite of their efforts. A child is often not in a position to take or encourage the recommended action, and this can lead to unresolvable fear. People will probably always get cancer. It cannot always be prevented.

Finally, the good news. European Cancer Year has created an awareness and opportunity for the introduction of cancer education which is unparalleled. It has never come before and it will probably never come again. Trials and evaluations of any new approaches are crucial. It is vital for us to seize this chance now to present the case for cancer education in schools to governments, Ministries of Education, local education authorities, teacher training institutions, headteachers and teachers.

References

1 Charlton, A. (1986) *The many opportunities for cancer education in schools*, paper presented at the 14th International Cancer Congress, Budapest, Hungary.

2 Draper, G. J. *et al.* (1980) *Childhood Cancer in Great Britain: Incidence, Mortality and Survival*, Studies on Medical Population Subjects, Office of Population Censuses and Surveys, HMSO, London.

3 Charlton, A., Pearson, D., Morris-Jones, P. H. (1986) Children's return to school after treatment for solid tumours, *Soc. Sci. and Med.* **22**, 1337–1346.

4 Ruddon, R. W. (1981) *Cancer Biology*, Oxford University Press, Oxford.

5 Doll, R. and Peto, R. (1981) *The Causes of Cancer*, Oxford University Press, Oxford.

6 Kahn, H. A. (1966) *The Dorn study of smoking and mortality among US veterans: report on eight and one-half years of observation*, National Cancer Institute Monograph, Bethesda.

7 Charlton, A. (1984) The Brigantia Smoking Survey: a general review. *Public Education about Cancer*, UICC Technical Report Series **77**, 92–102, International Union Against Cancer, Geneva.

8 Dobbs, J., Marsh, A. (1985) *Smoking among secondary school children 1984. An enquiry for the DHSS*, HMSO, London.

9 Goddard, E., Ikin, C. (1987) *Smoking among secondary school children 1986. An enquiry for the DHSS, Welsh Office and Scottish Home and Health Department,* HMSO, London.

10 Aaro, L. E., Hauknes, A., Berglund, E. L. (1981) Smoking among Norwegian Schoolchildren 1975–1980, II. The Influence of the Social Environment, *Scand. J. Psychol.* **22**, 297–309.

11 Charlton, A. (1986) Children who smoke, *Health at School* **1**, 125–127.

12 Evans, R. I. *et al.* (1981) Social modelling films to deter smoking among adolescents: a three year follow-up of an education programme for youth, *J. Appl. Psy.* **66**, 399.

13 Porter, A. (1982) Disciplinary attitudes and cigarette smoking: a comparison of two schools, *Brit. Med. J.* **286**, 1725.

14 Cooreman, J., Burghard, G. and Perdrizet, S. (1987) L'adolescent et le tabagisme, *J. Med. Strasbourg* **9**, 483–486.

15 Reid, D. (1985) Prevention of smoking among school children: recommendations for policy development, *Health Ed. J.* **44**, 3–12.

16 Rutter, M., Maugham, B., Mortimore, P., Ouston, J., Smith, A. (1979) *Fifteen Thousand Hours: Secondary Schools and Their Effects on Children*, Open Books, London.

17 Charlton, A. (1986) Children's advertisement awareness related to their views on smoking, *Health Ed. J.* **45**, 75–78.

18 Aitken, P., Leathar, D., O'Hagan, F. J. (1985) Children's perceptions of advertisements for cigarettes, *Soc. Sci. and Med.* **21**, 787–797.

19 Piepe, A., Emerson, M., Crouch, S. (1977) *Mass Media and Cultural Relationships*, Saxon House Press, Farnborough, UK.

20 Wake, R., McAlister, A., Nostbakken, D. (eds.) (1982) *A Manual on Children and Smoking*, IUCC, Geneva.

21 Lewit, E. M., Coate, D., Grossman, M. (1981) The effects of government regulation on teenage smoking, *J. Law and Econ.* **24**, 545–573.

22 Charlton, A. (1984) Children's opinions on smoking, *J. Royal Coll.Gen. Prac.* **34**, 483–487.

23 Charlton, A. (in preparation) Uptake of smoking by 12 and 13-year-olds.

24 Waterhouse, J., Muir, C., Shanmugaratnam, K., Powell, J. (eds.) (1982) *Cancer Incidence in Five Continents*, IARC, Lyon.

25 Boyd, J. T., Doll, R. (1964) A study of the aetiology of cancer of the cervix uteri, *Brit. J. Cancer* **18**, 419.

26 Charlton, A. (1983) Young people's knowledge of the cervical smear test, *Soc. Sci. and Med.* **17**, 235–239.

27 Chamberlain, G. (1981) Aetiology of gynaecological cancer, *J. Roy. Soc. Med.* **74**, 246.

28 Buckley, J. D., Harris, R. W. C., Roll, R., Vessey, M., Williams, P. T. (1981) Case-control study of the husbands of women with dysplasia or carcinoma of the cervix uteri, *Lancet* **2**, 1010.

29 Robinson, J. (1982) Cancer of the cervix: occupational risks of husbands and wives and possible preventive strategies. *Preclinical Neoplasia of the Cervix*, proceedings of the Ninth Study Group of the Royal College of Obstetricians and Gynaecologists, J. A. Jordan, F. Sharp, A. Singer (eds.) 11–27, RCOG, London.

30 Doll, R. (1979) Nutrition and cancer: a review, *Nutr. Cancer* **1**, 35–45.

31 Taylor, M. T., Mardle, G. D. (1986) Smoking and drinking among 16-year-olds, *Hlth. Ed. J.* **45**, 136–139.

32 Thompson, E. (1978) Smoking intervention programmes 1960–1976. A review. *Am. J. Publ. Hlth.* **68**, 250–257.

33 Fishbein, M. (1976) Attitude and prediction of behaviour, in M. Fishbein (ed.) *Reading in Attitude Theory and Measurement*, Wiley, New York.

34 Charlton, A. (1979) Cancer and cancer education: opinions of some secondary school teachers in northern England, *Hlth. Ed. J.* **38**, 77–83.

35 Charlton, A. (1979) An evaluation of two different approaches to teaching about cancer in secondary schools, *Int. J. Hlth. Ed.* **22**, 42–48.

36 Queen Wilhelmina Fund (1988) *Karin ... en 50,000 anderen*, Konigen Wilhelmina Fonds, Amsterdam.

37 Charlton, A. (1988) *Cells, Cancers and Communities*, Stanley Thornes Ltd, Cheltenham, UK.

38 Charlton, A. (1983) Assegai: teaching about cancer in general studies, *Int. J. Hlth. Ed.* **1**, 67–73.

39 International Union Against Cancer (1988) *Cancer Education in Schools: Guidelines for Teachers*, IUCC, Geneva.

Chapter 4

EDUCATING HEALTH WORKERS AND HEALTH POLICY MAKERS

Summary

Health workers and health policy makers give low priority to preventive activity, especially in the field of cancer prevention. Their training is often very inadequate in this area, and their attitudes towards preventive work are frequently negative.

Health policy makers need more education in activities relevant to the prevention of cancers. In addition:

- they should make sufficient funds available for preventive work
- they should ensure that the staff and facilities they have direct control over are able to work in a 'healthy health service'. This is important intrinsically, and also sets a good example to the rest of the community about the priority given to preventive work.

Paper 4.1: *The Role of Cancer Education* Dr. E. Milly L. Haagedoorn

Paper 4.2: *Practical Policies for Screening for Early Detection of Cancers* Professor Jocelyn Chamberlain

Educating health workers in the prevention of cancers

At the Colloquium, the working group that was discussing the education of health workers and health policy makers held the opinion that preventive work by health workers in the field of cancer prevention is underdeveloped and often accorded low status and poor levels of resourcing. Similarly, health policy makers, and even cancer societies and organizations, apparently give low priority to preventive activities. It is easy for decision makers to favour the more immediately appealing specialities of curative medicine or basic scientific types of research work.

Many other aspects of cancer work also seem to suffer from low status and poor resourcing within health authority budgets. Within the European Community, cancers are the second largest cause of death after coronary heart disease. Approximately three quarters of a million people in the EC countries die from a cancer each year and it has been apparent for some time that many of these deaths are preventable. However, many aspects of cancer work do not appear at present to have the priority that they deserve. One example of this is in the teaching and training of health workers about cancers and how they can be treated and prevented. The recent report by the Commission of the European Communities and the European Organization for Research and Treatment of Cancer (EC/EORTC, 1988), which reported the result of surveys of medical schools throughout the European Community, summarized its findings in this way:

> Undergraduate cancer education in Europe is:
>
> - inadequate in terms of lack of clear objectives, curriculum design and coordination;
> - widely variable between countries and between schools in individual countries;
> - lacking in practical clinical training with excessive reliance on formal lectures; poorly represented in examinations and rarely examined separately (at any stage in the undergraduate curriculum); lacking in teaching in important areas, such as cancer screening and pain control. There is still a lack of chairs in oncology in European medical schools;
> - discordant in terms of what teachers consider to be important and what students actually experience.

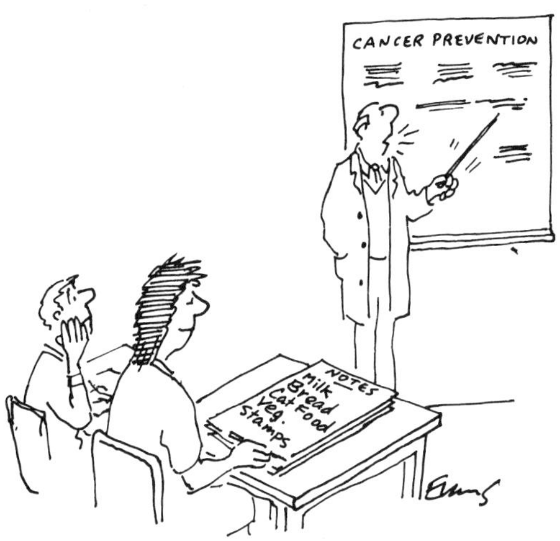

EXCESSIVE RELIANCE ON FORMAL LECTURES...

Often the experience of health workers as they undergo training can be very negative as regards the development of their attitudes towards cancer prevention. Their training often involves work with patients who are suffering from one of the cancers at an advanced stage, or during terminal care. Without access to people who have recovered from cancer, or indeed without knowledge of cancer-prevention activities in the community, their attitudes are often found to be negative towards acceptance of facts about cancer prevention. When the curriculum includes time spent with cancer societies, or with associations of cancer patients, as described in a project in Holland (Buitenhuis *et al.*, 1989), their attitudes and outlook regarding cancers and people developing one of the cancers, improved.

Expanding the target audience

The Colloquium working group decided that it is important to expand the notion of who actually acts as a health worker when thinking about a target audience for information about the prevention of cancers. It is no longer adequate to restrict our plans for the education of health workers to the traditional groups such as doctors and nurses. Many other groups in all countries now act as health workers in a broad sense, and we should expand our efforts to include the following groups of people when devising educational activities to change attitudes, knowledge and practices:

- traditional groups of health workers;
- all other health service workers;
- health policy makers inside and outside the health service itself;
- teachers and influential people or groups within the community;
- cancer organizations, societies and leagues.

The curriculum for training health educators is explained in Chapter 3.

Health policy makers

One important group of people who require education are the health policy makers. These influential people, at all levels of decision making, need to be re-educated so that the prevention of cancers receives its fair share of resources allocated in an appropriate manner. It is vital that the people taking decisions about health-related issues know the most recent facts about the preventability of the various cancers and how their decisions can affect the incidence of cancers within their community. It is important to think about an educational input to policy makers at all levels in such a way as to affect the total decision-making climate and ensure that decisions are taken that positively reflect the accumulated knowledge about the preventability of cancers.

Political parties

Political parties have an important part to play in nominating many of the people appointed to decision-making bodies, and they should be included as a target for educational activity on health-related issues. Many political parties have interest groups and lobbying organizations concerned with health issues and they should be approached through educational activities designed to show how cancers can be prevented. Ideally a cross-party commitment to a long-term project that can be established over several electoral periods is required. See, for example, the Swedish project described in Chapter 7 by Holm and Haglund (Paper 7.1). In the field of preventive health activities, there are key programmes that should not be jeopardized by inter-party arguments.

Cancer organizations

All the countries of the European Community have organizations specifically concerned with various aspects of cancer. Many of them are charities and receive funds, donations and legacies to enable them to work in the cancer field. The patterns of their work are very different; many are concerned with the relief of suffering for people who have cancer and provide money or equipment to make the illness more bearable. Other organizations use their funds to sponsor research into cancer-related problems. Often this involves specialist laboratory work, or detailed clinical trials of particular therapies. In recent years, more and more of these organizations have been concerned with educational activities. They provide educational material and information for people with a particular cancer and for their relatives. However, the participants of the Colloquium working group felt that only a small amount of the budgets of such organizations, and a relatively minor proportion of their total energy, is usually focused on preventive work.

Any educational activities that are designed to promote the prevention of cancers should include some attempts to educate the cancer societies themselves, so that a greater proportion of their activities are allocated to preventive work. Cancer societies are often very influential as opinion leaders within society. They are frequently responsible for large budgets and in many cases they have considerable leverage within the media. Some conscious increase of resources and effort towards the prevention of cancers would be beneficial and would help to create a positive climate for all other cancer-prevention activities.

As with the other sectors where change is required, it is important to understand the ways in which the policy of the cancer organization is made and to target the key committees and individuals with the information they require to bring about changes in policy. Often cancer organizations and cancer leagues, because of their comparative independence and flexibility, can develop innovative projects and schemes before the statutory services are able to change. The value of these pilot projects is immense, and preventive activity by cancer organizations can be especially valuable because of the impact that high profile, innovative schemes can achieve. Coupled with the excellent contacts with the media that many of these societies enjoy and the direct contact with large numbers of the general public who are involved in the society's activities, the societies offer the opportunity to become a powerful force for preventive work.

Health workers need education at every stage

Health workers throughout the structure of traditional health-care organizations need education about the prevention of cancers at all stages of their training and their subsequent careers. Undergraduates of all the professions within the health service need full education about the preventability of cancers and this educational effort should be continued into postgraduate and continuing educational activity to include doctors, nurses, dentists, pharmacists, social workers, physiotherapists, psychologists, dieticians and nutrition workers, and all health service employees.

Further consideration also needs to be made of health workers outside the particular structures of the health service itself. Certainly teachers within the educational system can be thought of as health workers.

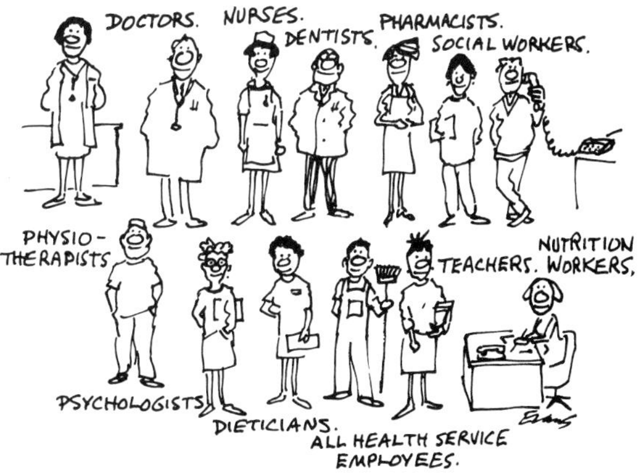

SOME TARGETS FOR CANCER PREVENTION EDUCATION

Targeting decision makers

Educational activities at all levels should be targeted on the most influential decision makers within the organization. It may be possible to identify the key person, or the key groups of people who seem to be the most powerful when it comes to shaping policy and the ethos of the organization.

Within the health policy sphere, it is often medically qualified doctors who remain influential at all levels of the decision-making process, and this should be recognized when specific educational activity is designed for policy makers. Doctors are often used as advisors and employed as health authority officers. For this reason, educational activity targeted at doctors may be especially effective under the current decision-making structures and processes.

The messages

The basic educational messages to be put across in all the activities designed for such an expanded target audience remain quite simple. Although the method of getting the message across will vary from group to group, depending on the educational situation, the basic elements that should be transmitted remain the same:

1 Many cancers can be prevented by appropriate action at a variety of levels.

2 Health workers have an important role to play in preventive work at all levels. They should use their influential position to good advantage.

3 Some cancers can be cured ... and the prognosis for many is getting better all the time.

4 Many people with cancer live a good quality life. This can depend on the support and care they receive.

5 For cancer-related work to be successful, multi-professional and team working is necessary, especially in the prevention of cancers. Doctors and nurses cannot do it alone.

6 Workers and patients need a healthy health service.

A healthy health service

Health services are major employers and the buildings and services which are organized for health activities are used by a large proportion of the general public. Health policy makers, who are concerned with the implementation of health policy in wider society, should consider the ways in which the people and facilities under their more immediate control might be changed to produce a healthy health service.

There are many ways in which health services could provide a healthy environment for the people working within them, and for the people attending for help. The overall impact of this on public awareness would be very considerable and would act as a major demonstration to the public at large of the importance of action to prevent cancers. While health-service premises and health-service employees remain unchanged, this major educational opportunity is being lost and may even be promoting a negative image. Although there are some examples of health authorities attempting to put their own house in order and promote a healthy environment on their own premises, the general picture throughout Europe was still thought to be rather poor.

The working group formulated some ideas that should be implemented within all health-service establishments:

1 A movement towards smoke-free health

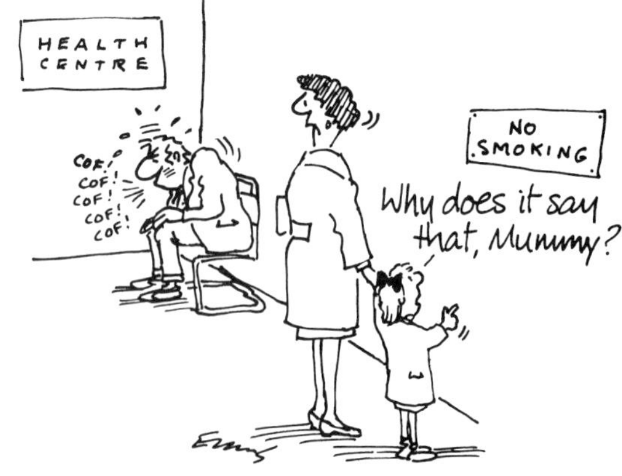

establishments. Hospitals and health centres should develop policies that move them towards being entirely smoke free.

2 There should be no sales of tobacco on health-service premises, either for health-service employees, or for people attending for treatment.

3 Tobacco use should be accepted as an addiction and a full range of therapy and counselling for staff should be available to help them overcome their problem.

4 A food policy should be implemented for attenders and employees that takes into account the latest recommendations for the prevention of diet-related diseases.

5 A policy on alcohol use within health-service premises should be developed. This issue is highly culture specific; for example, in some European Community countries, alcohol is served to patients in hospital with their meals, while in other countries no alcohol is allowed on hospital premises.

In these ways, the health services can fully discharge their responsibilities as employers and act as a powerful influence over the rest of society. If health services and health-service employees do not set a positive example, then it is hard to see how their other educational activities can possibly be effective.

Strategies for the implementation of health policy

The Colloquium working group considered that the implementation of the ideas for preventing cancers can be grouped under the following strategies:

- educational strategies;
- pricing strategies;
- provision strategies.

Education about the nature and function of each of these strategies is needed by health workers and health policy makers.

Educational strategies

Direct education of the whole range of health workers and health policy makers is necessary to widen the scope of the general health-education message so that it includes the cancer-prevention messages we outlined earlier. Most of the desired educational messages have already been listed in earlier parts of this chapter. However, it is important for people who wish to implement strategies for the prevention of cancers to recognize that education should be a two-way process. At the same time that cancer activists are attempting to teach, for example, health policy makers about the importance of cancer prevention, they should also be learning themselves about the ways in which health policy makers go about their tasks. Only through learning about decision-making structures and the organization of power and control can health activists discover the ways in which they might be able to favourably influence policies and the allocation of resources. The educational process also has to be targeted carefully to ensure that the messages get through to the key people within each part of the decision-making structure.

Educational activity can also be indirect. For example, policy makers might not be used to responding to overt educational activity, such as seminars or workshops, but could learn effectively if they are asked to express their beliefs and priorities about the prevention of cancers. By establishing their views on the subject, and then by requesting that these views are reflected in terms of practical policy, it may be possible to have a major effect on management education.

Whenever educational activities are carried out, a number of key elements need to be developed. The ten most important questions that need to be answered before any educational activity in the field of cancer prevention is undertaken are discussed by Dr. E. Milly L. Haagedoorn in Paper 4.1, *The Role of Cancer Education.*

Pricing strategies

The use of pricing strategies obviously depends on the type of health-service finance system that is in operation. Throughout Europe, many different methods exist to collect funds for use within the health service sector. Some of the following pricing strategies may be appropriate under particular funding arrangements.

Patients may be stimulated to attend preventive health activities if:

- they are very cheap or entirely free;
- they get cheaper curative care only if they have also undertaken certain preventive activities;
- other services, such as life insurance, are cheaper if they have attended preventive sessions or have a healthier life style, for example, do not smoke;
- they are threatened with sanctions, for example, the withdrawal of certain state benefits, if they don't attend.

Governments can stimulate preventive activity through:

- the heavy taxation of harmful activities;
- the subsidization of healthy foods and other products;
- the establishment of a separate fund for preventive activities, either from the extra taxation from harmful activities or from other forms of revenue collection.

It is important that the general public understand the function and importance of these measures so that they can support the governments and politicians attempting to implement these policies.

Provision strategies

Health policy makers should provide certain facilities to ensure that preventive activity is possible and can be undertaken effectively. For example, they could provide:

- better information and accurate statistics about health and illness (cancer registries are especially important in this context);
- role models for other large organizations and employers to follow—this will include working towards a healthy health service in the ways already outlined;
- appropriate screening services for all the relevant sections of the population that are their responsibility, including their own employees.

Many more types of services that are relevant to the prevention of cancers will be considered in Chapter 7 and in the accompanying papers (see particularly Paper 7.2 by Martin Moreno). This chapter considers the need for the provision of integrated activity across several sectors, not just within the health sector itself.

One example where detailed examination of all three strategies should be considered when implementing health-service policies is in policies for the establishment of screening services for the early detection of cancers.

The provision of screening services

One very important area health workers and policy makers need additional education about is screening for early detection of cancer. Too often they assume that screening is unproblematic and valuable. But, as Chamberlain points out in Paper 4.2, screening programmes are often introduced without adequate attention to basic principles.

When drawing up practical policies for screening for the early detection of cancers, it is essential that policy makers take decisions about the use of money and other resources on a rational basis. The main elements in the development of a rational policy, as described by Chamberlain, are:

1 Policy makers should take decisions on the establishment of screening programmes in the light of a full appraisal of the balance between the benefits of the programme and its costs and disadvantages.

2 The benefit of any programme should ideally be measured by a reduction of mortality consequent upon the introduction of a screening programme. However, other interim measures can be used, such as:

- an increasing yield of the specific cancer being screened in the population with the service;
- a shift in the stage distribution of cancers detected—in other words, cancers are being found earlier;

- screen-detected cases should be found to live longer than symptomatic cases.

A number of other strategies are now accepted as ways of showing whether screening saves lives, but at all times it is important also to consider the costs and disadvantages of screening. These include the financial costs of the programmes themselves, but also some assessment of the adverse side effects of screening. This is best assessed with randomized control trials comparing unscreened groups with the screened population. Although it might theoretically be possible to weigh up the benefits of screening for any particular cancer against the disadvantages and costs, and express this in some common unit, in practice this has never been achieved. Screening programmes continue to be introduced often with little or no proof of their effectiveness or without an appreciation of their true costs or disadvantages.

In conclusion

In this chapter we have explored the education and training that health workers require at all stages in their basic education and post-qualification period. We have shown the need for an expanded target audience, all of whom need to understand more about the preventability of cancers. In this way, increasing educational activity can help to create the climate in which policy decisions can be taken positively to bring about a reduction in the future incidence of cancers.

References

EC/EORTC (1988) report: *A Curriculum in Oncology for Medical Students in Europe*, EC/EORTC, Brussels.

Buitenhuis, E. C., van der Ploeg-Aarnout, A. J., Jongsma-Ebbelink, M., Haagedoorn, E. M. L. (1989) A result of student interaction with volunteers of a reach-to-recovery group, *J. of Cancer Ed.* **14**, supp. 1.

Paper 4.1

THE ROLE OF CANCER EDUCATION

Dr. E. Milly L. Haagedoorn
Cancer Education Program Director, Groningen University Hospital, Division of Surgical Oncology, Groningen, The Netherlands

Introduction

Although cancer prevention and detection programmes are adequately prepared and executed, we are frequently confronted with the fact that public compliance with cancer-prevention and detection techniques has not achieved optimal status. Little attention has been given so far to the underlying reasons. From the educational viewpoint, there are some reasons why most current cancer-prevention and detection activities are prone to failure. These are:

- misconceptions about cancer in the community (among health care professionals as well as among the public)
- unfamiliarity with educational techniques.

The impact of misconceptions about cancer among health-care professionals

A recently published report of the European Community (EC), prepared in cooperation with the Education Branch of the European Organization for Research and Treatment of Cancer (EORTC) and with deans of several European medical schools, summarizes the outcome of several studies on undergraduate cancer education in European medical schools[1]:

Undergraduate cancer education in Europe is:

- **inadequate** in terms of lack of clear objectives, curriculum design and coordination
- widely **variable** between countries and between schools in individual countries
- **lacking** in practical clinical training with excessive reliance on formal lectures; poorly represented in examinations and rarely examined separately (at any stage of the undergraduate curriculum); lacking in teaching in important areas such as cancer screening and pain control. ...
- **discordant** in terms of what teachers consider to be important and what students actually experience.

A major potential consequence of inadequate cancer education in medical schools is the important negative impact on health care. Primary-care physicians who have not been involved during their medical-school training in adequate cancer-education programmes might never have reached their potential skills and interest in cancer care, including cancer prevention and cancer control. Also, during their medical training, medical students and residents are usually confronted with advanced cancer cases; they are seldom involved with prevention, early detection or with cured patients in the outpatient clinics[2,3]. Negative attitudes, including fatalism and cynicism about cancer care and the value of prevention and early detection, usually are the result, and are thus incorporated into the habits of practising physicians. The avoidance or abandonment of cancer patients and cancer care, often subconsciously, is the result[4]. Love and Robinson describe such pessimism among non-oncologic-trained health professionals regarding the curability of any cancer[5].

Acknowledgement

The author wishes to thank Dr. J. Oldhoff (Professor of Surgery, Division of Surgical Oncology, Groningen University Hospital) and Dr. W. Bender (Director, Centre for Medical Education Research and Development, Groningen Faculty of Medicine) for their careful reading of this paper, their corrections and advice which was gratefully received.

Since the deficiency in undergraduate cancer education in many medical schools in Europe has been identified, a pressing need is recognized to ensure that the newly qualified doctors have the necessary positive attitude toward cancer, and possess the skills and knowledge required to participate in cancer prevention, cancer control and in cancer care in general[1]. Robinson states[6]:

> The teaching of medical students is of great importance because the future generations of doctors need to know that:
>
> 1 Cancer is a curable disease depending on the site and stage at diagnosis.
> 2 Cancer can sometimes be prevented.
> 3 Early detection of cancer increases the chances of cure.
> 4 Care for patients and family can improve quality of life.
> 5 The physician has an important role in Public Cancer Education.

In a guest editorial in the *Journal of Cancer Education,* Love stresses the fact that the increasing cancer-prevention services call for modification of continuing medical education[7].

The EC/EORTC report provides guidelines for a curriculum in oncology for medical students in Europe. However, although such a curriculum in oncology does provide cancer education guidelines, such a curriculum will still be part of the curricular structure of each individual medical school. Traditional curricular structures are most frequently teaching oriented, indicating another important deficiency in traditional medical-school education.

Unfamiliarity with educational techniques

In 1973 the World Health Organization stated in an introduction to the WHO Public Health Paper no. 52, *Development of Educational Programmes for the Health Profession*:

> Until recently, medical faculties concerned themselves mainly with what is taught and little with how it is taught or what is done with the knowledge acquired.

This statement could have been written in 1989. There are changes, but they are evolving extremely slowly. During the last two decades, educational science has become more and more involved in medical education. Professional educationists are trained in the development of education programmes and in educational measuring techniques (assessment and evaluation techniques), thus opening the door to educational research in biomedicine. With the introduction of professional educationists in the teaching of health-care professionals, a new and important area in health-care education is evolving, which has led to the establishment of some Centres for Medical Education Research and Development within medical schools. However, this is not yet the common picture in Europe.

It should be realized that medical doctors are not primarily trained to be educators. The majority of medical doctors do not have qualifications in educational theory and practice; the majority of medical doctors do not have skills in education programme development and in assessment and evaluation techniques. Moreover, medical professors are seldom appointed because of their skills in teaching, but are appointed because of their skills in patient care or biomedical research. However, it is no longer acceptable that medical-education programmes are set up without the involvement of professionals in medical education, education development and education research.

Planning a cancer-education prevention plan, course or curriculum

In planning a cancer-education prevention or detection plan, we should ask ourselves the ten questions to be asked when planning any educational activity, as described by Harden[9]:

1 What are the needs in relation to the product of the education programme?
2 What are the aims and objectives?
3 What content should be included?
4 How should the content be organized?
5 What educational strategies should be adopted?

6 What teaching methods should be used?
7 How should assessment be carried out?
8 How should the details of the curriculum be communicated?
9 What educational environment or climate should be fostered?
10 How should the process be managed?

These ten questions can be used as a basis for the development of any educational activity, and for every level of target groups. Of course the setting up of a cancer-prevention course for the public is dependent on cultural and socio-economic factors, which will be different from country to country, and between different socio-geographic regions within one country[10]. Nevertheless, the ten questions can be a basis for any educational activity anywhere in the world. The detailed planning will always have to be a project that requires a team effort from within a socio-geographic region and may well have different components in different regions.

It is evident that there is no universal way to outline detailed cancer-education activities. But the general principles, based on educational strategies, should prove useful in any environment. The ten questions will be discussed including several examples of different levels of cancer education.

Question 1: What are the needs in relation to the product of the cancer-education activity?

One specific item of this first issue for cancer-prevention and detection programmes is fundamental and is nearly always forgotten. As an important part of the cancer-prevention and detection activities to be set up, we need to ascertain what the public already knows about the specific problem that we want to tackle.

A major task in cancer-prevention and detection programmes is assisting the public in modifying those behaviours which put them at risk. Biomedical knowledge may be able to target behaviours to be changed, but it fails as a guide for generating procedures to produce change[11]. Modifying human behaviours is a complex process. People protect their health according to how they understand and interpret illness threats. Their perceptions may or may not correspond with current medical knowledge. Cancer, perhaps more than any other group of disease, is prone to the interfering effects of fear, fatalism and misconceptions. Inaccurate beliefs about causation may lead to changes in life style inappropriate to cancer control. The common view that cancer, like most diseases, has an acute onset, might for example be an underlying reason why public compliance with breast-cancer screening programmes often does not meet the professionals' expectations. Hidden erroneous concepts or images of cancer within the community provide a poor basis for effective long-term risk-reduction activities[12].

Hence an important step in a specific cancer-prevention and/or detection programme must be educational research to detect erroneous ideas on the topic in the community. To get full cooperation from the community, educational research must be followed by an adequate public cancer-education activity based on correcting the erroneous ideas and providing additional relevant information. Hirschman and Leventhal emphasize that making misconceptions explicit and correcting them facilitates clear communication which lays the groundwork for instituting changes through the use of detailed action plans[11].

Question 2: What are the aims and the objectives?

Aims should describe why a specific cancer-prevention or detection programme is set up and what end result is aimed for. Any educational programme starts with writing explicit objectives for whatever population is involved. The UICC Technical Report Series, vol 44 (1979) provides good examples of writing objectives for different target groups in cancer-prevention and control programmes[4].

Educational objectives are frequently confused with teaching activities. Describing teaching activities is not the same as describing educational objectives. The latter describe in detail the things that the learner will be able to achieve and/or to do by the end of the educational programme.

Question 3:
What content should be included?

Once the decision of a subject is reached, the question of the extent or depth of coverage must be determined. For instance, in a cancer-education course for medical students, it is not enough to tell them that smoking is bad for the health of their patients and the community. The content of such a cancer-education course improves when the course provides the students, for example, with action plans on how to help their patients in smoking cessation[13].

Question 4:
How should the content be organized?

Once the content components are determined, it must be decided how the different subjects will be grouped and in what order. In the case of a cooperative cancer-education action, it should also be decided which teachers of what disciplines should be responsible for covering specific topics (physician? nurse? behavioural scientist? educationist? dentist? clergy?).

Question 5:
What educational strategies should be adopted?

For cancer-prevention plans there are several options.

1 Public education with action plans for the whole nation.
2 Small groups, for example classroom teaching about cancer for young children.
3 Action plans for educating high-risk groups.
4 Individual education (learner centred): for example, a physician or a nurse teaching a woman breast self-examination during physician/patient or nurse/patient contacts in the medical office (or in a screening clinic). The primary care physician (including physicians working for insurance companies, physicians in the workplace setting, physicians in the army/navy/airforce, and dentists) in the ambulatory setting is an important link in delivering the necessary education for cancer-prevention and control procedures to large segments of the population[14].
5 The education can be problem solving or information gathering. Problem solving aims for the learner to acquire knowledge and skills through tackling problems: for instance, teaching young women breast self-examination, and teaching men testicular self-examination. Within information-gathering education, the emphasis is on the presentation of the information.

Question 6:
What teaching methods should be used?

This issue presents two decision areas. Firstly, learner grouping (nationwide); smaller groups with learner/teacher interactions; individual (patient/physician or patient/nurse contacts). Secondly, the use of teaching tools (printed text, audio-visual materials, models). The choice of teaching tools is important. As Harden describes:

> The educational value of a method is dependent as much on how the method is used as on the choice of the method. A good audio-visual programme is almost always better than a bad lecture, and vice versa.

The choice of the method should reflect:

- the course aims and objectives
- the availability of local facilities
- staff experience with a chosen technique.

Question 7:
How should assessment be carried out?

This is the field where the professional medical educationist has a task. It is a very difficult area in which physicians are not usually trained. Newble and Cannon state that the quality of many assessment and evaluation procedures set up by physicians leaves much to be desired because medical teachers most frequently do not measure what is supposed to be measured[15]. In medical education research, as in other biomedical research areas, measuring instruments are used. A sound measuring instrument is valid (it measures what it is supposed to measure) and it is reliable (it produces consistent results).

Gallagher and co-workers demonstrate how

difficult the area of medical-education measuring techniques is in 'Evaluating the cancer education program: examining a range of approaches'[16]. Commonly found deficiencies in programme evaluation in cancer education are described, and several strategies for avoiding and overcoming these deficiencies are discussed.

Harden concentrates in 'Approaches to research in medical education' on answering the question of what research in medical education actually is, and what it can offer[17]. Different possible approaches to research in this field are discussed.

Question 8: How should the details of a specific cancer-prevention and/or detection plan be communicated?

Two target groups are to be addressed.

Firstly, details of the plan have to be communicated to the staff responsible for teaching. This should be left to the discretion of local officers. Methods of communication are, for example, the presentation of the aims and objectives, or by means of syllabi with a timetable.

Secondly, we must not forget that the details of the plan must also be communicated to the public. To set up a good cancer-prevention and detection programme the public must become partner in the prevention activities. This can only be accomplished when people feel personally involved; hence the necessity for adequate comprehension of cancer risks, prevention and detection measures, and knowledge of the possibilities of cure.

Question 9: What educational environment or climate should be fostered?

The climate of the educational environment is very important and should not be underestimated. It may have profound effects on the outcome of the education plan. For instance, launching a cancer-prevention plan from within a cancer hospital might frighten people away, whereas launching the plan from within a 'neutral' setting might serve to encourage people to participate.

Question 10: How should the process be managed?

In educational management it must be clear who is responsible for planning, and who is responsible for implementation and monitoring. Educational management is the field of the professional educationist.

Summary

It has been identified that cancer education in European medical schools is inadequate and insufficient. Recently a directive for a curriculum in oncology for undergraduate medical education has been published by the EC/EORTC.

Medical education is not the same as (traditional) medical teaching. Professional educationists are trained in programme development and in educational research strategies. The setting up of an education programme follows educational theory and practice lines. Professional educationists should be involved in setting up cancer-education (prevention and detection) plans.

Educational approaches for prevention and detection programmes will be inadequate and will perhaps fail if the social beliefs and institutions of the target groups are not understood.

The public must become partner in cancer-prevention and detection activities and this can be achieved by means of adequate education on risks, prevention and detection measures, and on the possibilities of cure.

References

1 EC/EORTC (1988) *A Curriculum in Oncology for Medical Students in Europe,* Brussels.

2 Bakemeier, R. F. *et al.* (1981) *Cancer education survey: final report, Cancer Education in US Medical Schools,* vol. 6. DHHS publ. no. 81-2260. National Institute of Health, Bethesda, Maryland.

3 Haagedoorn, E. L. (1985) Aspects of cancer education for professionals, thesis, Groningen.

4 Hill, D. J., Heffernan, M. W., Rice, D. I. (eds.) (1979) *Involving Doctors in Health Education about Cancer*, UICC Technical Report Series, vol 44, Geneva.

5 Love, R. R. and Robinson, E. (1988) Educational objectives for a cancer control course for Israeli medical students, *J. of Cancer Ed.* 3, **2**, 109–110.

6 Robinson, E. (1988) Teaching oncology to medical students in Israel, *J. of Cancer Ed.* 3, **2**, 107–108.

7 Love, R. R. (1988) Increasing cancer prevention services calls for modification of continuing medical education, *J. of Cancer Ed.* 3, **2**, 71–73.

8 WHO Public Health Paper no. 52 (1973) Development of Educational Programmes for the Health Profession, World Health Organization, Geneva.

9 Harden, R. M. (1986) Ten questions to ask when planning a course or curriculum, *Med. Educ.* **20**, 356–365.

10 Fink, D. J. and Sheehan, H. E. (1988) Cancer prevention and detection: an overview of variables influencing adoption and practice, *Cancer* **61**, 2391–2395.

11 Hirschman, R. S. and Leventhal, H. (1983) The behavioural science of cancer prevention, in S. B. Kahn *et al.* (eds.) *Concepts in Cancer Medicine*, Grune and Stratton Inc., New York.

12 Sternburg, J. K. (1983) Identification and management of risk factors for cancer, in S. B. Kahn *et al.* (eds.) *Concepts in Cancer Medicine*, Grune and Stratton Inc., New York.

13 Gritz, E. R. (1988) Cigarette Smoking: the need for action by health professionals, *Cancer Journal for Clinicians* **38** 4, 194–212.

14 Williams, P. A. and Williams, M. (1988) Barriers and incentives for primary care physicians in cancer prevention and detection, *Cancer* **61**, 2383–2390.

15 Newble, D. and Cannon, R. (1983) *A Handbook for Clinical Teachers*, MIT Press Ltd, England.

16 Gallagher, R. E. *et al.* (1986) Evaluating the cancer education program: examining a range of approaches, *J. of Cancer Ed.* 1, **3** 141–151.

17 Harden, R. M. (1986) Approaches to research in medical education, *Med. Educ.* **20**, 522–531.

Paper 4.2

PRACTICAL POLICIES FOR SCREENING FOR EARLY DETECTION OF CANCERS

Professor Jocelyn Chamberlain
Cancer Screening Evaluation Unit, Institute of Cancer Research, Sutton, Surrey, England

Introduction

The purpose of screening for early detection of cancer is to interrupt the natural history of development of a cancer, and thereby to prevent it from progressing to a more advanced stage and ultimately to death. As a means of cancer control, screening is a third-best solution. The ideal is primary prevention (for example, avoidance of cigarette smoking, immunization against hepatitis B) and second best is an effective treatment to cure all cases (for example, treatment of testicular cancer). It is only where these alternatives are not available (sadly, this applies to most of the common cancers in the western world) that screening may be applicable.

The principal reasons for suggesting that screening falls short of an ideal method of control are two. Firstly, it implies subjecting very large numbers of well people to a medical procedure which, for the vast majority, will not do them any good, and may do them some harm. Secondly, because the growth rates of most cancers are variable, it is unlikely that screening can favourably influence all cases. At one end of the growth rate distribution, the cancer may be progressing so quickly that it has already metastasized before being detectable by screening, while at the other extreme, the cancer may be so slow-growing that it would still be curable even if left undetected until it gave rise to symptoms. Hence early detection by screening can only alter the prognosis for cancers with growth rates between these two extremes.

A further relevant point in considering the natural history of presymptomatic cancer is that various degrees of cellular abnormality can often be identified histologically, with an apparent progression from mild to moderate to severe dysplasia, to carcinoma-in-situ, to frankly invasive cancer. In screening for cancers of several sites, it is found that many more people are identified with the earlier abnormalities than one would expect to progress to invasive cancer, which leads us to the implication that many of these early abnormalities are not progressive.

Tests, such as the cervical smear, which can identify these very early changes, have the advantage that they can arrest a tumour before it becomes invasive, and hence not only reduce mortality, but also a great amount of morbidity. Against this must be set the disadvantage that they overdiagnose many people with non-progressive lesions. Overdiagnosis applies not only to pre-invasive disease; it can also be a problem with the invasive stage of some cancers. For example, one study of screening for neuroblastoma in infancy[1] reported a yield of 20 cases per 1000 screened, twice the expected cumulative life-time incidence of this tumour.

In considering practical policies for screening, it is important that health authorities should strike a balance between the benefits of a particular screening programme, and its costs and disadvantages. The principal benefit is, of course, a reduction in the number of people who die from the cancer, although other benefits can also be identified, such as a reduction in the number of patients requiring radical treatment, a reduction in the costs of any treatment necessary, and, for screened subjects who are found negative, reassurance that they do not have cancer.

On the costs side of the balance, the principal factors to be evaluated are the excess physical and psychological morbidity caused to people with false positive results needing diagnostic work-up, the similar morbidity to patients over-diagnosed as having early cancer, the financial and resource costs of the whole programme, and any hazards that are attendant upon the screening test itself.

Evaluation of benefits and costs

Measurement of a reduction in mortality consequent upon a screening programme is a daunting task requiring study of very large numbers of subjects over several years. Nevertheless, it cannot be too strongly emphasized that screening should not be introduced as a service until the results of such research are available.

In the following discussion of different stages in the measurement of the benefit of screening, it is assumed that any research studies maintain the highest available standards of population participation, test sensitivity, and the other factors influencing the quality of the programme discussed in the section on quality assurance of screening services below.

There are three interim measures of the impact of screening which can be assessed on relatively small numbers, relatively soon after the introduction of a screening programme. All of these are necessary measures but on their own they are insufficient to prove that screening is actually saving lives.

The first is the yield of cancer detected. On first screening a population, if the test is reasonably sensitive, it will detect a higher prevalence of cancer than the expected incidence of cancer in that population. For example, mammographic screening for breast cancer in women aged 45 to 64 can be expected to find five cancers per 1000 women screened[2], whereas the expected annual incidence, from cancer registry data, is only about 1.6 per 1000. This suggests (but does not prove) that screening is detecting cancers that would not otherwise present with symptoms for two to three years. In subsequent screening rounds, the yield of cancer should fall back to approximately the expected incidence level, but the cancers should all be at an earlier stage.

A shift in the stage distribution is the second measure of the impact of screening. Current studies of colorectal cancer screening[3], for example, show that the proportion of Dukes' Stage A cancers found at screening is over 50%, whereas in a similar unscreened population, it is only 10%. This clearly shows that the test (faecal occult blood) is able to detect cancer at an early stage.

The third of these interim ways of evaluating screening is a comparison of survival of screen-detected cases with symptomatic cases. It has been shown, for example, that the five-year survival of lung cancers found by screening is 40%[4], very much better than the 5% five-year survival of cases presenting symptomatically. Because such survival comparisons are the usual method of evaluating therapeutic procedures, it is often assumed that longer survival proves the value of screening. There are a number of reasons why such an assumption is invalid.

Firstly, survival is measured from the time of diagnosis, and screening automatically advances the date of diagnosis by a time interval known as the lead time. Therefore, even if the date of death were not altered, a patient with screen-detected cancer would have lived longer after diagnosis than a similar patient whose cancer was not diagnosed until it became symptomatic.

Secondly, the case-mix of presymptomatic cancers found at screening is likely to contain a disproportionate number of slow-growing cases because fast-growing cancers go through the phase when they are detectable but presymptomatic too rapidly for all to be detected by screening unless the latter were repeated very frequently. Hence screen-detected cases are biased towards more benign tumours with longer survival. Overdiagnosis of non-progressive disease clearly introduces an extreme form of the same bias.

Finally, as with most preventive services, the people who participate in screening programmes tend to be better educated and more health-aware than those who do not participate; this implies that, even if screening were not available, participants would notice and seek help for their symptoms at an early stage and hence have a better prognosis than non-participants. This selection of good-prognosis cases into the screened group is clearly seen in recent studies of breast-cancer screening in which mortality from breast cancer in non-participants is 1.5 to twice that of an unscreened control group[2].

If yield, stage and survival are insufficient to prove that screening saves lives, how can this question be answered? A number of research strategies have been devised, all of which share the common principal that they compare the risk of dying from the cancer concerned in a population for whom screening has been available and in a similar unscreened population. Inevitably, it will take several years after introduction of screening for its effect on population mortality to become apparent, and the size of population required to demonstrate a reduction in a relatively small risk is always large[5]. These constraints of having to include a large population, who have been screened for a long time, serve to explain our present inadequate knowledge of the effect of screening for many cancers.

Retrospective studies of the effectiveness of screening have been done in two ways. The first is by comparing trends in mortality between similar populations with and without screening programmes over a period starting before introduction of the screening programme and continuing for several years thereafter. This method has been successfully used to demonstrate the effectiveness of cervical screening in several Scandinavian countries[6,7].

Another retrospective method which is being used increasingly is the case-control study. Cases are people who have died of cancer which was diagnosed after introduction of the screening programme; controls are age-matched living people from the same population. The screening history up to the date of diagnosis of the case is noted for both cases and controls. From this, it is possible to draw up a table showing numbers of cases and controls screened and unscreened, and thereby to derive an estimate of the chance of a screened person dying, relative to that of an unscreened person. This odds ratio shows the relative protection conferred by screening; it is free from lead-time bias of slow-growing tumours which affect survival comparisons, but retains the selection bias of including more good-prognosis cases in the screened group. Hence, case-control studies tend to overestimate the effectiveness of screening. They are, however, very useful for comparing the effects of different screening policies, such as variations in the age group screened or the frequency of screening[8].

In general, prospective studies, despite their size and duration, are preferable for the initial evaluation of a screening programme. Ideally, they should be designed as randomized controlled trials in which a defined population is randomly allocated to a study group which is provided with screening, and a control group which is not. In both groups, all cancers diagnosed after the start of the trial are noted, regardless of whether they are diagnosed by screening or by symptomatic presentation. All deaths among these cancers are also recorded over a period of several years, and this enables a valid comparison of cumulative mortality rates between the study group and the control group.

The study group deaths include those among non-participants in screening, and hence may underestimate the reduction in risk which screening may confer on an individual person; nevertheless, the results of such a comparison clearly show what the likely public health impact of population screening will be. The classic example of research of this sort is the trial of breast-cancer screening in the Health Insurance Plan of Greater New York[9], but subsequently similar randomized controlled trials have been set up in order to evaluate other cancer-screening programmes.

Another form of prospective evaluation is a non-randomized comparison between areas providing or not providing screening[10]. Although much less satisfactory in their statistical validity, such trials may be all that is practical for evaluating early-detection programmes, such as that for melanoma, which depend upon public education campaigns.

Measurement of the disadvantages and costs of screening can be partly derived from routine recording of the screening and diagnostic follow-up process, but may also require *ad hoc* studies, for example to investigate anxiety induced by the programme, or to investigate its financial costs. It is best to assess the adverse side-effects of screening within a randomized controlled trial in order that the prevalence of these effects in an unscreened control group can also be determined.

Without knowledge of, for example, the number of benign biopsies in the control group, the extent of excess biopsies resulting from false positive results of screening cannot be measured. Moreover, the only way of measuring the extent of overdiagnosis is by comparing the cumulative life-time incidence of the cancer in the population offered screening, with that in an unscreened population. It may be more reliable to conduct such a comparison in a controlled trial, rather than relying on routine cancer registration data to be representative of an unscreened population.

In an ideal situation (never so far achieved in practice) the benefit of screening for a cancer should be weighed against its disadvantages and costs expressed in some common unit. This would give policy makers an explicit valuation of the screening programme in terms of cost units per year of life gained. This would enable them to decide how much, if any, investment to put into it.

In the case of cervical-cancer screening, the first programme to be widely implemented, no evidence on either benefits or costs was available, and programmes were introduced mainly because both public and profession thought that it must be a good thing. Doubt about its efficacy remained for many years, leading to low levels of participation, which then further compounded the problem of evaluation.

More recently, breast-cancer screening is being introduced in a more controlled form based on the knowledge of potential benefits and costs derived from controlled trials; however, the precise level of both benefit and cost varies from programme to programme, which emphasizes the need for each new programme to be carefully monitored. Despite the experience of cervical-cancer screening programmes being inefficiently introduced without evaluation, various other cancer-screening programmes are being provided as a service with no proof that they are effective and little or no idea of their costs.

Present evidence on benefits of screening for cancers of different sites

Table 4.1 summarizes the present evidence. From this it is apparent that screening programmes for cancer of all these sites have succeeded in meeting the first three criteria for evaluation, but that, for most of them, there is still no confirmatory evidence that screening saves lives.

The case of lung-cancer screening provides a salutary warning. Although fulfilling the first three criteria, screening by chest X ray and sputum cytology, even when repeated as frequently as four-monthly, has failed to reduce mortality. One randomized controlled trial in England[11], a second in the United States with a seven-year follow-up[12], and a case-control study in East Germany[13] have all found that the risk of dying of lung cancer is no different between screened and unscreened groups. What appears to be happening is that screening is detecting relatively slow-growing cancers which would not lead to death within the ensuing seven to ten years; but is failing to detect the fast-growing cancers which arise as 'interval cases' in the interval after a negative screen and before the next routine screen is due, and which rapidly prove fatal.

Cervix

It is now clear from numerous retrospective studies, that cytological screening of cervical smears can reduce both the incidence of invasive cervical cancer and mortality from it. Scandinavian studies have shown how trends in both incidence of[6] and mortality from[7] cervical cancer have fallen in countries without such programmes. Several case-control studies have

Table 4.1 Summary of present evidence on the benefit of screening for cancer of various sites

	Necessary but Insufficient Evidence			Sufficient Evidence			
				Reduction in mortality shown by			
	Increased yield at Ist screen	Shift to earlier stage-distribution	Better survival of screen-detected cancers	Comparison of mortality trend	Case-control study	Prospective geographical comparison	Randomized controlled trial
Lung	Yes	Yes	Yes	Not done	No benefit	Not done	No benefit
Cervix	Yes	Yes	Yes	Yes	Yes	Not done	Not done
Breast	Yes	Yes	Yes	Not done	Yes	Yes	Yes (2/3 trials show benefit)
Colorectal	Yes	Yes	Yes	Not done	In progress	Not done	In progress
Stomach	Yes	Yes	Yes	Yes	Yes	Not done	Not done
Bladder	Yes	Yes	Yes	Not done	Not done	Not done	Not done
Melanoma	Yes	Yes	Yes	Not done	Not done	Not done	Not done
Neuroblastoma	Yes	Yes	Yes	Not done	Not done	Not done	Not done
Ovary	Yes	Yes	Not yet done	Not done	Not done	Not done	In progress

shown consistently that the risks of developing invasive cancer are reduced in women who have been screened, compared to those unscreened, and that these differences persist even when adjusted for differences in aetiological factors between screened and unscreened groups[14].

The situation regarding evaluation is not static, however, since an underlying trend towards increasing incidence of disease in recent generations, possibly associated with sexually transmitted viral infections, has led many gynaecologists and cytopathologists to lower their criteria for distinguishing positive smears from normals, and to recommend intervention by colposcopy for women with minimal cellular abnormalities. Further research is needed to provide evidence on the costs and benefits of using different cut-off points of degree of dyskaryosis to intervene.

Breast

There has been more evaluative research on screening for breast cancer than for any other cancer site. Three randomized controlled trials have so far been published[15,16,17], and several others are still in progress. There have also been three case-control studies[18,19,20], a prospective geographical comparison[2] and a similar comparison of observed and expected mortality rates in an uncontrolled study[21].

The first two of the randomized trials, with follow-ups of respectively 18 years and nine years, have shown mortality reductions of around 30% in the population offered screening, with the reduction persisting, albeit reduced to about 23%, right up to 18 years from entry. The third randomized trial showed no mortality reduction up to nine years, although a small, statistically insignificant reduction in the tenth year. All three case-control studies showed a 50% to 65% reduction in the risk of dying in screened women compared to unscreened. The two non-randomized prospective comparisons showed mortality reductions of around 20% after six to seven years of follow-up.

On balance, therefore, the evidence points to the fact that screening can detect a proportion of breast cancers sufficiently early to alter their otherwise fatal progress. Several of the prospective trials have also shown that the unwanted side-effects of screening can, with high-quality diagnostic procedures, be kept to a minimum.

One important aspect of breast-cancer screening requiring further education is its effectiveness among women screened under the age of 50. All of the studies mentioned above have shown a mortality reduction in women aged 50 or over when first screened, but there has been a consistent failure to demonstrate the same for women aged under 50 during the first years of follow-up. With longer follow-up the New York HIP study has shown a reduction in deaths among women aged 40 to 49 at entry, although the younger the woman, the longer it took for the reduction to appear, and at no time has it reached a level of statistical significance.

Because the numbers of deaths among young women is so low, a very large sample size is required in order to give the trial sufficient power to demonstrate a significant reduction. None of the studies carried out so far has included enough women under 50. Another contributing factor is the lower sensitivity of screening in pre-menopausal women, implying that screening needs to be repeated among young women more often than it does among those over 50[22].

Colorectal cancer

This cancer is very common in Western countries, but mortality rates have remained more or less constant over the past few decades. There is therefore great interest in screening to determine if detection and removal of presymptomatic (Dukes Stage A) cancers could result in a greater proportion of cures. Moreover, there is much circumstantial evidence that many cancers are preceded by dysplastic adenomatous polyps. Identification and removal of these might therefore be expected to reduce subsequent cancer incidence.

Various research studies have shown that screening meets the first three criteria of increased yield, altered stage distribution and improved survival, but none has so far shown a mortality reduction. Randomized controlled studies are currently in progress in the US[23], Sweden[24], Denmark[25] and the UK[3], and a case-control study (personal communication) is in progress in the Federal Republic of Germany, where faecal occult blood screening has been widely used for many years.

The results of the various evaluation studies can be expected to emerge within the next five to seven years. Those wishing to set up service screening programmes would be well advised to defer decisions until there is evidence from these trials on the benefits and costs.

Stomach cancer

Screening for stomach cancer has been widely used in Japan, where this cancer is very common. As with cervical cancer, no prospective evaluation has been done. Despite many years of experience, there is still doubt about the contribution of screening to falling mortality rates. Retrospective comparisons of mortality trends between intensively screened and less intensively screened populations show an improvement in the well screened group. A case-control study has similarly shown benefit. However, screening has been taken up selectively by well educated people of high socio-economic groups who, over recent years, have also adopted a more Western diet, and whose incidence of stomach cancer has been rapidly declining. It is still unclear how much of the fall in stomach-cancer mortality can be attributed to falling incidence, and how much can be attributed to screening[26].

Bladder

Screening for bladder cancer by urinary cytology has been applied to high-risk groups, such as those exposed to industrial carcinogens, or to chronic schistosomiasis infection. Although fulfilling the first three criteria for evaluating screening, there has so far been no research on the effect of screening on mortality[27].

Melanoma

Early detection of melanoma by self-examination is widely encouraged, and intensive education programmes to achieve this end have resulted in a large proportion of early-stage melanomas presenting to dermatologists[28]. The incidence rates of melanoma have recently been increasing in many parts of the world, particularly where fair-skinned people have had greater exposure to sunlight. Mortality rates have also been increasing, more so in men than in women.

So far the main suggestion of the impact which early detection may have on mortality from melanoma comes from Queensland in Australia. Although the incidence trend there continues to rise, mortality has levelled off, implying that more cases are now being cured than formerly[29]. Another small study from the US has shown that the incidence of advanced stage melanoma has fallen following an education campaign for early detection.

Neuroblastoma

This is the only childhood tumour for which screening has been applied. Studies in Japan have shown that testing six-month-old infants by measurement of vanillyl mandelic acid (VMA) in urine has resulted in detection of early-stage neuroblastoma with good survival. The intention of screening is that a single test will detect all cases which would not otherwise present until later in childhood; in general, the older the child at diagnosis, the worse the prognosis. So far, however, no evidence has been presented to show that the incidence of neuroblastoma at older ages, nor the mortality, have been reduced as a result of screening.

Ovary

Screening for ovarian cancer by ultrasound, or by serum levels of a monoclonal antibody, CA 125, have shown that it is possible to detect ovarian cancer at an early stage, although at the price of a large number of false positive results. A feasibility study for a randomized controlled trial is just starting in the U.K.

From the foregoing brief review of the current evidence on benefits of cancer screening, it is apparent that there are only two sites—breast and cervix—for which screening services can at present be justified. For lung cancer, screening is almost certainly not worthwhile. Further research is required for all remaining sites, and it is therefore incumbent on health authorities considering implementation of screening programmes for these other cancers that they do so only in a way which will permit evaluation of their effects, preferably using a randomized controlled trial design.

Quality assurance of screening services

Whether provided as a service, or as part of a research project, there are various aspects of a screening programme which need to be monitored in order to maximize the benefits and minimize the costs of screening. The principal factors influencing the size of benefit achieved are as follows: participation in screening by the target population, efficient follow-up of all abnormals; and adequate treatment of all cancers detected. The principal factors influencing cost are as follows: resource cost of the screening test; safety of the screening test; ambience of the screening and diagnostic follow-up process.

Participation

It should always be clear, both to the public and to health professionals, exactly which groups of people the screening programme is intended for. In practice, age and sex are the only two risk factors used to define the target population. Many breast-cancer screening programmes, for instance, are limited to women aged over 50 because of the current lack of evidence showing the effectiveness in women screened below this age; whereas for cervical-cancer screening, it is usual to include all women from 20 years up to 65 to 70.

The best method of achieving high participation by the target population is unquestionably personal invitations to be screened, preferably coming from the individual's GP, and preferably accompanied by a specific appointment to attend (where relevant). As well as obtaining high participation, a personal invitation system has the additional advantages that it allows the screening workload to be controlled, and allows non-participants to be identified so that further personalized efforts to recruit them can be made. A system for inviting each person is dependent upon a population register and this is not available in every country.

In the absence of a register and invitation system, measures to ensure high participation include education of relevant doctors to take opportunities for either doing the screening test themselves (for example, cervical smears) or referring eligible people to a screening clinic (for example, mammography); provision of well advertised screening clinics (for example, mobile clinics visiting workplaces); and media advertising. Efforts to educate the public in the value of screening should be based on research findings on the beliefs, attitudes and health behaviour of the target population, particularly focusing on the reasons why people are reluctant to be screened. Sample surveys of the target population show that screening tests based on self-examination rates are lower.

Sensitivity of the screening test

A completely sensitive test is one which will pick up 100 per cent of the cancers (or precancers) present in the screened population—i.e. a test which gives no false negative results. There are problems in defining false negatives to cancer screening but, by convention, they are taken to be synonymous with cancers presenting symptomatically after a negative screen—so called 'interval cases' because they are diagnosed in the intervals between screens.

One way of measuring sensitivity is to express the number of screen-detected cases as a proportion of the sum of screen-detected cases and interval cases. A preferable measure, that is only feasible if the expected incidence of the cancer in the absence of screening is known, is to express sensitivity as the proportion of the expected incidence which does not present as interval cases (E - I/E where E is the expected incidence and I is the incidence of interval cases). This shows the proportion of cancers that are expected to arise in the next year (or two years, etc.), whose diagnosis has been advanced by screening.

In order that a screening programme can monitor its sensitivity, it is important that it has a system for finding out about all interval cancers diagnosed in the screened population. This can be achieved by regular matching of the screened population against new cancer cases diagnosed in all histopathology laboratories serving the catchment population, and/or against the local cancer registry. The principal means of maintaining high sensitivity is to ensure that all screening staff engaged in taking tests and in interpreting them are adequately trained and regularly receive feedback on their performance, as well as ensuring that all equipment passes regular quality control tests.

Sensitivity can be improved by lowering the cut-off point for distinguishing negative cases from positive cases requiring diagnostic work-up. Indeed, fear of false negative results underlies the current shift in cervical-cancer screening towards referring cellular abnormalities showing only mild dyskaryosis, or even only evidence of human papilloma virus infection, for investigation by colposcopy. Altering cut-off levels in this way inevitably decreases specificity, and therefore requires an explicit decision on whether the marginal gain in sensitivity achieved justifies the extra costs.

Specificity of the screening test

A test which is completely specific correctly classifies all people without neoplasia as negative—that is, it gives no false positive results. Specificity is measured by the proportion of negative results among all people without neoplasia. Another commonly used indicator of the problem of false positive results is the predictive value of a positive test—that is, the proportion of all positive tests which are true positives.

False positives are a cost to the people concerned in terms of the unnecessary anxiety they cause and, if invasive procedures such as biopsy are required to establish that cancer is not present, physical morbidity as well.

Screening programmes should therefore be organized to keep the level of positive results at as low a level as is compatible while maintaining reasonable sensitivity. For programmes such as mammography screening for breast cancer, some authorities recommend a back-up 'second-stage screening' clinic to sort out women requiring biopsy from those who do not, without referral to hospital.

Frequency

The frequency with which routine re-screening should be repeated depends upon the distribution of growth rates of the tumour concerned. Obviously, the more often screening is repeated, the less likely the occurrence of interval cases, but one gets progressively diminishing returns in cancer yield from shortening the interval between screenings. For example, in populations with a Western-Europe-type incidence of invasive cervical cancer, it has been shown that screening once every ten years would halve the expected incidence of invasive cancer; every five years would reduce the expected incidence by 84%; every three years by 91%, and every year by 93%[8].

Efficient follow-up of people with abnormal test results

It seems self-evident that screening cannot succeed unless action is taken to diagnose and treat all abnormalities uncovered. Nevertheless, failure to follow up milder degrees of abnormality has been shown to be an important reason why some screened women go on to develop invasive cervical cancer[30].

Screening programmes can largely overcome this problem if a fail-safe warning is built into the record system so that, if confirmation of diagnosis or continuing follow-up is not received within a defined time after an abnormal test result, an alert is raised and the person who performed the screening test is made responsible for contacting the screened subject.

Adequate treatment of screen-detected cases

Similarly, all neoplasia found at screening should be appropriately treated. This is not usually any problem, although there may still be a need to compare the long-term results of alternative treatment strategies for very early disease. For example, it is not yet known whether adjuvant radiotherapy or endocrine therapy is required in addition to surgery for minimal breast cancer. The long-term effectiveness of laser eradication of cervical intraepithelial neoplasia, compared to other forms of cautery or surgery, is likewise unknown. Ideally these uncertainties should be resolved by randomized controlled trials.

Cost of the screening test

Not surprisingly, the principal component of the resources required for a population-screening programme is the cost of the test itself. In calculating the cost, it is important to include all the clerical costs of recruiting subjects into the screening programme, as well as the professional staff costs of performing the test and interpreting its result. So far, automated interpretation has not proved feasible for cancer screening, although if biochemical tests such as VMA analysis for neuroblastoma, or CA 125 for ovarian cancer, are shown to be valuable, autoanalysis may help to reduce costs.

Throughput of subjects being screened

The unit cost per person screened can be minimized by ensuring that both staff and equipment are used to their fullest capacity. Another means of reducing cost is to screen for more than one condition at the same attendance at the screening clinic, so that some administrative costs, and personal costs to the subject, are shared between screening for different conditions.

Safety of the test

A test which in itself carries any substantial risk of morbidity is obviously unsuitable for application to symptomless people. Of tests used for early detection of cancer, the greatest concern expressed has been about the radiation hazard of mammography. However, with the radiation doses used in film-screen combinations of current mammography practice, the risk of inducing breast cancer by radiation is orders of magnitude less than the chances of reducing mortality. Other potentially dangerous tests which may be used for screening include flexible sigmoidoscopy for colorectal cancer, and barous meal X ray for stomach cancer. Since the benefits of screening for these conditions are still unknown, it is not possible to compare risk and benefit.

Anxiety

Cancer screening in itself may provoke anxiety. To minimize this adverse effect, screening should be organized so as to emphasize that it is examining well people, not patients. Prompt notification of results also helps to minimize anxiety. Anxiety is inevitable among people with positive screening results and, since many of these will be false positives, it is important to keep this unnecessary anxiety as low as possible. Provision of nurses, trained in all aspects of the programme and with counselling skills, may be useful.

Ongoing evaluation

The information gained from evaluative studies provides a useful starting point for drawing up a practical policy for screening, and also suggests certain minimum targets which should be met, for example on participation rates, sensitivity and specificity. A well organized, preferably computerized record system is an invaluable aid to managers of screening programmes, not only for servicing administrative and clinical aspects, but also for ongoing routine statistical monitoring, with feedback to all those providing the service. The record system should include a means of reliably capturing data on all cancers diagnosed among the target population (whether detected by screening or diagnosed as internal cases or as non-attenders), and all deaths among patients whose cancer was diagnosed after the start of the programme.

The achievements and the costs of the programme can thus be monitored (aided by *ad hoc* sample surveys for some aspects), and possible improvements in the screening service can be evaluated. In assessing the impact of changes in screening policy, it is important to assess the marginal costs and benefits of the proposed change. Theoretical calculations, for example, suggest that in the United Kingdom, a change from five-yearly to three-yearly screening for cervical cancer would cost an additional £183 000 for each case of invasive cancer prevented, and changing from three-yearly to annual screening would cost £11 000 000 per extra case prevented[31]. These calculations could more usefully be expressed as costs per extra year of life gained, adjusted also for changes in the quality of life, but the requisite data are not available.

Expressing the balance between the benefits and costs of screening programmes in such a way enables policy-makers to make informed decisions, initially on whether or not to start a cancer-screening programme, and subsequently on changes that can be made to improve its efficiency. Moreover, the value of resources expended on the screening programme can also be compared with their value for alternative purposes.

References

1 Sawada, T., Kawakatu, H. and Sugimoto, T. (1987) Screening for neuroblastoma, *Lancet* **2**, 1204.

2 UK Trial of Early Detection of Breast Cancer Group (1988) First results on mortality reduction in the UK trial of early detection of breast cancer, *Lancet* **2**, 411–416.

3 Hardcastle, J. D., Armitage, N. C., Chamberlain, J., Amar, S. S., James, P. D. and Balfour, T. (1986). Faecal occult blood screening for colorectal cancer in the general population, *Cancer* **58**, 397–403.

4 Fontana, R. S., Sanderson, D. R., Taylor, W. F., Woolner, L. B., Miller, W. E., Muhm, J. R. and Uhlenhopp, M. A. (1984) Early lung cancer detection: results of the initial (prevalence) radiologic and cytologic screening in the Mayo Clinic Study, *Am. Rev. Respir. Dis.* **130**, 561–565.

5 Moss, S. M., Draper, G. J., Hardcastle, J. D. and Chamberlain, J.(1987), Calculation of sample size in trials of screening for early diagnosis of disease, *Int. J. Epidemiol.* **16**, 104–110.

6 Hakama, M. (1982) Trends in the Incidence of Cervical Cancer in the Nordic Countries, in *Trends in Cancer Incidence, Causes and Practical Implications*, K. Magnus (ed.) 279–292, Hemisphere Publishing Corporation, Washington, D.C..

7 Laara, E., Day, N. and Hakama, M. (1987) Trends in mortality from cervical cancer in the Nordic countries, associated with organized screening programmes, *Lancet* **1**, 1247–1249.

8 Day, N. E. (1986) The Epidemiological Basis for Evaluating Different Screening Policies, in *Screening for Cancer of the Uterine Cervix*, M. Hakama, A. E. Miller and

N. E. Day, 199–209, IARC Scientific publ. no. 76, International Agency for Research on Cancer, Lyon.

9 Shapiro, S.(1984), Strax, P. and Venet, L. (1966) Evaluation of periodic breast cancer screening with mammography, J. Am. Med. Ass. **195**, 731–738.

10 UK Trial of Early Detection of Breast Cancer Group (1981) Trial of Early Detection of Breast Cancer: Description of Method, *Brit. J. Cancer* **44**, 618–627.

11 Brett, G. Z. (1969) Earlier diagnosis and survival in lung cancer, *Brit. Med. J.* **4**, 260–262.

12 Fontana, R. S., Early Detection of Lung Cancer: The Mayo Lung Project, in *Screening for Cancer* P. C. Prorok and A. B. Miller (eds.), UICC Technical Report Series no. 78, 107–122.

13 Ebeling, K. and Nischan, P. (1987) Screening for lung cancer: results from a case-control study, *Int. J. Cancer* **40**, 141–144.

14 Berrino, F., Gatta, G., d'Alto, M., Crosignani, P. and Riboli, E. (1986) Efficacy of Screening in Preventing Invasive Cervical Cancer: a Case-Control Study in Milan, Italy, in *Screening for Cancer of the Uterine Cervix*, M. Hakama, A. E. Miller, and N. E. Day (eds.), 111–123, IARC Scientific publ. no. 76, International Agency for Research on Cancer, Lyon.

15 Shapiro, S., Venet, W., Strax, P. and Venet, L. (1988) *Periodic Screening for Breast Cancer*, The Johns Hopkins University Press, Baltimore.

16 Tabar, L., Gad, A., Holmberg, L. H., Ljungquist, U., Fagerberg, C. J. G., Baldetorp, L., Gröntoft, O., Lundström, B., Manson, J. C., Eklund, G., Day, N. E. and Petterson, F. (1985) Reduction in mortality from breast cancer after mass screening with mammography, *Lancet* **1**, 829–832.

17 Andersson, I., Aspegren, K., Janzon, L., Landberg, T., Lindholm, K, Linell, F., Ljungberg, O., Ranstam, J. and Sigfusson, B. (1988) Mammographic screening and mortality from breast cancer: the Malmö mammographic screening trial, *Brit. Med. J.* **297**, 943–948.

18 Verbeek, A. L. M., Hendriks, J. H. C. L., Holland, R., Mravunac, M., Sturmans, F. and Day, N. E. (1984) Reduction of breast cancer mortality through mass screening with modern mammography, *Lancet* **1**, 1222–1224.

19 Collette, H. J. A., Day, N. E., Rombach, J. J. and de Waard, F. (1984) Evaluation of screening for breast cancer in a non-randomised study (the DOM project) by means of a case-control study, *Lancet* **1**, 1224–1226.

20 Palli, D., Rosselli del Turco, M., Buiatti, E., Carli, S., Ciatto, S., Toscani, L. and Maltoni, G. (1986) A case-control study of the efficacy of a non-randomised breast cancer screening program in Florence, Italy, *Int. J. Cancer* **38**, 501–504.

21 Morrison, A. S., Brisson, J., Khalid, N. (1988) Breast Cancer Incidence and Mortality in the Breast Cancer Demonstration Project, *J. natl. Cancer Inst.* **80**, 1540–1547.

22 Tabar, L., Fagerberg, G., Day, N. E. and Holmberg, L. (1987) What is the optimum interval between mammographic screening examinations?, *Brit. J. Cancer* **55**, 547–551.

23 Mandel, J. S., Bond, J., Snover, D., Williams, S., Bradley, M., Walker, C., Schumann, L. M. and Gilbertsen, V. (1988) The University of Minnesota's Colon Cancer Control Study, in *Screening for Gastrointestinal Cancer*, J. Chamberlain, and A. B. Miller (eds.), 17–24, Hans Huber Publishers, Toronto, Canada.

24 Kewenter, J., Bjork, S., Haglind, E., Smith, L., Svanvik, J. and Ahren, C. (1988) Screening and Rescreening for Colorectal Cancer, *Cancer* **62**, 645–651.

25 Kronborg, O., Fenger, C., Sodergaard, O., Pedersen, K. M. and Olsen, J. (1987) Initial mass screening for colorectal cancer with fecal occult blood test, *Scand. J. Gastroenterol.* **22**, 677–686.

26 Oshima, A. (1988) Screening for Stomach Cancer: The Japanese Program, in *Screening for Gastrointestinal Cancer* J. Chamberlain and A. B. Miller (eds.) 65–70, Hans Huber Publishers, Toronto, Canada.

27 Prorok, P., Chamberlain, J., Day, N. E., Hakama, M. and Miller, A. B. (1984) UICC Workshop on the Evaluation of Screening Programmes for Cancer, *Int. J. Cancer* **34**, 1–4.

28 Mackie, R. M., Elwood, J. M., Hawk, J. L. M. (1987) Links between exposure to ultraviolet radiation and skin cancer, *J. Roy. Coll. Phys.* **21**, 91–96.

29 Holman, C. D. J., James, I. R., Gattey, P. H. and Armstrong, B. K. (1980) An analysis of trends in mortality from malignant melanoma of the skin in Australia, *Int. J. Cancer* **26**, 703–709.

30 Ellman, R. and Chamberlain, J. (1984) Improving the effectiveness of cervical cancer screening, *J. Roy. Coll. Gen. Practit.* **34**, 537–542.

31 Smith, A. and Chamberlain, J. (1987) Managing cervical screening, *Information Technology in Health Care* **4**, B.2.7.8, 02–12.

Chapter 5

EDUCATING BUSINESSES ABOUT CANCER PREVENTION

Summary

Businesses have received too little attention from agencies whose aim is to reduce the risks of cancers. Many businesses have the power to influence cancer rates, either directly, through the safety of the product and the workplace or by promoting harmful products such as tobacco, or indirectly, by manipulating or restricting the purchasing choices that customers make.

Attention must be focused on the relationship between businesses and governments so that positive pressure is exerted through education, pricing, taxation, subsidies, provision and regulation policies to ensure that the healthier choices for businesses are also profitable choices. The relationship between businesses and their customers should also be considered and, where necessary, policies should be enacted to ensure that healthier products are available, people can afford them and they are fairly advertised.

Introduction

The discussion and the conclusions that follow are the result of a very lively and committed working group 'brainstorming' about how best to influence businesses, in what directions and with what strategies. The wider impact of businesses on health is an area that few health professionals and educators have studied in depth and little has been written on the subject. The working group were, therefore, taking an important step in thinking about businesses and cancer prevention in a systematic and innovative way. In order to focus the discussion more sharply, part of the time was spent on working through two case studies chosen by members of the group: the food business and the tobacco business.

Which businesses do we want most to influence?

Several groups of businesses were identified:

1 businesses whose manufacturing process generates or uses carcinogens in a manner that is hazardous to the workforce and possibly also to the local community.

2 businesses whose workplace increases the risk of cancers developing among workers because the environment itself is unhealthy in particular ways; for example, workers may be exposed to tobacco smoke for long periods, or required to remain sedentary, or have an inadequate choice of nutrition available to them in workplace restaurants.

3 businesses whose product is known to be directly carcinogenic to a significant proportion of its consumers; the most important example is the **tobacco business**, but the **alcohol business** could also be cited.

4 businesses whose product is known to be associated with certain health risks or health benefits for the consumer, which probably include changes to the risk for certain cancers. The **food business** in all its many forms belongs to this category.

5 businesses who provide a service (rather than a consumer product) that directly or indirectly affects the risk of developing a cancer. For example, direct risks may be incurred by users of the **transport business** and the

leisure business (for example, in cinemas and restaurants) from exposure to tobacco smoke. Risks may be influenced indirectly by the **media business** through the advertising of products; the promotion of certain sorts of life style in commercials, plays and films; and the manner in which health-related news is reported (or ignored). Cancer risks may also be influenced by the **insurance business**, through the differential pricing of policies and benefits for individuals who make certain choices in their life style—for example, not to smoke or not to become obese.

Selecting strategic targets

It is unrealistic to expect to approach *every* business with an influence on cancer prevention. Therefore *strategic targets* must be selected. In order to select wisely, we must first ask *who* makes the choices for us about what we can buy or what we are provided with and then consider *where* those choices are made for us. Using these questions as our framework, the working group identified the following as the two most important groups of strategic targets:

- major **multinational corporations** who manufacture many diversified products with an impact on health. Examples include: the tobacco companies; the alcohol companies; the large manufacturers of processed cereals and breads (for example, Kelloggs, Sofrapain); the agri-chemical business, who influence what farmers can grow with the help of fertilizers and pesticides.

- major **consumer businesses** who can, by their purchasing power, influence the availability and quality of products for the whole population. Examples include: supragovernmental organizations such as the EC, who influence the choices made by primary growers of agricultural products, such as grain, tobacco, butter and beef, and who 'consume' surpluses by buying them at favourable rates; government departments who purchase raw and processed foodstuffs for consumption by millions of people throughout Europe in the canteens and restaurants of government offices, in schools, hospitals, prisons and the armed forces; major supermarket chains, who choose which products to stock on their shelves; and national chains of 'fast-food' outlets (e.g. Macdonalds).

The aim should be to make *gradual* changes to the availability and composition of products at a *national* level. The greatest impact on health will be made by small changes in the consumption of common products, rather than in the provision of a few healthier alternatives that reach only a small section of the population.

Educational strategies: getting the message across to businesses

Four 'Golden Rules' should be kept in mind when designing strategies to raise the health-consciousness of selected businesses:

1 Effective educational strategies cannot be designed by health professionals and educators unless we know much more about how the chosen businesses function; detailed 'insider knowledge' is required.

2 The scientific evidence with which we attempt to convince businesses of the need for change must be very good indeed, or our educational messages will not be believed.

3 Cancer prevention is only one goal in a much wider set of aims to improve health in Europe; the managers of businesses do not have time to absorb separate messages about cancers, heart disease, etc. and we must therefore construct integrated health messages.

4 Never underestimate the power of businesses to defend their own interests.

Intervention at strategic levels

Businesses should not be seen as separate entities—they interact with each other in complex ways. Therefore, the entire production process from raw materials to the sale of the final product must be examined to see if there are *strategic levels* within this process that are particularly amenable to change. For example, one business might be most influenced by the availability or price of its raw materials, so the strategic level at which influence could be exerted most productively would be the grower or supplier of raw materials. The strategic levels identified by the working group were:

- supply of raw materials;
- research and development;
- processing;
- packaging;
- distribution;
- advertising;
- sales.

Identification of the most effective strategic level at which to exert positive pressure for change could result in individual businesses making a significant contribution to reducing cancer risks. The contribution might take various forms, for example, by:

- reducing exposure of the workforce to occupational carcinogens;
- making the workplace healthier through anti-smoking policies and the provision of healthier working practices and healthy food in on-site restaurants;
- purchasing healthy ingredients from suppliers of raw materials;
- manufacturing a safe and healthy product;
- delivery systems that ensure the product can be sold in a safe condition;
- marketing and labelling policies that inform the customer truthfully and clearly about the contents of the product;
- pricing policies that bring healthier products within the purchasing power of most people;
- offering a choice of healthier products so that the customer does not have to sacrifice variety for health.

Educating the strategic gatekeepers

At each level of each business there are key individuals who hold particular power in their organization, either through their position in the hierarchy or through their personal qualities and influence. These are the **strategic gatekeepers** who have the greatest ability to change the ways in which the business is run. We must attempt to identify these gatekeepers and to make personal contact with them. In order to influence them most effectively, we must identify who from among the ranks of health promoters is the person (or pressure group) that is most likely to succeed.

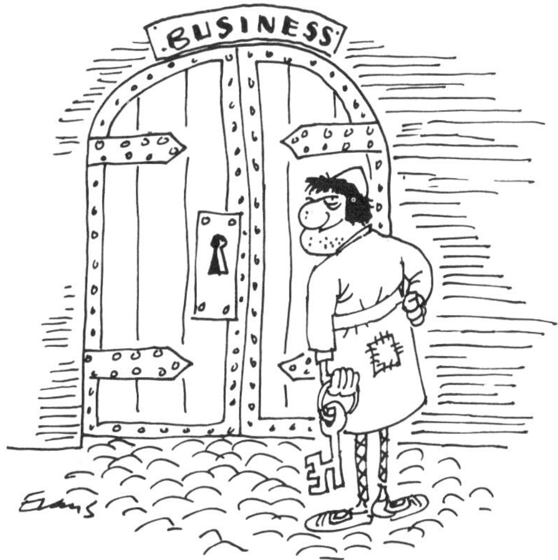

IDENTIFY THE 'STRATEGIC GATEKEEPER'...

The choice of who approaches the strategic gatekeepers of business will depend on many things. Within each country, the choice may be limited by certain cultural expectations, for example, that doctors are the most (the only?) respected advocates for health issues. There may be certain 'experts' who have received sufficient media exposure in their own country to ensure that their views will carry weight in the business world. Alternatively, the most productive educator might be someone with similar skills to those of the strategic gatekeeper: for example, a fellow-scientist; an expert in using the media; a senior academic who has managerial responsibilities; or an active member of a Trade Union in one of the health professions.

Trades Unions and local workers committees are often powerful strategic gatekeepers. They were given particular attention by the working group, who recognized the potential power of organized labour to initiate and maintain constructive changes in the businesses that employ their members. Traditionally, Trades Unions have concentrated their attention on eliminating direct hazards in the workplace, including occupational carcinogens. This role remains an extremely important one.

However, Trades Unions have generally been slow to seize opportunities to improve the health of their members in other ways. Indeed, they have often opposed the introduction of anti-smoking policies. Trades Union representatives and negotiators are strategic gatekeepers who could, with effectively designed education and assistance, influence both the quality of the *working environment* for their members and the quality of the *product* for their customers. Part of the educational message to Trades Unions should focus on the immediate local benefits to be gained from becoming involved in wider health issues, for example, a healthier workforce with lower rates of sickness absence.

Product diversification

Where possible, workers must be reassured that their jobs are not jeopardized by switching the output of their business to healthier products, and management must be convinced that there are adequate profits to be made from marketing them. (The recent huge success of low alcohol beers and wines in the UK was cited as an example of the healthier product making even greater profits than the products that it replaced.) However, the working group recognized that there is far more potential for product diversification in (say) the food industry than within the tobacco industry. All tobacco products are dangerous to health, so there is no scope for switching to a 'healthy' cigarette. Tobacco companies have diversified into other business interests, for example, the insurance industry, but this does not safeguard the livelihoods of tobacco growers nor the livelihoods of those employed in the manufacture and sales of tobacco.

The food business: a case study

The working group chose to look more closely at the food business so that specific issues could be more readily discussed and understood within the framework of a concrete example. The choice was shaped primarily by the extent to which epidemiological research has revealed an association between diet and certain cancers. Conservative estimates associate about one-third of preventable cancers with diet (see Doll, Keynote Address) and in certain countries the estimate may rise as high as 50 per cent (Doll and Peto, 1981). A second reason for choosing the food business as a case study was the level of controversy and debate that exists about the precise components of the diet that either promote cancers or protect against them. The working group were not seeking an easy task.

A major advantage of making the food business a prime target for education about cancer prevention is that we can approach the strategic gatekeepers with two very positive messages:

1 Production of healthier foodstuffs need not cause a significant upheaval in the day-to-day running of the business. Health experts have the necessary knowledge to assist individual companies in developing healthier but attractive and profitable alternatives to existing products; existing manufacturing processes can often be adapted to new products and the same workforce can be retained.

2 The components of a healthy diet that will reduce the risks of cancers are, as far as we know at present, the same as those recommended to reduce the risks of

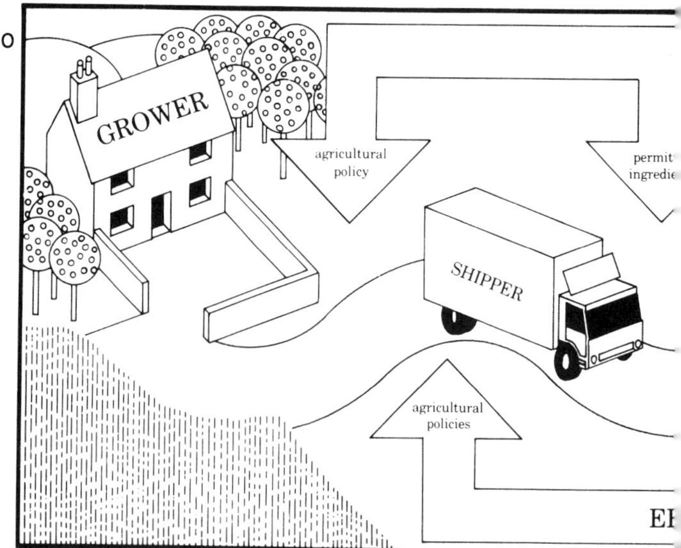

cardiovascular disease, certain non-malignant diseases of the gut (diverticular disease, ulcerative colitis) and maturity-onset diabetes. Thus, changes to the nutritional composition of certain widely consumed products or prepared meals (e.g. in workplace canteens) can be expected to have a significant impact on local or even national morbidity and mortality. The food business and its shareholders could find this an attractive image to promote.

Certain key areas of the food business merit special attention (see Figure 5.1). They are: marketing strategies and accessibility of the product; pricing strategies; labelling policies; provision of raw materials and new technology; influencing the bulk-buyers; government and supragovernmental intervention to improve national diets; and evaluation of outcome. The working group considered each of these important areas.

Marketing strategies and accessibility

In certain product areas, there has been a tangible measure of financial success for businesses in marketing higher-fibre, lower-fat products and products with reduced or absent preservatives, artificial colouring and flavours. (The working group commented that a reduction in the use of preservatives may actually *increase* the risk of gut cancers by increasing the content of carcinogen-forming moulds in food.) Many of these products are widely available and bear recognized 'big-brand names' (e.g. Walls low-fat sausages; Kelloggs All Bran; Flora polyunsaturated margarine).

However, there is still a general tendency for healthier products to be advertised, distributed and priced in ways that direct sales to the more affluent sections of the population. These products are frequently unavailable in small local shops where people on lower incomes are often forced to buy their food; supermarkets may choose not to stock them, preferring to stick to the tried and tested profitable brands. Supermarkets are increasingly moving to the outskirts of towns, where land is cheaper, but they (and their healthier products) are then only accessible to customers who can afford a car. Supermarkets that do stock so-called 'health foods' have a tendency to hide them away in a small specialized section and then they become hard to locate in the vast halls. Furthermore, advertising may serve to promote the image of healthier brands in ways that will appeal to more affluent customers and will discourage those on lower incomes.

Figure 5.1 Intervention is possible at many points along the food production chain.

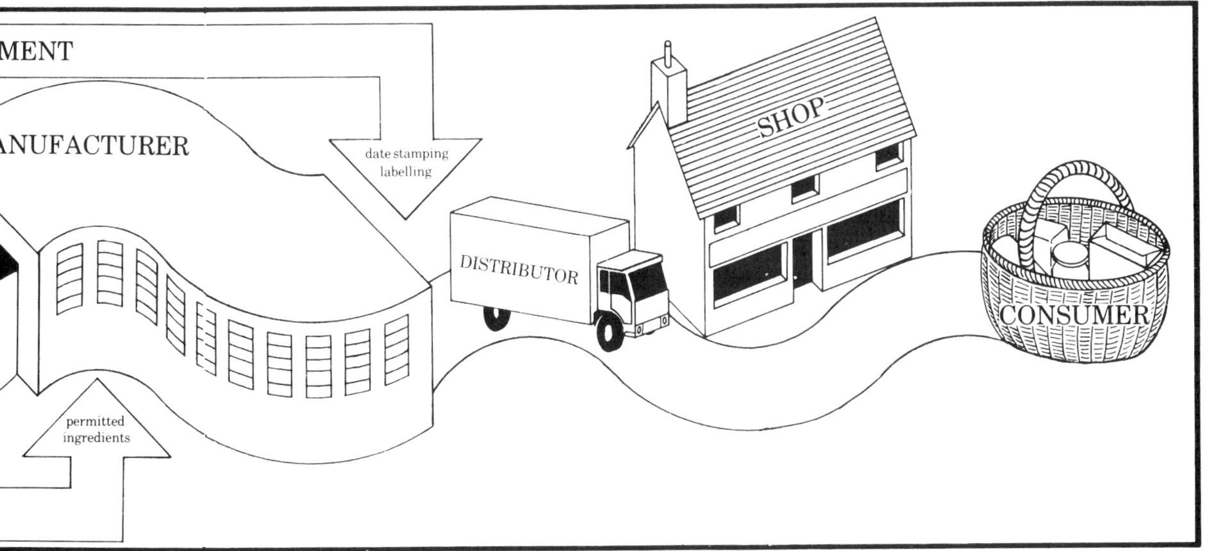

All these elements combine to reinforce the dependency of the least affluent members of society on the very products that are most likely to damage their health. Businesses must be persuaded to make healthier products more attractive and accessible to a wider range of shopkeepers and a wider range of customers.

Pricing strategies

The accessibility of healthier products is strongly influenced by price. Businesses could choose to subsidize the price of healthier products during the initial period of marketing when sales are low. A price subsidy could even continue if the production costs of the healthier product remain higher than its less healthy rivals. However, businesses are not famous for their altruism. It is more likely that pressure to promote a better diet for the population as a whole will come from pricing strategies that are reinforced at a government or supragovernmental level. Subsidies to growers could be altered in favour of (say) lower-fat meat or dairy produce, or higher-fibre cereals. Price support for these products would encourage their purchase, especially by those on lower incomes.

Labelling policies and the need for consistency

Businesses must be educated about the need for a fair and consistent labelling policy. The increasing level of trade between member states of the European Community (which will rise even faster after trade barriers are abolished in 1992) is a strong argument in favour of standardized food labelling. This is an issue that must be tackled at government and EC level; businesses cannot be expected to agree a policy amongst themselves.

The working group identified two major problems that will have to be overcome before an agreed European policy on food labelling can be enacted. First, the experts are still not in agreement about the health risks associated with certain foods or dietary additives such as salt, vitamins, etc. Second, the meaning attached to certain terms is culture-specific; 'fats' may mean hard fats such as butter in one country and olive oil in another. Despite these problems, the effort should be made.

Terms such as 'high fibre' or 'low fat' are meaningless unless the customer knows:

- the precise composition of the fat or fibre;
- the absolute content in grams;
- the recommended safe levels of consumption.

However, we cannot expect the general public to become experts in dietetics. What is required is a labelling system for certain agreed nutritional components, such as fibre and fats, that will enable customers to see at a glance whether the product conforms to certain standards (see Figure 5.2). The messages on current labels tend either to be misleadingly bland, or are so technical that they are useless to the general public.

Labelling issues are not simply confined to what is printed on packaging; the labelling of shelves in shops and supermarkets, and the 'emotional labels' attached to products by the advertising media must also be considered.

Moreover, health experts must put their own house in order! The labels that we attach to certain foods in the health advice that we issue to the general public is sometimes misleading or ambiguous. Three examples were cited from the European Code Against Cancer:

- **Moderate your consumption of alcoholic drinks.** The usefulness of this advice is compromised by the absence of any guidance about safe limits for individuals.

- **Frequently eat fresh fruits and vegetables.** The emphasis on 'fresh' produce may be unnecessary and counterproductive. Increasing the total intake of fruits and vegetables—whether fresh, frozen or tinned—would be beneficial in the diet of many sections of the population, particularly those on lower incomes in urban environments. Fresh produce may be unavailable or too expensive. It may also contain concealed hazards not found in frozen or tinned equivalents. Examples of concealed hazards are pollutants from fungicides and other agri-chemicals used to keep the produce 'fresh', or the fall-out from

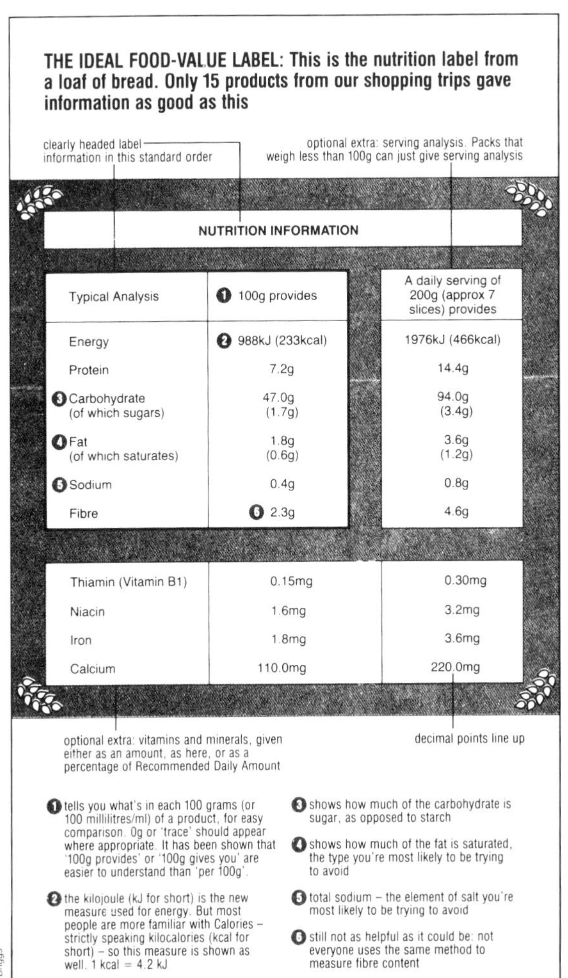

Typical Analysis	(1) 100g provides	A daily serving of 200g (approx 7 slices) provides
Energy	(2) 988kJ (233kcal)	1976kJ (466kcal)
Protein	7.2g	14.4g
(3) Carbohydrate (of which sugars)	47.0g (1.7g)	94.0g (3.4g)
(4) Fat (of which saturates)	1.8g (0.6g)	3.6g (1.2g)
(5) Sodium	0.4g	0.8g
Fibre	(6) 2.3g	4.6g
Thiamin (Vitamin B1)	0.15mg	0.30mg
Niacin	1.6mg	3.2mg
Iron	1.8mg	3.6mg
Calcium	110.0mg	220.0mg

Figure 5.2 This label for packaged bread has several good points but may still appear too technical for some customers.

atmospheric pollution (traffic fumes, industrial waste, radioactive particles), which is more likely to contaminate fresh foods during distribution, storage and in open storefronts.

- **Limit your intake of fatty foods.** This advice suffers from the lack of detail about safe limits and, perhaps more importantly, from the lack of specificity in the composition of the fat. There is no evidence that the intake of olive oil should be limited, and there is clear evidence that polyunsaturated oils and fats are significantly less harmful to health in general than are the hard fats. The link between cancers and dietary fats (as opposed to obesity) has been called into question by several epidemiological studies, although the association with cardiovascular disease is accepted.

Provision of raw materials and new technology

If product diversification is to take place, then the food business will need supplies of new raw materials (e.g. higher-fibre cereals). The scientific and technical community can help in several ways, all of which require funding support either from governments or from the business community itself. Important contributions could be made by:

- giving research priority to the development of new strains of 'healthier' crops and livestock that will thrive in existing agricultural conditions;
- developing new, safe agricultural chemicals to increase the yields of healthier crops;
- developing new feedstuffs for livestock, which produce lower fat carcasses and dairy products;
- developing technology that will assist the conversion of existing factories and machinery to the manufacture of the new products, and for the processing of new products.

Influencing the bulk-buyers

This is a vitally important part of the overall strategy to provide Europeans with a better quality diet. If government departments, the major multinationals, supermarkets and fast-food chains could be persuaded to tender for bulk purchases of foodstuffs on the basis of *health* as well as *price*, then the availability of a healthier diet for the whole population will increase. Such a change in policy would have a direct effect on the quality of food delivered to government employees, schoolchildren, hospital patients, the armed forces, prisoners, etc; and on the individual customers buying from major retailers.

But the *indirect* effects are likely to be even more profound. The choice of raw materials purchased by these bulk-buyers has enormous influence on what primary producers can afford to grow, and hence on the composition of their entire agricultural output. If, for example, high-fat or low-fibre raw materials became much less profitable because the bulk-buyers withdrew their purchasing power, then those raw materials would decline in production. They could be substantially replaced by more profitable, healthier alternatives with a knock-on effect across the whole spectrum of the food business.

Government and supragovernmental intervention to improve national diets

The foregoing discussions point clearly to the need for government funding and legislation to assist in altering the composition of European diets. Although the details will vary from country to country, governments and supragovernmental agencies can assist the reduction of diet-related cancers in many ways. The working group identified several examples:

- funding research into the interaction of nutrition and health, the development of new strains of crops and livestock, and new agri-chemicals;

- collaborating with the scientific and medical community to establish dietary standards and thresholds of safe consumption and promoting public knowledge of these standards;

- regulating government purchasing and processing of foodstuffs to the agreed standards; improving the quality of government-funded catering would have a major impact on diet-related diseases, including certain cancers;

- developing a fiscal policy that includes health promotion as a primary goal; such a policy would use various financial instruments such as taxation, subsidies and price support to ensure that healthier choices become available to the grower, the manufacturer and the customer;

- developing and enforcing consistent and understandable labelling policies—on food products, on the shelves and in advertising;

- acting as a watchdog over advertising to ensure that the old unhealthy products are not sold in disguise;

- acting as a watchdog over exporters in order to ensure that the old unhealthy products are not being dumped abroad. The Third World countries are particularly vulnerable to this form of exploitation.

Evaluation of outcomes

The outcomes of implementing any part of the above strategies must be properly evaluated. There are several dimensions to evaluation in both the short and longer term:

- Sales statistics and profit margins on healthier new products must be collected by the health promotion community (as well as by the business concerned). These data will represent an important tool in persuading rival companies to change.

- Trends in key indicators of health must be monitored carefully in association with changes in diet. Evaluation should not rely on national data alone; the diets of individuals must be monitored over long periods.

- The composition of existing products must be monitored for changes, both in terms of healthier ingredients and to ensure that new hazards do not creep in!

- The effects on employment in all parts of the food chain must be evaluated. Governments and businesses will not support policies that result in avoidable job losses.

- The effects of product alteration must be evaluated outside the chosen industry, particularly among the small processors (i.e. if the large businesses take all the 'good' food, what happens to the 'left-overs'?)

- Indirect adverse consequences for health must be monitored; for example, new production processes may result in an increase in environmental pollution or in the use of fossil fuels.

- Food policy changes in the EC must be monitored for their effects on other economies, especially in the Third World, both in terms of the import of raw materials and the export of processed foodstuffs.

The tobacco business: a brief consideration

Several of the arguments and issues raised in the foregoing discussion on the food business apply to the tobacco business and will not be repeated here. However, there are certain fundamental differences that must be addressed if any impact is to be made on tobacco consumption in EC member states. The most critical difference is encapsulated in the view that very little can be achieved with the collaboration of the tobacco business itself. As a consequence, reliance on government intervention will be commensurately greater than in the food business.

However, the case is undeniable that reducing tobacco consumption will substantially reduce the incidence of the most important causes of morbidity and mortality in the European population. There is no room for equivocation—the experts are in agreement.

In brief, the strategies that could be adopted to reduce tobacco consumption are:

- Regulate sales through direct legislation, with special emphasis on legislation to protect the young purchaser; penalties for breaches of the law should be prohibitive and rigorously enforced; sales in hospitals should be banned altogether (see the discussion of the 'healthy health service' in Chapter 4).

- Regulate advertising, both direct and indirect (for example, through sports promotion, on clothing, the packaging of other products in facsimiles of tobacco packages, etc).

- Regulate price by manipulating taxation.

- Regulate tar content and consider creating a price advantage for lower-tar brands in the form of reduced taxation.

- Regulate the sales, advertising, price, etc. of smokeless tobacco. There is a real danger that the tobacco business will attempt to increase consumption to compensate for falling demand (in some countries) for smoking tobacco.

- Regulate the size of health warnings on tobacco packages; warnings should appear on the front of the package and be as large as the brand name and logo.

- Encourage the adoption of anti-smoking policies in public buildings, on public transport and in workplaces. It is up to the health promotion experts to educate and get the message across; we already have examples of good practice that we can draw on and successes to publicize.

- Provide appropriate help for smokers who want to quit.

- Increase the level of education about the dangers of smoking, especially in schools.

- Consider alternative products and uses of land for those people whose livelihood depends on tobacco.

- Monitor the export of European tobacco products to other countries. We have a responsibility not to export our ill-health, but the signs are that new markets in the Third World are being exploited.

- Collect all available data about smoking-related deaths. The example was cited of the State of Oregon in the USA, which has recently introduced legislation requiring medical practitioners to record on death certificates whether or not smoking was a contributory cause of death.

- Encourage each other as experts in the field of cancer prevention to take a more active role in demanding progress in reducing the incidence of smoking-related deaths. The evidence has been available for many years, yet progress has been slow in some areas and non-existent in others.

Conclusion

Businesses of many kinds could make a contribution to the overall aim of the European Commission to reduce deaths from cancers by 15 per cent by the year 2000. They are unlikely to make the necessary changes without pressure being exerted on them from three major directions:

- from above, through supragovernment and government legislation and the manipulation of fiscal policy;
- from below, through the choices of product bought by consumers at all levels of spending power;
- from inside the business itself, through workers at all levels in the industry as well as the strategic gatekeepers who have been persuaded by our educational efforts that a safer product from a safer workplace is in the interests of all.

Reference

Doll, R. and Peto, R. (1981) The causes of cancer: quantitative estimates of avoidable risks of cancer in the United States today, *J. natl. Cancer Inst.* **66**, 1191–1308.

Chapter 6

THE ROLE OF GOVERNMENTS AND SUPRAGOVERNMENTAL ORGANIZATIONS

Summary

The policies and actions of governments set the agenda and create the climate in which all other work concerned with the prevention of cancers takes place. The policies of all branches of government have a bearing on health issues, not just the health ministries themselves. For this reason, multisectoral activities are especially important.

Specific government activity is required in the following ways:

- improved registration and statistics on cancers;
- setting an example as employers and controllers of public places;
- control over harmful products and processes;
- positive use of taxation and fiscal policies to promote healthy options;
- development and financing of screening policies;
- research policy development;
- improved health-service finance and the development of preventive activities;
- international and inter-governmental coordination of activities;
- control over the export of carcinogenic hazards and products, in particular to Third World countries.

Paper 6.1: *Cancer Prevention and the European Community* David Sweet

Paper 6.2: *Developing Effective Policy for the Prevention of Cancers* Dr. Hans H. Storm and Dr. Ole M. Jensen

Paper 6.3: *Policies for Reducing Smoking-Related Cancers* Michael Wood

Paper 6.4: *International Union Against Cancer (UICC) Programme on Smoking and Cancer* Professor Michael Kunze

The role of governments

At the Lisbon Colloquium, one group met to discuss the role of governments and supra-governmental organizations in preventive action to reduce the death rate from cancer throughout Europe. This chapter represents a report of their discussions and the discussion papers that were provided for all participants before the Colloquium.

Governments, through their direct and indirect actions and policies, help to create the setting in which all other activities are undertaken to bring about a reduction in the rates of cancers. Thus, participants at all the other levels in the movement to prevent cancers perform their activities in a climate which is to some extent determined and controlled by government policy and action.

This does not necessarily mean that activity at governmental level is the most important part of the work to prevent cancers, but that all the people involved in the struggle to prevent cancers at whatever level they are active should be aware of the ways in which government activity provides the general social, political and economic setting in which their activities take place. People who are actively engaged in activities to prevent cancers need to learn the ways in which their governments and policy makers go about their tasks and thus to find ways in which to influence their decision-making. This education is a two-way process; cancer-prevention workers need to be educated in some detail about the ways in which policies are determined, and at the same time they need to provide education for the policy makers on the facts and details about a variety of cancers and the ways in which they can be prevented.

We must bear in mind that all governments are subject to a variety of other pressures that may tend to work against health-related targets. It will not be just the health lobby that is attempting to put across their message. Often very powerful pressure groups will be similarly engaged in attempting to produce policies that maintain the status quo, or to actively promote their own interests, which may not necessarily be formulated to produce a positive health effect. Examples of this can readily be found in the ways in which governments determine the tax on tobacco products. It can also be assumed that in most instances the powerful pressure groups, perhaps representing commercial interests, will have made considerable efforts to understand the process of government decision-making and may be prepared to spend enormous resources to educate, or influence, those decision-makers within government.

Governments often seem to develop a very short-term view of their role, and develop policies which seem immediately attractive to the people they rely on for votes in the near future. These short-term measures, which may be superficially attractive and prevent upset and disturbance in a political sense, can often be identified as being neutral or negative to the health of the people. The emphasis on short-term solutions and immediate political expediency is a significant barrier to the types of long-term planning and policy development that is essential in relation to health goals regarding cancer prevention. Positive policies that could bring about reductions in the incidence of cancers may not be popular, and may be politically difficult to implement.

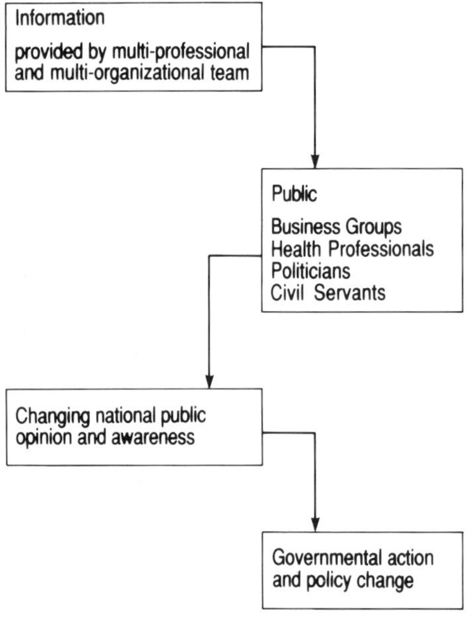

Figure 6.1 Achieving governmental action

It is important to recognize that many different ministries will be involved in the determination of the policies that may ultimately affect the levels of health in any particular state. It is important not to simply focus on the Ministry of Health when attempting to introduce health-related policy changes. In fact, the Health Ministries may have a comparatively minor role to play in bringing about the changes that would ultimately affect the cancer levels in any particular population.

Later in this section, we will look at examples where other Ministries' policies will be affected, for example the Finance Ministry, when attempting changes to fiscal policy to favour healthy behaviour, or the Ministry of Agriculture when attempting to bring about particular changes in food production and distribution. The role of the Ministry of Education will naturally be crucial when discussing ways in which early education of school pupils should be encouraged to put across health-related messages and actively change the knowledge and attitude levels within any population regarding the prevention of disease.

It can be seen that health-related policies need to be an important component of all policy making throughout the spectrum of government ministries, and that the planning for positive health can not be left as the sole concern of any single Ministry. Indeed, the lack of a coordinating approach throughout all ministries in government was identified by the Colloquium as a significant problem in all European countries and a major constraint to the development of effective preventive activity.

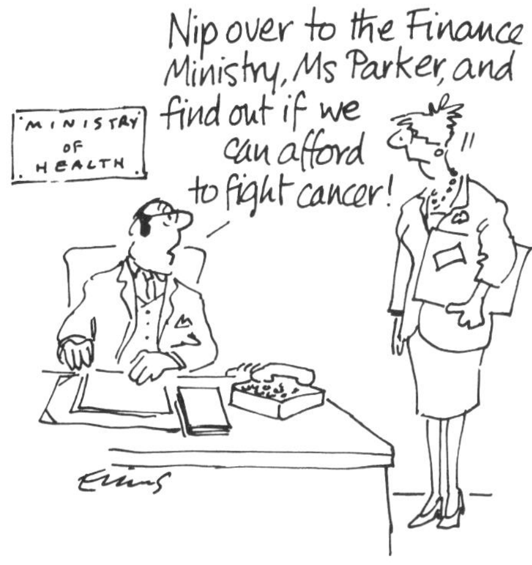

Supragovernmental organizations

The group at the Colloquium also thought that it is increasingly important to recognize the role of supragovernmental organizations in the determination of policies that might affect health levels within any given country. In the European context, this obviously means that an understanding is necessary of the way in which the Commission of the European Communities works. In Paper 6.1, David Sweet describes the ways in which the European Commission works on a number of programmes and projects which are designed to bring about the reduction of death from cancers throughout the countries of the European Community. He also outlines ways in which an understanding of the structure and function of the various departments (directorates) of the Commission can be used to influence decisions, such that policies which bring about positive health results can be implemented across the board.

What should governments be persuaded to do?

1 Improved cancer registration and statistics

Good statistics about the incidence and mortality from all cancers are a vital foundation of any programme of cancer prevention. In Paper 6.2, Hans Storm and Ole Jensen discuss the pressing need for improved statistics to be collected by specialized cancer registries. Basic data on cancer incidence and mortality is needed both for uncovering the causes of human cancers and to monitor and evaluate the effects of any preventive measures that are implemented. In their paper, Storm and Jensen claim that only Denmark and the United Kingdom have adequate population-based cancer registration, and, using figures taken from other published work, demonstrate that only one-third of the entire population of the European Community member states is covered by adequate cancer registration.

The establishment of specialized cancer registries should be one of the first stages in any government's policy on cancer prevention.

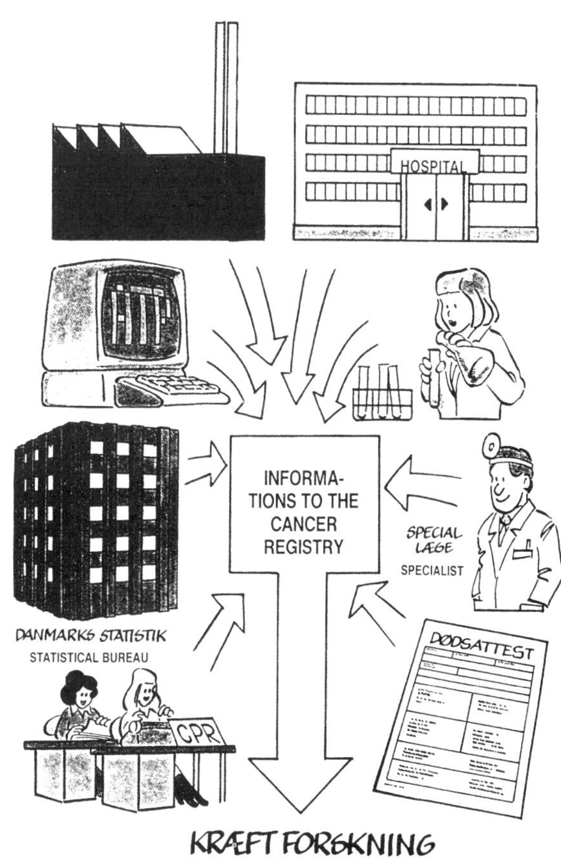

from the Danish Cancer Society Annual Report 1987

This will allow for the effectiveness of all the other policies to be gauged. The actual systems used to establish registration should also be compatible with those in use in other countries so that comparative work between countries can also be undertaken.

The way in which statistics about cancers are used by governments is also of vital importance. The information collected should be used to inform members of the general public about the current state of knowledge regarding cancer prevention and should be presented to them in a relevant and accessible form. The statistics are also important for policy makers at all levels and they should be prepared and disseminated in a form that is both useful and accessible to all those involved.

2 Setting an example

Governments are major employers and are responsible for large numbers of public buildings and places open to members of the general public. For this reason, it is important that where governments are directly responsible for the facilities, positive health policies are enforced, and that these are made explicit. For example, non-smoking policies should be enforced in all ministry buildings and healthy fresh food should be readily available in all government-controlled eating places. The educational value of this type of exercise is enormous and visibly demonstrates the importance that is attached to the health messages that are promoted in more traditional health-education campaigns.

In the same way, it can be shown that where prominent individuals in government, or high levels of decision-making in other spheres, disregard health messages, this can seriously undermine work done elsewhere in the service. General practitioners, and nurses, are perhaps the key role models as far as the general public is concerned. They must be seen to model the behaviour they hope to encourage their patients to adopt. It is therefore particularly discouraging that a special survey of GPs in Europe in 1988[1] revealed that:

> In the European Community more than one third (36%) of doctors smoke; only 10% in the UK, as a result of various anti-smoking campaigns conducted by the British Medical Association, but 39% in Portugal and in Greece, 41% in Italy and 45% in Spain.
>
> Other European surveys show that in several countries, the proportion of GPs who smoke is greater than in the population as a whole. This is the case in Italy and even more so in Portugal.

3 Coordination of messages and activities

In many ways, the build up of knowledge about the prevention of cancers involves complex research and intricate specialized concerns; however, the messages that need to be put across to the general public always need to be clear and straightforward. It should be the role of government to attempt to coordinate the activities of the various groups and departments involved in cancer-prevention activities and ensure that they all present similar messages to the general public. The major groups may be professional groups, cancer societies and workers directly employed by the government itself. It is important that all these groups are perceived by the general public to be putting across a coherent and unified set of messages that can be acted upon in the real world by ordinary citizens in their everyday circumstances.

This is not solely the concern of government; other organizations have their part to play. For example, in the United Kingdom, as in many other European countries, there are a large number of cancer societies and organizations; perhaps they could examine for themselves whether their functions and messages could be simplified and made more effective if they were united, perhaps under the banner of a single Europe-wide Cancer Society?

The best process for this coordination and cooperation may well be through the formation of a structure that allows interaction and collaboration between these various agencies; one possible structure that has been successful in some European countries is the establishment of expert committees, formed by members of all the important organizations involved in cancer prevention, which collect all the available evidence and come to some consensus view on the latest developments. When such a consensus has been developed, then it is the role of the expert committee to advise the government on policy and to formulate the messages that can be promoted to a wider audience. Obviously where further research is needed before such a consensus can emerge, then it is their responsibility to advise the government on the need for such further research.

4 Control measures

Governments have the power to control a considerable number of the factors that are important in determining the health status of their populations. This is especially true in the field of cancer prevention, and a number of examples can be found where governmental control could be used to reduce some of the adverse factors. It is also true that some of the governments in Europe, inside and outside the EC, have been enormously active in this respect, while others have been slow or even reluctant to use their powers to achieve health-related aims. In many of the countries of the EC, examples of some positive controls can be found that are designed to protect the general population, or specific groups, from the future development of a number of cancers.

Within each country it can be seen that certain control measures are actively pursued, while others are comparatively underdeveloped. It is also apparent that supragovernmental activity by the European Community as a whole could be important in harmonizing many of these controls throughout Europe.

Examples of governmental controls

- product controls (controls over manufacture, import and distribution of harmful products)
- controls to protect workers in particular industries
- radiation controls
- food purity controls (controls over pesticides etc.)
- controls over advertising and sponsorship of harmful products.

5 Taxation and fiscal policies

Governments have enormous power to adjust the prices of particular products and services through the use of taxation. There is increasing realization of the importance of this mechanism in the promotion of products that may produce a positive health benefit, and the reduction of consumption of potentially harmful products. In the field of cancer prevention, the products that can be manipulated in this way are alcohol, fresh fruit and vegetables and of course tobacco. In Paper 6.3, Michael Wood outlines the ways in which tax and price policies for tobacco products can play an important part in reducing smoking levels. Price is a major determinant of smoking levels. In those countries where price is low, consumption is high, and vice versa.

Most governments feel that taxation of tobacco products is an important part of their fiscal policy; they enjoy large revenues from this source and may therefore be reluctant to pursue too vigorously policies that may reduce this income; price rises, through tax increases, could also add to the cost of living index and create additional inflationary pressure. However, it is important for people concerned with reducing the incidence of cancer within any population to counter these arguments with the facts and figures that show the importance of price increases in real terms on the levels of smoking, especially amongst young people who are particularly price sensitive.

Taxation policies can be used to promote low-tar tobacco products and bring about a reduction in consumption of the most harmful high-tar products. Similarly, low-alcohol drinks can be promoted through positive taxation policies. The variations in tobacco-taxation policies throughout Europe are being examined by the Commission of the European Communities; their aim is to align taxes on tobacco upwards when trade barriers are eliminated before the end of 1992.

6 Screening policies

The issue of screening for the early detection of cancers was discussed in Chapter 4. Policy at governmental level also needs to be clear on this issue. Where screening can be shown to be effective, it should be promoted and supported as part of government-level policy; funding should be made available for the screening and for research and continuing evaluation of the services at a national level.

However, in cases where the screening of particular cancers has not yet been shown to be effective, then national policies should be held back until the results of research and pilot projects become available.

7 Research policy development

Governments have an important role in determining priorities for research within their countries. There is increasing need for some of the research effort that has been expended on the *treatment* of cancers to be diverted into areas which can inform about the *prevention* of cancers. It is also apparent that international effort is required, and that national research policies should arise as a result of multinational collaboration.

Where epidemiological research is involved, it is important to use the diversity of life styles throughout Europe to throw light on the factors causing particular cancers.

8 Health service development

In many European countries, the health services are still mainly designed to treat disease episodes when they arise. For the emphasis to move to prevention of disease, careful thought and planning needs to be given to the structure of health services and the development of teams that can effectively undertake appropriate preventive work.

Preventive work demands organization, planning, resources and trained personnel. Although much of the emphasis in this section has focused on activity in wider spheres, work within the health service itself is still important when it comes to the prevention of cancer. Governments need to ensure that sufficient funds are available to the health service to develop the teams that are necessary to carry out preventive work at a local level.

9 International and intergovernmental activity

The desirability of intergovernmental activity in the realms of research activity has already been mentioned. In addition, there are other areas where cooperation and coordination between national governments is important. The tax-free concessions on alcohol and tobacco products enjoyed at international ports and airports promote a message that is opposed to basic health-education campaigns and there are plans to phase sales of these products out through multinational agreement.

Other areas where multinational cooperation is important include:

- the upward alignment and harmonization of tobacco taxation;
- the standardization of health warnings on tobacco products;
- the international moves towards low-tar tobacco products and the banning of high-tar products;
- the international banning of the sale of tobacco products to children;
- the regulation and restriction on the promotion of tobacco products;
- international pressure to reform agricultural policies towards the production and subsidization of healthy food products;
- improvement of multinational research on diet and cancer and the development of more sophisticated epidemiological research throughout Europe;
- international agreements on improved labelling for foodstuffs to inform consumer choice;
- improved information on carcinogenic materials and international registering of information and research findings;
- international legal measures to protect workers from carcinogenic substances;
- international protection against ionizing radiation, and the development of international standards of exposure and permissible levels in foodstuffs, etc.

The European Commission is already active in many of these areas, but pressure needs to be maintained on individual governments to ensure that these international directives are actually enforced within each country.

10 Governmental control over the export of hazards

The export of carcinogenic hazards remains a real possibility. Even governments diligently performing all their national responsibilities may simply be exporting their cancers overseas. This is especially important in the context of the developing nations, where controls may not be so strict. It can be seen that if a particular manufacturing process is prohibited, or strictly controlled within one country, because of the carcinogenic risks involved, it may be possible for unscrupulous manufacturers to switch production to a developing nation where controls are less rigid.

Damn! They've tightened up the asbestos regulations! Switch production to Brazil!

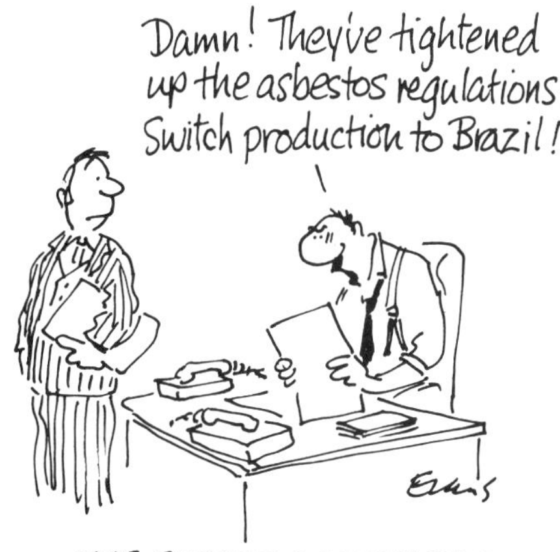

THE EXPORT OF HAZARDS...

The workers in this industry, or the people in the surrounding districts, may be exposed to carcinogenic hazards that would not be allowed in countries where stricter controls exist. The need for control and sanctions over companies acting in this way is important when it is seen in the international context of reducing the total burden of cancer throughout the world.

Similarly, the export of harmful products to countries where few controls exist should be prevented by active campaigns and forceful international action. There is considerable recent evidence of efforts by cigarette manufacturers to promote sales within developing nations because of the decline in sales in health-conscious European and North American markets.

The need for integrated activity

In this section, we have included many ideas from the Colloquium group for action at governmental level. However, for a significant number of cancers to be prevented, there is an overwhelming need for activities towards this goal to be coordinated and integrated with each other. For example, in Paper 6.3, *Policies for Reducing Smoking-Related Cancers*, Michael Wood identifies ten crucial areas where action is required to control tobacco production, sales, promotion and use. Without such comprehensive and integrated activity, the chances of success may be dramatically reduced and the effort reduced to a disorganized mixture of pragmatic and ineffective measures.

The ten points he lists and discusses add up to a really effective and comprehensive campaign to meet the stated objectives. These are:

1 Control of advertising and promotion.

2 Effective government health warnings.

3 A low-tar/nicotine policy.

4 Tax and pricing policies.

5 Alternative economic policies.

6 Policies to protect young people and prevent the onset of smoking.

7 Policies to protect non-smokers by:

(a) restrictions on smoking in public places

(b) restrictions on smoking in the workplace.

8 Policies to control production and promotion of smokeless and other new forms of tobacco and/or tobacco substitutes.

9 A levy on tobacco of at least 1% to fund health-education programmes.

10 Development of health-education and public-information programmes and the training of health professionals to provide practical help in giving up smoking.

Similar integrated action is proposed by Michael Kunze in his description of the UICC programme on smoking and cancer (Paper 6.4). In an interesting development of ideas, he details the Charter Against Tobacco for Europe which stresses the rights of individuals with respect to pollution by tobacco smoke. It could be argued that adoption of this charter by national governments would involve them in ensuring that these rights were actually upheld for their citizens.

Radiation, cancer and government policy

Excess radiation causes a variety of different cancers. In Paper 2.2, John Kaldor and Elisabeth Cardis describe these cancers. Government policy and action is necessary in the areas listed below, especially in view of the widespread public concern on this subject:

- Regulation and control is necessary at governmental level because action can not be left to individuals or individual companies to control the potential problems.
- International cooperation is important because of the global nature of some of the radiation hazards, for example the fall-out from the Chernobyl disaster.
- An enormous amount of additional research is needed before certainty on the exact levels of the hazard from different forms of radiation can be determined. This will involve international collaborative research.
- The secrecy surrounding much of the radiation issue, presumably because of the use of radioactive products by the armed forces, is not helpful to the scientific effort to discover the effects of radiation. The excessive secrecy that surrounds radiation issues can work against the best interests of the general public and the speed of dissemination of information.
- Even where the hazards of radiation are known it should be recognized that enforcement of control measures by government agencies can be problematic.

Diet, cancer and government policy

The Colloquium considered that there is a need for much more government-sponsored and international collaborative research in this area. In Paper 2.4, *Diet and Cancer: a sobering look*, Eyvind Thorling states: '... even though a large amount of information is already at hand on the topic, we are still not ready for giving specified, detailed or quantitative advice to the general public.' However, he does report a major conference that has made a list of seven recommendations which would impinge on government policy on food production, distribution and pricing.

- The intake of saturated and unsaturated fat should be reduced in those countries where fat constitutes more than 30% of total food energy.
- A varied diet should be eaten containing different types of vegetables and fruits, especially green leafy and root vegetables and citrus fruits.
- Foods rich in complex carbohydrates should be eaten.
- Appropriate body weight should be maintained.
- A low-salt diet should be consumed.
- Fresh or minimally processed foods should be used.
- Alcohol should be drunk only in moderation, if at all.

It can be seen that within each part of this list of recommendations there is scope for some government activity, both to disseminate this information to their people and to stimulate changes in the directions recommended by appropriate food policy and subsidy and taxation structure. Specific messages and recommendations about the prevention of cancers must be seen in a context of other health-promotion messages concerning the adoption of a healthy life style. These are, in fact, identical with the action that needs to be taken to prevent coronary heart disease. The actions and messages about prevention of cancers in no way replace or contradict other messages relating to the overall context of the need for a healthy diet.

This information is highly culture specific. Each government must make recommendations that are relevant to its own population. Even within Europe, there are enormous variations in patterns of food intake. The traditional diet in many of the Mediterranean countries has a total fat intake that is well below the recommended amount and a mixed diet that already performs well against these dietary recommendations. The message for those governments might well be to encourage their populations to continue to eat their traditional diets, and to resist change towards western European or transatlantic types of eating habits and overconsumption.

Priorities for government action

What then should a government do to help prevent cancers? Our conference in Lisbon produced a list of actions:

1 **Eliminate all forms of tobacco advertising and promotion in all EC countries within five years.**

2 **Increase taxation on all tobacco products.**

3 **Place prominent labels on the front of every packet of tobacco. These should say '*Smoking causes cancer.*'**

4 **Ban alcohol on television in a fashionable or promotional atmosphere.**

5 **Encourage and fund relevant research on the prevention of cancers, especially international and collaborative research.**

6 **Develop and fund comprehensive cancer registries in every European country.**

7 **Promote positive messages for healthy life styles and cancer-prevention messages as one part of these.**

8 **Stop duty-free sales of tobacco and alcohol at international airports and other outlets within Europe.**

These recommendations from the Lisbon Colloquium could be called **The Lisbon Declaration**. Although many of the recommendations relate to the traditional targets of tobacco and alcohol, the importance of action on a broad front to prevent cancers was strongly advocated.

References

1 This survey was carried out by 12 national institutes grouped in 'The European Omnibus Survey' (Brussels), including NORMA in Porgugal. As quoted in B.A.S.P. (Belgian Association for Smoking Prevention) Newsletter 4, L. Joossens (ed.), April-May 1989.

Paper 6.1

CANCER PREVENTION AND THE EUROPEAN COMMUNITY

David Sweet
Commission of the European Communities, Brussels

A personal paper especially commissioned for this book at the request of the participants at the Lisbon Colloquium.

This paper is intended to provide a very brief 'user's guide' to the way the institutions of the European Community work with reference to the Europe Against Cancer Programme. It is a personal view and does not necessarily express the official opinion of the community.

Institutional overview

It is unfortunately necessary for anyone who wishes to influence or work within the context of a Community Programme to have at least some idea of the institutional structure involved. Put very simply, there are two bodies with executive powers, the Commission and the Council, and two with consultative rights, the Parliament and the Economic and Social Committee (ESC). In theory, the Commission (constituting career international civil servants) initiates policy, the Parliament (elected members) and ESC (nominated representatives, e.g. employers, unions) give opinions on it, the Council (Ministers and committees of civil servants) decides and the Commission executes it.

The important point to remember is that the Commission is limited, firstly by the legal basis of the Treaties, and secondly, by what the Council may be expected to approve. This has particular relevance to health issues because health is not an objective of the Treaties—rather it is a constraint on other actions: in other words, actions to build a Common Market and European unity must not tend to reduce the level of health protection that is available. The position of occupational health is different, incidentally: the improvement of working conditions and occupational health is an explicit objective set out in the Treaties.

The roles of the Parliament and the ESC deserve a brief mention. Both are to be consulted on most issues (virtually all concerning health and social questions). However, the influence of the Parliament has been increasing markedly in recent years, and the Commission and even the Council will very often take account of amendments to measures passed by the Parliament. In addition, the Parliament has a limited power to increase funding for certain actions, and this has been used to the advantage of the Europe Against Cancer Programme in the past. Finally, if the Parliament is opposed to a measure, it is difficult, though not impossible, to enact it. (Outright opposition to a measure proposed by the Commission is extremely rare.) The ESC, on the other hand, has seen its significance reduced as the significance of the Parliament has increased. Its role is primarily to bring expert, and interested, scrutiny on draft measures, but the status of its members as representatives of interests means that the opinions are only given the weight that the recipients choose to give them. For example, the ESC opinions on the draft Directives on labelling and tar content of tobacco products were heavily influenced by the fact that the rapporteur was an employers' representative with links with the tobacco industry.

From idea to action: the process of gestation

The policy of the European Community, as developed by the Commission, will begin with an idea. This idea, more or less relevant to the Treaty of Rome, might come from a Commissioner, a national Minister, but it is most likely from a Commission official. If the political winds are favourable, it could then be worked into a proposal normally requiring funds, or a legal decision, or both. Advice will be taken, almost certainly, from an existing or newly created group of experts who may well be national civil servants. The proposal will then be circulated to interested Directorates General* (e.g., Agriculture, Internal Market, for actions relating to tobacco) and submitted to the Commission (i.e. the Commissioners) for approval.

At this stage, and strictly speaking only now, it is published as a draft Decision, Directive or other legal instrument (briefly and very approximately, Directives impose an obligation on Member States to incorporate the relevant legislation into national law; Decisions impose policy on the Commission; other instruments, such as Resolutions and Recommendations, carry no legal obligations). The draft is submitted to the European Parliament, to the Economic and Social Committee and, most importantly, to the Council.

The Council will establish an *ad hoc* working party, composed of national civil servants with a representative of the Commission, which will examine and discuss the proposal line by line. During this stage intensive negotiations take place and it becomes clearer which points may be genuinely unacceptable to a Member State and which are being used as bargaining counters for this or another proposal. It is during this stage, therefore, that the opportunity for effective external influence is most apparent.

The subsequent progress of the proposal depends heavily on whether the proposal is accepted as falling under the scope of the Single European Act and the Internal Market† (1992 legislation) or not. If it does, and so far all the tobacco-related proposals have been accepted under this heading, then unanimity is not necessary and it is unlikely that any one Member State will be able to block progress for long, unless it is the current President of the Council (this position revolves every six months; the major power involved is that of setting timetables and agendas of meetings). In addition, the role of the Parliament becomes more important since if it amends a proposal, and the Commission accepts the amendment, then the Council can only overturn that amendment by a unanimous vote, though it can still reject the measure altogether.

When the Presidency feels that a proposal has been sufficiently studied in a working group, then it may appear on the agenda of a meeting of the relevant Council of Ministers (Health in this case). Here it will, if at all controversial, again be discussed exhaustively and possibly amended. Typically agreement is not reached on the first appearance and it is necessary to send the measure back for further discussion. Eventually, it will reappear on the agenda of a later Council meeting on the relevant topic (usually health). Incidentally, Health meetings are taking place every six months at present, which is considerably more often than in the past, primarily due to the AIDS problem.

***Directorates General** are equivalent to Ministries, and are divided into (often semi-independent) Directorates. Each Commissioner is responsible for one or more Directorates General. He is assisted by his *Cabinet*—half a dozen 'high fliers', mostly of his own nationality, who, individually and collectively, have considerable influence on the development of proposals.

†The Single Act and the Internal Market
The signing of the Single Act, a series of amendments to the Treaty of Rome, brought about a considerable change in the procedures of the Community. Previously, unanimity was the rule in almost all areas of activity, which meant that one strongly dissenting Member State could effectively block any measure. Now, however, if a measure is agreed as falling within a defined scope, basically of actions necessary to complete a frontier-free Europe by 1992, then a qualified majority is all that is necessary to pass it. The powers of the Parliament are also increased for these measures. That is the reason why many of the measures proposed under the Europe Against Cancer Programme are actually formulated in such a way as to appear to be promoting the free movement of tobacco or tobacco advertising. The reasoning is that if a certain level of protection is imposed by one Member State, then it is necessary either for that state to restrict the import of non-conforming products, which would infringe the rules on free movement of goods, or for the same level of protection to be applied throughout the Community, which is generally the chosen path.

The progress through Parliament is also affected by the status of the measure vis a vis 1992. The procedure is more complicated, but basically the proposal will be allocated to a Committee which will appoint a rapporteur. He or she will prepare a report for the Committee which will form the basis for discussion of the measure. Amendments may be proposed by the Committee, but only the full Parliament can actually adopt the report with or without amendments. Discussions by the Committee are public and outside experts or the Commission may be invited to give evidence.

Pressure points

What then are the conclusions for a campaigner. Firstly, it is no use pressurizing the Commission to take action which does not lie within its power, or competence. To take an extreme example, the Commission cannot introduce a proposal to ban smoking, except by consenting adults in private, because such a measure has not been imposed in any Member State, meaning it would be new legislation and not harmonization. Even if such a law did exist in one country, it is very doubtful whether it could be argued to have a significant influence on trade. On the other hand, if smoking at the workplace were to be banned in one Member State on the grounds of preventing occupational exposure to carcinogens, then there could well be a legal basis for extending this protection to workers in other countries. Even then, however, it is not enough only to put pressure on the Commission. Such a measure could only be passed if there were the basis of a consensus of national governments behind it.

Suppose that the conditions expressed above are satisfied: one country has banned smoking at work and the Commission has been persuaded that there is a chance of success for a Directive imposing the same rules throughout the Community. The proposal would be prepared by the Health and Safety Directorate in consultation with (mainly Government appointed) occupational safety experts in the Community. If there seemed a reasonable prospect of progress, a proposal would then be submitted to the Commission for a draft Directive, after explicit consultation with other Directorates General. At this stage, therefore, the most effective pressure would be on senior Commission officials in the relevant areas, *and* on the national Ministries.

If the draft is accepted and published by the Commission, it is time to bring on the major campaign at the ESC, and to find a reasonably favourable rapporteur at the Parliament to ensure that MEPs are made aware of the positive arguments, and are not too swayed by the opposition, and most importantly, at the level of national administrations, to encourage the participants in Council working parties not to take too negative an attitude. Here a coordinated, though not necessarily uniform, European campaign can be most effective, especially if at least one or two Governments can be persuaded openly to support the measure. Pressure needs to be maintained at the Commission to ensure that its resolve does not weaken, but it should be realized that after publication of a draft measure, progress is largely out of the Commission's hands. National interest, twelve times over, becomes the key.

Paper 6.2

DEVELOPING EFFECTIVE POLICY FOR THE PREVENTION OF CANCERS

Dr. Hans H. Storm and Dr. Ole M. Jensen
Danish Cancer Registry, Institute of Cancer Epidemiology, Copenhagen, Denmark

Cancer prevention is the joint responsibility of the individual and the community. The community has a major responsibility in synthesizing the scientific experience on risk factors for cancers, and transforming the result into regulatory actions and/or education of the individual. The informed person can then choose to reduce his or her exposure to various identified risk factors. The noble goal set forth by the World Health Organization in the Alma-Ata declaration on Health for All by the year 2000 (WHO, 1978), and the EC objective of reducing cancer mortality by 15 per cent by the same year, cannot be met without close collaboration and understanding by governments and populations.

The term prevention can be divided into primary prevention and secondary prevention. **Primary prevention** is concerned with the elimination or modification of risk factors to prevent the development of cancer, and should be the ultimate goal for our efforts. This was clearly stated by Sir Thomas Adams who, in the 17th century, said: 'He is a better physician that keeps the diseases off us, than he that cures them being on us. Prevention is so much better than cure, because it saves the labor being sick.'

Secondary prevention involves treating people when they have become ill as well as screening apparently healthy people to detect preclinical or symptomless cancers at an early stage, when treatment is more likely to be effective. While individuals benefit from early treatment, a number of potential side effects of screening programmes should not be overlooked, including unnecessary examination and the unnecessary treatment of non-fatal cases.

There are many aspects to consider when developing an effective cancer-control policy. When the goal is a reduction in cancer mortality, a cancer-control programme must focus on:

1 known risk factors for cancer—in order to establish a cancer-prevention policy on a rational basis;
2 early detection of cancers—where such an effort has been shown to lead to a reduction in mortality;
3 optimal treatment—with the aim of curing patients who have contracted the disease.

The registration by a cancer registry of all cancer cases arising in the population, together with parallel information on mortality, is an essential part of any rational programme in cancer control (Muir, 1985). The cancer registry provides basic information on the burden of cancer in the community, as well as the data that is needed to uncover the causes of cancer and for evaluation of the steps that can be taken to control the disease.

The burden of cancer

The Danish Cancer Registry provides information on the number of cancer cases and risks by type in the community (Danish Cancer Registry, 1988; IARC, 1987). This immediately highlights areas where efforts should be concentrated, both in terms of using current knowledge on risk factors for a given cancer to achieve prevention with a significant impact on public health, and in terms of research. Only incidence statistics provide the information on where such actions would be most cost effective, and thereby lead to the maximum reduction in human suffering.

Table 6.1 shows that information on the incidence of cancer is available for only a few populations in the European Community (Coleman and Démaret, 1988). It can be seen that adequate population-based cancer registration exists only in Denmark and the United Kingdom, while around 10 per cent of the population is covered in most other countries. In Belgium, registration is higher at 97 per cent, but still considered incomplete. Based on the information from these Cancer Registries, it has been estimated that approximately 1.2 million new cancer cases arise in the EC countries every year, excluding non-melanoma skin cancer (Coleman and Démaret, 1988).

The Cancer Registry also provides information on the importance of cancer by site. In Denmark, the most common cancer among men is lung cancer, followed by cancers of the skin, prostate, bladder, and colon. Among women, breast cancer is the most frequent, followed by cancers of the skin, lung, and ovary. Tumours of these sites alone in men and women respectively account for more than half of all tumours of that given sex (Danish Cancer Registry, 1988). The detailed registration of cancer also makes it possible to determine the cancer occurrence according to such characteristics as age, occupation, and geographical region. It is clear that in Denmark, as well as elsewhere in the EC, lung cancer is the major problem among men, and breast cancer among women. Preventive actions which lead to even a small proportional reduction in the risk of cancer of these sites would have a major numerical impact on the total cancer occurrence in the community.

Combined with mortality statistics, information on cancer incidence gives us the possibility of calculating the years lost in the population due to death from specific causes (assuming that the death rate of the cancer patient is otherwise similar to that of the general population). In Queensland, Australia, the average number of years of life lost from brain cancer, leukaemia and melanoma exceeded 20 years on average, whereas those lost from lung, prostate and stomach cancers were less than 14 years. Cancers of the lung, large bowel, breast, stomach and prostate are, in terms of numbers, the top five causes of death by cancer in Queensland. When combining the number of years of life lost and the number of cases of a

Table 6.1 Estimated annual number of new cancer cases (excluding skin cancer) in 10 member states of the European Community 1982–1985. Rates per 100 000 male–female ratio, population size and coverage by general registries by country

Country	No. of cases per year	Male–female ratio	Rate per 100 000	Population size	Average coverage by registration %	No of general registries
Belgium	28 936	1.0	293.8	9 848 647	97	1
Denmark	20 306	1.0	396.9	5 115 605	100	1
FRG	152 661	0.7	247.7	61 637 600	19	3
France	174 217	1.3	320.6	54 346 000	11	12
Ireland	9 310	1.0	270.4	3 443 405	16	1
Italy	213 194	1.2	381.2	55 928 500	9	7
Netherlands	49 259	1.1	339.7	14 500 000	11	7
Portugal	20 460	1.0	208.1	9 833 014	2	2
Spain	103 066	1.3	273.5	37 682 355	14	7
United Kingdom	216 266	0.9	383.9	56 337 909	100	18
Total	987 675	0.9	320.0	308 673 035	33	59

From: Coleman and Démaret, 1988

given cancer, lung, large bowel and breast cancer are still the top three on the list, but leukaemias and brain cancers now rank fourth and fifth, stomach sixth and melanoma seventh, as shown in Table 6.2 (Queensland Department of Health, 1985). This measure is also highly relevant for setting priorities for preventive actions.

Basic population statistics

Reliable population statistics are one of the cornerstones of cancer registration, as well as cancer mortality figures. The composition of the population by age, sex, residence, occupation and other variables must be known in order to calculate true rates of incidence and mortality. If the information on the population, either derived from censuses, or from a central population registration, as is the case in Denmark, can be linked to cancer incidence and mortality data, at the level of an individual, a very important source of data will be available for the evaluation of risk factors and cancer patterns. Basic population statistics, and forecasts on future development in age and sex structure of the population, based on previously compiled information, are very important when evaluating the incidence over years, and when projecting cancer trends into the future.

Trends and projections

Many years of registration enables the evaluation of trends in incidence (Hakulinen *et al.*, 1986), as well as mortality, and gives unique possibilities for predicting the importance of cancer of various sites in the future. Figure 6.2 shows the trends in incidence for selected cancer sites in Denmark since 1943 among males and females. It is obvious from the decreasing trend in incidence that stomach cancer is no longer a high priority area for prevention in Denmark, and indeed this cancer may well disappear spontaneously from the list of the most common cancers. However, research is still needed to understand why stomach cancer is declining, since we do not fully understand all the risk factors in operation (Jensen, 1982).

Lung cancer shows a trend clearly in the opposite direction. A dramatic increase has been observed during the past 45 years for men and, during the last decades in particular, for women also. Lung cancer is, therefore, in both

Table 6.2 Relative importance in terms of number of deaths and years of life lost by cancer site, Queensland, Australia, 1982. Ranks in parentheses.

Site	% of all cancer deaths	(Rank)	Average years of life lost	(Rank)	Potential years of life lost	(Rank)
Lung	22	(1)	13.8	(7)	10 678	(1)
Large bowel	13	(2)	14.4	(6)	6 964	(2)
Breast	7	(3)	19.7	(4)	5 242	(3)
Stomach	6	(4)	12.6	(8)	2 073	(6–7)
Prostate	6	(5)	8.4	(11)	1 788	(9)
Pancreas	4	(6)	12.4	(9)	1 963	(8)
Leukaemia	4	(7)	23.3	(2)	3 429	(4)
Brain	3	(8)	26.0	(1)	2 856	(5)
Melanoma	3	(9)	21.4	(3)	2 073	(6–7)
Bladder	3	(10)	11.4	(10)	1 091	(11)
Ovary	2	(11)	19.1	(5)	1 626	(10)
Other	27		–		16 782	
Total	100		–		56 565	

From: Queensland Department of Health, 1985.

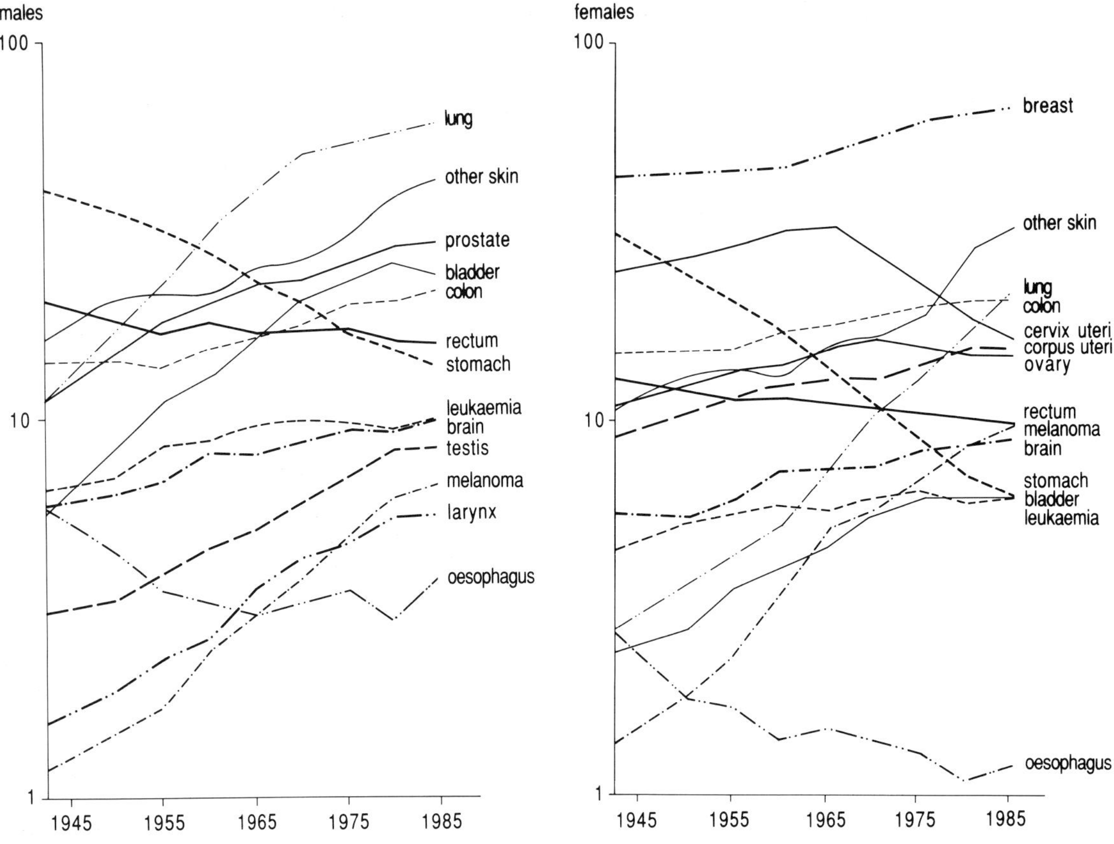

Figure 6.2 Incidence rates of cancer in Denmark 1943–1985

sexes, an area of the highest priority for prevention. This can to a large extent be achieved by reducing tobacco smoking, which for almost 40 years has been a well known risk factor for lung cancer (Doll and Hill, 1950).

Recently, a sharp increase has been observed in the incidence of melanoma skin cancer and a parallel increase in the mortality rates. As with lung cancer, the increase in malignant melanoma of the skin is linked to birth cohorts—a generation effect—where the risk for one generation is five to six times higher than the risk for the preceding one (Østerlind *et al.*, 1988). This indicates that the overall incidence will probably increase in the future, making this cancer an important area for research and intervention.

Projections, based on known trends, can be carried out taking both the predictive changes in the cancer rate and the population composition into consideration. Projections will indicate what the cancer pattern is likely to look like in the future. If knowledge of risk factors is available, the potential impact of various preventive strategies can also be forecast; for example, Hakulinen and Pukkala (1981) estimated the trend in lung cancer incidence in Finland which would result if various proportions of the population stopped smoking. It is thus possible to plan ahead and allocate resources in the best possible way to fulfil the task of diminishing the cancer burden.

Mortality

Mortality statistics represent a very important international data source. In most countries, the statistics are compiled according to World Health Organization standards. It is a universal comprehensive registration which places the problem of fatal cancers in an overall context with other fatal diseases. It is possible, for example, to evaluate cancer mortality according to site, sex and age at death, as well as according to other variables collected.

As with the incidence information, mortality statistics should be compiled on the basis of records of identifiable individuals in order to facilitate links with other data sources (for example, cancer incidence data and exposure data) for the purpose of aetiological research and evaluation of screening programmes. It is a prerequisite of any survival analysis that at least the date of death can be linked to the incidence data information for a given individual.

Mortality is an indicator of the success of both primary and secondary prevention taken together. It has therefore been the obvious choice as the overall measure in EC cancer-control efforts. Today the situation within the EC differs from country to country. In many member states, data are collected anonymously, making it impossible to validate stated death diagnosis, and discarding linkage possibilities completely. Thus research and evaluation of prevention is impossible at a scientific level. Mortality statistics, method of compilation, and use of data linking individual patients should be a policy of all governments who wish to ensure the success of cancer-prevention programmes.

Monitoring of cancer

Registration of all cancer cases and cancer deaths in the population is also necessary for the surveillance of the effectiveness of primary preventive measures, or early detection undertaken as part of a cancer-control programme. This would seem obvious but is rarely implemented.

The effectiveness of screening for pre-cancerous lesions of the cervix uteri has been clearly demonstrated from incidence trends in the Nordic countries (Hakama, 1976). In Denmark, a rapid decrease in incidence was demonstrated, in particular in areas where organized screening programmes have been implemented (Lynge, 1983), as a result of the basic cancer-registration system which has been used for monitoring the effect of the screening programme. Furthermore, appropriate registration of cancer incidence data also provides clues to the identification of high-risk groups, such as for which age groups a screening programme should be offered.

Conclusion

Studies on cancer incidence and mortality have assisted in identifying risk factors for the most common cancers (Clemmesen, 1965). Those factors which are most clearly determined are the life-style characteristics of smoking, alcohol intake, sexual behaviour and reproductive history, as well as exposure to occupational carcinogens, X rays, drugs and sunlight. There are also strong indications that diet may play a role for many cancers (Doll and Peto, 1981). The magnitude of the cancer problem, the cancer patterns, and groups of persons at high risk, have been identified in areas where cancer registration is working adequately.

Mortality statistics are essential to evaluate the combined effect. Linking individual data to other data sources can shed light on risk factors for cancer. While individual rights to privacy must of course be observed when compiling records, confidential access to such data for medical research purposes should be available for the benefit of the community. Such possibilities exist in the United Kingdom and Denmark, as well as the other Nordic countries, and no abuse resulting from it has ever been recorded.

A basic requirement for the development of an effective policy for the prevention of cancer in the EC is the reliable registration of all cancer cases with information compiled in such a way that it corresponds to other demographic data sources and allows for comparisons to be made among the various countries. For the successful implementation of prevention programmes, and for these programmes to prove effective, reliable cancer statistics based on good cancer registries are essential.

References

Clemmesen, J. (1965) Statistical studies in the etiology of malignant neoplasms, *Acta Path Microbiol. Scand.*, vol i, suppl. 174.

Coleman, M., Démaret, E. (1988) Cancer registration in the European Community, *Int. J. Cancer* **42**, 339–345.

Danish Cancer Society, Danish Cancer Registry (1988) *Cancer incidence in Denmark 1985*, Danish Cancer Society, Copenhagen.

Doll, R., Hill, A. B. (1950) Smoking and carcinoma of the lung. Preliminary report. *Brit. Med. J.* **2**, 739–748.

Doll, R., Peto, R. (1981) The causes of cancer: quantitative estimates of avoidable risk of cancer in the USA today, *JNCI* **166**, 1193–1308.

Hakama, M. *et al.* (1976) Effect of a mass screening program on the risk of cervical cancer, *Am. J. Epid.* **103**, 512–517.

Hakulinen, T., Magnus, K., Malker, B., Schou, G., Tulinius, H. (1986) Trends in cancer incidence in the Nordic countries. A collaborative study of the Nordic cancer registries, *Acta Path Microbiol. Scand.* suppl.

Hakulinen, T. and Pukkala, E. (1981) Future incidence of lung cancer: forecasts based on hypothetical changes in the smoking habits of males, *Int. J. Epidemiol.* **10**, 238–240.

Hakulinen, T., Pukkala, E., Hakama, M., Lehtonen, M., Saxen, E., Teppo, L. (1981) Survival of cancer patients in Finland 1953–73, *Ann. Clin. Res.* **13**, suppl. 31.

International Agency for Research on Cancer (1987) *Cancer Incidence in Five Continents*, C. Muir, J. Waterhouse *et al.* (eds.) volume v, IARC, Lyon.

Jensen, O. M. (1982) Trends in the incidence of gastric cancer in the five Nordic countries, in K. Magnus (ed.) *Trends in Cancer Incidence*, Hemisphere Press, New York.

Lynge, E. (1983) Regional trends in incidence of cervical cancer in Denmark in relation to local smear-taking activity, *Int. J. Epidemiol.* **12**, 405–413.

Muir, C. S., Démaret, E. (1985) The Cancer Registry in Cancer Control: An Overview, in *The Role of the Registry in Cancer Control*, M. Parkin, G. Wagner, C. S. Muir (eds.) International Agency for Research on Cancer, publ. no. 66, IARC, Lyon.

Queensland Department of Health (1985) The Queensland Campaign for Cancer Prevention, Cancer Epidemiology and Prevention Unit, Brisbane.

World Health Organization (1978) Alma-Ata 1978: Primary Health Care, WHO, Geneva.

Østerlind, A., Engholm, G. and Jensen, O. M. (1988) Trends in cutaneous malignant melanoma in Denmark 1943–1982 by anatomic site, *APMIS* **96**, 953–963.

Paper 6.3

POLICIES FOR REDUCING SMOKING-RELATED CANCERS

Michael A. Wood
Ulster Cancer Foundation, Belfast, Northern Ireland

Tobacco smoking is the largest single avoidable cause of ill health and premature death in Europe, where it is responsible for more than half a million deaths each year. For more than two decades, it has been clear that prevention of smoking would lead to substantial reductions in the death and misery associated with lung and other cancers, heart disease, bronchitis, emphysema and other conditions. Despite this knowledge, the problem of tobacco-associated disease has increased in many parts of the world. If we only consider the effects of smoking tobacco on the incidence of cancer, we can say that some 90 per cent of lung cancers, 50 per cent of cancers of the bladder and renal pelvis are due to cigarette smoking in men, plus a substantial number of cancers of the larynx, oesophagus, pharynx and pancreas. Cancers probably caused by smoking include cancers of the stomach, liver, nasal sinuses, cervix uteri, adeno-carcinoma of the kidney and leukaemia[1]. All in all it is now accepted that some 30 per cent of all cancers owe their origin to smoking.

When we include all the other diseases of the respiratory system caused by smoking, vascular disease, damage done to the foetus and complications in pregnancy, recent evidence of the effects of environmental tobacco smoke (which in addition to causing a substantial proportion of lung cancer cases in adult non-smokers, is also known to cause a greater frequency of respiratory infections and symptoms in children), and the new hazards arising from the introduction of smokeless tobacco products in a number of European countries, then surely we can legitimately paraphrase the UK Royal College of Physicians' 1971 Report and say that 'action to protect the public against the damage done by tobacco use would have more effect upon the public health than anything else that could now be done in the whole field of preventive medicine'.

But any consideration of policies to prevent smoking-related cancers must not only be concerned with the health issues; tobacco is also of major concern as a social and economic issue. The use of tobacco is still an established habit practised by millions of people in Europe. The social value of tobacco varies widely throughout the European region. In some groups, smoking and other forms of tobacco use are still accepted, and even seen as a desirable part of social life, whilst in others tobacco use is now strongly discouraged. Obviously such social influences will affect the individual choice of whether or not to take up the smoking habit and as a result there are wide variations in smoking prevalence amongst different social groupings.

Individual choices are, of course, strongly influenced by the powerful vested interests of the tobacco industry. Advertising and sponsorship of cultural and sporting activities reinforce the social acceptability of the product and also do much to undermine the effectiveness of the health messages which are intended to reduce the prevalence of smoking. Tobacco use is also a major economic issue, since tobacco is the most widely grown non-food plant in the world and provides employment and income to farmers, factory workers, the printing, packaging and advertising industries as well as being an important source of tax revenue to governments.

Measures adopted to deal with the tobacco problem must therefore be comprehensive and embrace all the issues outlined above. In order to be effective, such measures will need legislation by European governments.

The following are the main areas in which action is required to control tobacco production, sales, promotion and use, and should form part of a comprehensive tobacco-control policy:

1 Control of advertising and promotion.
2 Effective government health warnings.
3 A low-tar/nicotine policy.
4 Tax and pricing policies.
5 Alternative economic policies.
6 Policies to protect young people and prevent the onset of smoking.
7 Policies to protect non-smokers by:
   - restrictions on smoking in public places
   - restrictions on smoking in the workplace.
8 Policies to control production and promotion of smokeless and other new forms of tobacco and/or tobacco substitutes.
9 A levy on tobacco of at least 1 per cent to fund health-education programmes.

In addition, high priority needs to be given to the development of comprehensive health-education and public-information programmes and the training of health professionals and other key personnel to provide practical help in giving up smoking.

Current European initiatives by international governmental and voluntary agencies support these objectives, in particular the European Community's Strategy Document for 'Europe Against Cancer' and the World Health Organization Regional Office for Europe's five-year action plan for a smoke-free Europe[2].

The remainder of this paper summarizes the rationale for the comprehensive tobacco-control policy outlined. These summaries are largely based on the series of background documents prepared for the World Health Organization Regional Office for Europe's First European Conference on Tobacco Policy held in November 1988 in Madrid in association with the European Community, International Union Against Cancer and the International Agency for Research on Cancer[3–11].

Control of advertising and promotion

Why ban tobacco advertising? As Chapman says in *Pushing Smoke*[10]:

> Tobacco advertising promotes the idea that smoking is normal, good and glamorous. Tobacco advertising continually tells people that smoking is desirable. It undermines the credibility of government statements which say that smoking is bad for health. It is, therefore, incompatible with the government's wider smoking-control policy and leads to a widespread cynicism about health-education messages.

The tobacco industry's argument of course is that if it is legal to sell a product, then it should be legal to advertise it. This particular argument attempts to win sympathy by portraying the industry as the victim of an unjust principle. The argument is, however, highly misleading. It has been said that tobacco is the only legal product which is lethal when used as directed and it is certainly true to say that if tobacco was discovered today and an attempt made to place it on the market with all the knowledge that we have today about the attendant health risks, no government would permit it to be sold.

Advertising is one of the strongest weapons the tobacco industry has and it spends millions of pounds per year to lure consumers to its products. The power and pervasiveness of tobacco advertising which associates smoking with success, pleasure, relaxation etc. make it essential that it be banned in order to alter the environment in which young people grow up and to free them from the pressure to smoke. The argument that tobacco advertising only creates brand consciousness and does not influence the total demand for tobacco simply does not bear examination. Logically tobacco advertising will do at least four things:

1 influence smokers to change brands;
2 influence smokers to smoke more;
3 influence non-smokers to start smoking;
4 discourage or delay smokers from giving up the habit.

David Abbot, a leading British advertiser, has said:

> As an argument (that tobacco advertising is only aimed at brand switching and not at attracting new consumers) it is so preposterous, it is insulting ... to claim that cigarette advertising does not encourage smoking, flies in the face of all advertising knowledge and experience.

The experience in Norway, whose programme of legislation is considered an international model of smoking control, showed that in 1970, when the Norwegian Parliament decided to introduce a smoking-control programme that included a ban on all tobacco advertising and promotion, sales declined markedly. In 1975, when the Norwegian Tobacco Act came into force, a further decline in cigarette sales was experienced.

The minimal approach of an advertising ban is to prohibit the promotion of tobacco on television and radio. However, the ultimate aim should be to phase out all advertising and promotion including sponsorship by the tobacco industry and thus to remove totally the influence of the tobacco industry from society.

Effective government health warnings

In Europe, some 18 countries are known to require health warnings on cigarette packs. However, in many of these countries, the warnings have lost their impact through familiarity and are weak, stating merely that smoking may be dangerous to health. Twelve European countries require a statement of tar/ nicotine content and sometimes carbon monoxide emission of cigarettes. Rotational warnings are now being introduced by a number of European countries following the Swedish practice. Such notices change periodically and are more likely to draw the smoker's attention to the warning contained in them. Six European countries now use this type of warning. To be effective, health warnings should be included on all cigarette packs and other tobacco products and on such advertising as is permitted. These warnings should be rotated regularly and should take up a much larger area of the cigarette pack in order to be clearly identified and read by the smoker.

Low-tar and nicotine policies

It is generally agreed that there should be a move towards the reduction of the tar and nicotine in all cigarettes sold within the EC. The EC recommends that there should be a prohibition on sales of cigarettes with a tar content exceeding around 15mgs. by 1989 and 12mgs. by 1992[12]. Some difference of opinion exists, however, among experts as to whether low-tar/nicotine-level cigarettes actually provide any protection to the smoker since they say that smokers will only compensate by inhaling more deeply. On the other hand, most agree that a dose reduction by lowering tar in cigarettes smoked reduces the relative risk and that a low-tar/nicotine cigarette may also be less satisfying for the smoker and may therefore be a step towards cessation. However, all agree that there is no such thing as a safe cigarette.

Tax and price policies

Analysis of cigarette consumption in 19 European countries has shown that price is a major determinant of smoking levels in Europe[11]. Tobacco taxes are an attractive means of raising revenue because they are easily administered and politically acceptable. Increasing taxes on cigarette prices discourages smoking because the demand for cigarettes responds to changes in prices. Studies in a number of countries, including the United Kingdom and the United States, have shown that the demand for cigarettes varies inversely with price and the price response is higher for teenagers. Comprehensive analysis of tobacco-price policy in Finland found that substantial price increases may be necessary to produce a significant impact on prevalence[11].

A step that would make it easier to introduce regular and repeated increases in the price of tobacco products would be to exclude these products from the cost of living index. If this was done, increases in tobacco prices would not contribute to a rise in the index which in some countries is the basis for automatic wage rises.

The EC's Europe Against Cancer programme has identified the need to align tobacco taxes upwards among members of the EC. This would cause some cigarette prices to rise quite substantially in southern European countries. However, concern has been expressed that in the UK, Ireland and some Scandinavian countries, the effect of such harmonization would be to hold back potential price increases to enable other European countries to catch up with those who have higher prices. In general, it can be said, however, that any policy to raise real cigarette prices in any country will be an aid to public health and is likely to be particularly effective in deterring young people from taking up the smoking habit.

Alternative economic policies

Perhaps the greatest challenge to governments in their efforts to reduce the effects of tobacco smoking is to devise alternative economic strategies. Tobacco is the most widely grown non-food plant in the world and it seems that so long as the demand for tobacco continues to increase, farmers will have strong incentives to produce tobacco because of its profitability. Unless worldwide demand is restrained, it will be difficult to make tobacco less remunerative and to reduce production. The FAO predict that the world leaf tobacco output will increase annually by about 1.9 per cent to about 7.9 million tons in 1995 and about 8.5 million tons by the year 2000[13].

Quite apart from the income from cash crops worldwide, tobacco production and processing provides widespread employment to factory workers and the industry provides substantial support for the print and broadcast media. In addition, of course, it provides tax revenues to governments. However, there has perhaps been too little consideration of the debit side of the balance sheet. A number of studies carried out have identified some of the costs to society from tobacco production and use. A study conducted in Northern Ireland[14], the home of a substantial proportion of the UK tobacco industry's manufacturing process, showed quite clearly that when all the costs to society were considered (including health care costs, number of working days lost annually because of smoking, fires caused by tobacco use etc.), then there was a net loss to the community of around £103 million. When this was grossed up to UK figures, then the net loss was staggering. No attempt has ever been made to quantify in monetary terms the pain and suffering caused to individuals and their families as a result of smoking-induced diseases.

The following economic strategies have been identified as possible ways of reducing tobacco production and consumption:

1 the elimination of subsidies in tobacco production;
2 crop substitution and the phasing out of tobacco production;
3 the determination of alternative sources of government revenue.

The European Community is in a very strong position to make a major contribution to these strategies by harmonizing agricultural and economic policies among the members of the EC so as to promote public health objectives[4].

Policies to protect young people and to prevent the onset of smoking

The World Health Organization's Ten Countries Study[15] suggests that more than 60 per cent of children have tried smoking by the age of 15 and almost one-third of all young people will become smokers by the age of 18. Young people's actions reflect the attitudes, values and norms of the society in which they live. If young people see smoking as normal behaviour, and there are few environmental restrictions on where and when people can smoke, those who wish to behave as adults perceive smoking as one way of doing so. All actions taken by governments and other organizations to reduce smoking among the adult population, will also have some influence on young people.

The influence of advertising and promotion of tobacco products has already been discussed. There is indeed a growing body of evidence to show that advertising directly influences the decision to start smoking. The way in which smoking is more generally portrayed in society and in particular in the media through television and film drama may also influence young people Those who control the media should be made aware of their influence and the important role they have in presenting a more positive non-smoking image to young people.

Peer influence

Peer pressure has long been identified as a major factor influencing the smoking behaviour of young people. Young people who smoke usually smoke with friends; and most non-smokers have friends who do not smoke. Experimentation usually takes place in groups and peer approval is an important factor in the adoption of regular smoking for these reasons. Helping young people to develop the confidence and skills to resist the social pressure to smoke would help reduce the incidence of smoking in young people. Those from homes where no adults smoke or where parents are disapproving of smoking in their children are much less likely to become regular smokers; so influencing parental smoking and attitudes will also help to reduce smoking among young people[8].

Attitudes and beliefs

Knowledge and beliefs about smoking have been shown to be related to smoking behaviour. Young people who do not smoke usually hold negative beliefs about smoking, while adolescents who smoke usually have less knowledge of the health risks concerned. Health education should, therefore, emphasize the short-term effects of smoking on health and appearance as well as examining values and beliefs in relation to smoking[8].

The development of health-education programmes about smoking

The following factors are important considerations in the development of health-education programmes about smoking for young people:

1 Smoking-education programmes need to be relevant to the different developmental stages of smoking.

2 Smoking-education programmes need to address the social and environmental influences on smoking behaviour as well as improving knowledge about the dangers of smoking to health.

3 Programmes need to balance action directed towards supporting non-smokers as well as encouraging current smokers to stop and in some cases teaching 'how to stop' skills.

4 Programmes need to balance effort directed at individual young people with action to provide a more supportive environment for non-smoking.

Legislation to control sales of tobacco products to young people

In a number of European countries, sales of cigarettes to young people is illegal. The minimum age varies from one country to another. Clearly, a comprehensive smoking-control policy should prohibit the sales of tobacco products to young people (say) under 16 years of age and effective legislation should be introduced to ensure that these laws are obeyed. Unfortunately, in many countries where laws do exist to prohibit the sale of tobacco products to young people, the restrictions are ignored and young people are found to be able to freely purchase cigarettes from tobacconists. High prices, as we have seen, *are* likely to deter young people from purchasing cigarettes[11].

Policies to protect non-smokers by restrictions on smoking in public places and in the workplace

The evidence against Environmental Tobacco Smoke (ETS), the inhalation of which is known as 'passive smoking', is presented in the *US Surgeon General's Report on Passive Smoking*[16], the IARC report, *The Health Effects of Exposure to Environmental Tobacco Smoke*[17], and the *Fourth Report of the UK Government's Independent Scientific Committee on Passive Smoking*[18]. The importance of the passive-smoking issue is summed up by WHO Europe as follows:

> Non-smokers are also affected by the social consequences of tobacco. Although the risk to a non-smoker's health from breathing environmental tobacco smoke is small compared with direct smoking, the existence of this risk is real. Moreover, it has symbolic importance because it is a clear infringement of the non-smoker's personal liberty. When they smoke in public, smokers put not only their own health but also that of others at increased risk. This knowledge has created an entirely new argument in the debate about

the right of smokers versus those of non-smokers where clearly the latter's right not to have an increased health risk imposed on them might prevail.[2]

A draft Charter Against Tobacco for Europe produced at the WHO First European Conference of Tobacco Policy states that:

1 Fresh air which is free from tobacco smoke is an essential component of the fundamental right to a healthy and unpolluted environment.
2 All citizens have the right to smoke-free air in enclosed public places and transport.
3 Every worker has the right to breathe air in the workplace which is unpolluted by tobacco smoke.

The draft charter goes on to identify a number of strategies for the elimination of death and disability caused by tobacco smoking which includes:

1 the need to recognize and maintain the people's right to a smoke-free life (i.e. the fresh air norm) and
2 the need to establish in law the right to smoke-free common environments.

Clearly, any effective smoking-control policy today must recognize the right for non-smokers to breathe fresh air and to be protected from other people's cigarette smoking. This applies in all public places, all places of recreation, public transport and, most importantly, in the workplace. This right should also include the right of children to be free from tobacco smoke in the home!

Policy to control production and promotion of 'smokeless' tobacco and other new forms of tobacco or tobacco substitutes

The recent introduction of 'smokeless' tobacco to the United Kingdom markets and the establishment of a factory in Scotland to produce a product called 'skoal bandits' has emphasized the need for constant vigilance in monitoring the tactics of the tobacco industry, which is ever seeking new markets. Smokeless tobacco products are well established in some European countries and in the United States. Fortunately, the marketing of this product was a failure in the United Kingdom and the UK government are currently considering a total ban on the production and sale of smokeless tobacco products in the UK.

Bans on the importation and sale of smokeless tobacco have already been implemented in Hong Kong, Ireland, Israel and New Zealand. In countries where such products are permitted to be sold, health warnings should be required on all smokeless tobacco and on all new types of tobacco or tobacco substitutes introduced to the market and these should come under the same controls for advertising and promotion as existing tobacco products.

A levy on tobacco products to fund health-education programmes

A number of governments have now taken the step of allocating a proportion of their revenue from tobacco taxes to anti-smoking programmes. It certainly seems reasonable to use the income from tobacco products to help to combat the influence of the tobacco industry. The use of a levy to fund sponsorship of sporting and other events in the place of tobacco sponsorship is an attractive proposition and has been introduced successfully in the state of Victoria, Australia. The draft recommendations from the WHO Regional Office for Europe's Madrid Conference include the recommendation that a levy of at least 1 per cent of tobacco revenue should be made to fund specific tobacco-control and health-promotion activities.

Health-education and information programmes and help for smokers wishing to stop

Public education and information programmes designed to reduce the incidence of smoking by persuading those smokers who can easily stop smoking to do so, and non-smokers not to start, are of prime importance in any smoking-control programme. It is now recognized that in addition it is necessary to provide help for smokers who need support during the cessation process[19]. There is no wonder cure for smokers who wish to give up. For some it is apparently easy, for others exceedingly difficult. However, the vast majority of those who do succeed in stopping smoking do so on their own.

Public information programmes

The dividing line between public 'information' and 'education' programmes is somewhat blurred; however, they complement and reinforce each other. An ongoing public information programme will provide the background and social climate necessary for a successful public education programme. The mass media have played an important role in encouraging people to stop smoking. Successful smoking and health programmes involving mass-media campaigns include the UK's National No Smoking Day, now into its sixth year. Evaluation of this campaign in 1986[20] suggested that up to 50 000 smokers may have given up smoking permanently as a result of the campaign. Such campaigns provide reinforcement for smoking and health activities at local-community level, including those aimed at specific target groups. The importance of public information/publicity campaigns is that they help to keep the smoking 'issue' constantly in the public eye.

Public education programmes

Public education programmes about smoking should be designed to reach specific target groups. These will include young people at school, adolescents who have left school, high-risk groups (for example, young women) and other adult smokers. As well as including information about the harmful effects of tobacco use and its addictive nature, such programmes should also provide motivation to stop and teach 'how-to-stop' and 'how-to-stay-stopped' skills. They should also stress the positive image of non-smoking and the need for a non-smoking 'norm' in society in the light of new evidence on passive smoking.

Helping people to stop

The role of education about smoking is to persuade people to attempt to stop; their consequent success or failure will depend on their motivation, will power and knowledge of what is at stake as far as the health risks are concerned and the benefits of stopping. However, we still have much to learn about why people become dependent on tobacco, and why some smokers can stop with little effort while others cannot. In the UK, for example, about half of all smokers have given up in the past decade or so; of the half who still smoke, surveys show that at least two-thirds are reluctant smokers[21]. There are, in fact, many individual smokers who have not been able to respond to the challenge to break their dependence on nicotine. They need something more, and only intervention programmes which recognize the need for support during the cessation process, which teach 'how-to-stop' skills and deal with the problems of withdrawal, will meet the needs of this large body of dissonant smokers, many of whom may be heavier, more dependent smokers, and especially at risk from smoking-induced disease[22]. Thus it is crucial that smoking-control policies include the provision of support for those smokers who need help in stopping.

Obviously the greatest benefit to the largest number of smokers will be achieved by the widespread availability of such support. This can be provided by primary health-care professionals who are in a unique position to help many smokers to stop[23]. Health professionals have two important roles: to model non-smoking behaviour and to help their patients to stop. The UICC *Guidelines on Smoking Cessation*[19] states:

> Smoking cessation treatment is part of the duties of any health professional working inside or outside the hospital and in whatever specialty of medicine. It has importance in disease prevention, the treatment of disease and as part of a comprehensive rehabilitation procedure.

Training for health professionals in how to provide support and counselling for their patients and in the effective use of available pharmacological intervention is, therefore, a priority. Other 'stop-smoking' programmes, such as those in the workplace and those directed at adolescents, should also form part of an overall tobacco-control policy.

References

1 Doll, R. (1988) Tobacco Related Diseases, plenary address given at the WHO European Conference on Tobacco Policy, Madrid, November 1988.

2 WHO Europe (1988) *A Five Year Action Plan*, Smoke Free Europe, Copenhagen, November.

3 WHO Europe (1988) *The Physician's Role*, Smoke Free Europe 1, Copenhagen, November.

4 WHO Europe (1988) *Legislative Strategies for a Smoke Free Europe*, Smoke Free Europe 2, Copenhagen, November.

5 WHO Europe (1988) *The Evaluation and Monitoring of Public Action on Tobacco*, Smoke Free Europe 3, Copenhagen, November.

6 WHO Europe (1988) *Tobacco or Health*, Smoke Free Europe 4, Copenhagen, November.

7 WHO Europe (1988) *Helping Smokers Stop*, Smoke Free Europe 5, Copenhagen, November.

8 WHO Europe (1988) *Planning for a Smoke Free Generation*, Smoke Free Europe 6, Copenhagen, November.

9 WHO Europe (1988) *The Dying of the Light*, Smoke Free Europe 7, Copenhagen, November.

10 WHO Europe (1988) *Pushing Smoke*, Smoke Free Europe 8, Copenhagen, November.

11 WHO Europe (1988) *Tobacco Price and the Smoking Epidemic*, Smoke Free Europe 9, Copenhagen, November.

12 Commission of European Communities (1988) *Proposal for a Council Directive on the Approximation of the Laws, Regulations and Administrative Provisions of the Member States concerning the Maximum Tar Yield of Cigarettes*, 88/C48/10, February.

13 Malhotra, S. P. (1988) FAO, The Economic Significance of Tobacco and the Future Outlook, plenary address given at WHO European Conference on Tobacco Policy, Madrid, November.

14 Ulster Cancer Foundation (1986) *The Economic Consequences of Smoking in Northern Ireland*, November.

15 WHO Europe (1985) Health Behaviour in Schoolchildren: a cross-national survey, Copenhagen.

16 US Surgeon General, Report on Passive Smoking, Report of the Surgeon General, US Department of Health and Human Services, Maryland.

17 Riboli, E. (1988) The Health Effects of Exposure to Environmental Tobacco Smoke, IARC plenary address given at WHO European Conference on Tobacco Policy, Madrid, November.

18 Fourth Report of UK Government's Independent Scientific Committee on Passive Smoking (1988) HMSO, London.

19 Kunze, M. and Wood, M. (1984) *Guidelines on Smoking Cessation*, UICC, Geneva.

20 Linthwaite, P. (1986) National No Smoking Day 1986, *Hlth Ed. J.* **45**, 243–44.

21 UK National Opinion Polls, 1977–79.

22 Wood, M. A. (1986) Stop Smoking Campaigns—the need for more integrated strategies, *Hlth Ed. Res.* **1**, 4, 333–6.

23 Ramstrom, L., Raw, M., Wood, M. (eds.)(1988) *Guidelines on Smoking Cessation for the Primary Health Care Team*, WHO/UICC, Geneva.

Paper 6.4

INTERNATIONAL UNION AGAINST CANCER (UICC) PROGRAMME ON SMOKING AND CANCER

Professor Michael Kunze
Institute for Social Medicine, University of Vienna, Vienna, Austria

Philosophy of the programme

This programme offers:

1 an agreed international policy;

2 a discussion opportunity;

3 a focal meeting for national/regional groups;

4 expertise for:
   (a) analysis of local problems
   (b) establishment of opportunities
   (c) development of solutions and priorities.

UICC policy objectives regarding smoking control

1 achievement of lower smoking rates in all age groups of the population. This implies the application of whatever downward pressures on smoking rates are practical. These might include health warnings on packets, taxation manipulation, restrictions on smoking opportunities, encouragement of the rights of the non-smoker, as well as measures such as are involved in political, publicity and education programmes.

2 the encouragement of non-smokers to remain non-smokers. The emphasis of this programme is on youth.

3 the cessation of all forms of tobacco promotion.

4 those who have not yet stopped smoking, and therefore remain at high risk, should be encouraged to reduce, as far as possible, their exposure to harmful components of tobacco smoke.

5 to maintain liaison with other health organizations and authorities to ensure maximum effectiveness and avoid conflict of activities.

6 to achieve public health control of relevant industrial and environmental factors which contribute to lung cancer.

Charter Against Tobacco for Europe

First European Conference on Tobacco Policy in Madrid, November 1988

Fresh air which is free from tobacco smoke is an essential component of the fundamental RIGHT to a healthy and unpolluted environment.

Every child and adolescent has the RIGHT to be protected from all tobacco promotion and to receive all necessary educational and other help to resist the temptation to start using tobacco in any form.

All citizens have the RIGHT to smoke-free air in enclosed public places and transport.

Every worker has the RIGHT to breathe air in the workplace which is unpolluted by tobacco smoke.

Every smoker has the RIGHT to receive encouragement and help to overcome the habit.

Each citizen has the RIGHT to be informed of the unparalleled health risks of tobacco use.

State of the art of smoking cessation

Cessation now has enough scientific background to be implemented much more than before.

Cessation means offering a wide variety of techniques and methods for different target groups, different organizational structures with different levels of assistance for the smoker.

Many smokers do not need any help to stop smoking or only a little motivation, whereas others need a lot of assistance or formal treatment.

There are at least three groups of techniques:

- methods to help the already highly motivated, low-dependency smoker (mass-media-assisted techniques, simple brochures, self-help techniques)
- methods to help the motivated, rather highly dependent smokers (nicotine replacement therapy)
- basic to all the other intervention techniques are methods to create and maintain motivation (health education, public information, public education).

Chapter 7

THE NEED FOR INTEGRATED ACTION: EXAMPLES OF GOOD PRACTICE

Summary

The Lisbon Colloquium working groups frequently emphasized the need for integrated action when planning cancer prevention:

A All those who might be involved in policy development and planning—or whose activities might be affected by such plans—first of all need education about the urgent need for action to reduce the risks of cancers. In addition, all those who could promote (or impede!) such policies and plans should be involved at the earliest possible time in the development of the programmes.

B The implementation of plans can often place demands on a variety of service deliverers and plenty of preparation time is needed before the public programme is launched. Any health authority that has experienced the backlog of cytological investigations of possible melanomas that builds up after premature popular media coverage of 'how to examine your skin for suspicious moles' can vouch for the ill will and consternation that unplanned health education can generate.

C The opposition of those whose livelihood may be threatened by proposed behavioural change in the population must be taken into account. How can they be persuaded of the urgent need to reduce cancer risks? Can a benefit for them be built into the programme? What alternative pricing or legislative strategies may have to be invoked to make it easier for people to change their ways in the face of those who could be said to promote ill health?

D Health promotion programmes to prevent cancers must be able to prove that they work and should define the criteria by which they are prepared to be judged. They must have integrated plans for evaluation and an allocated budget to achieve this.

Integrated action

Integrated action involves the smooth working together of many parts. If the many parts (possible cancer-prevention activities) can be planned together, they can make an integrated (whole) programme. This programme can be more effective in action and outcomes than separate and possibly disorganized projects.

The Lisbon Colloquium attempted to model this integration by bringing together a wide range of equal but diverse experts to consider the issues involved in cancer prevention. Feedback after the Colloquium revealed that most participants found this stimulating and rewarding and the sheer volume of background discussion papers, discussion notes from the working groups and television interviews generated during the Colloquium convinced the organizers that the whole was indeed greater than its parts!

It became clear that, as in the Colloquium, the development of a cancer-prevention programme involves integrated teamwork. Though there may be elements of professional rivalry about the contributions of the separate expert domains, there was a shared commitment to protecting the health and well being of the community. At the Colloquium, funded as it was by the EC Europe Against Cancer project, a picture of the health needs of an integrated but diverse European community emerged.

Planned integration Such integration ought to be a key component of the development and delivery of cancer education programmes. Particular attention should be given to ensuring:

- multisectoral involvement in the development of the programme;
- delivery as part of health promotion and community development;
- implementation by multiprofessional teams;
- assessment by integrated evaluation;
- avoidance of analysis/paralysis.

1 Multisectoral involvement in the development of the programme

Integrated programmes usually require multisectoral involvement, with all interested parties working together.

Commitment to the need for action The demand for the development of a health policy for cancer prevention should not be seen as coming only from health experts. The report of a joint WHO/Welsh Heart Programme Workshop[1] points out that:

> Acquiring and maintaining support from politicians, the public and professionals is essential to the success of programmes in health promotion. Backing from one sector will influence the degree of support from other sectors. Professionals are more likely to support activities for which there is public enthusiasm; similarly, the public is more likely to endorse a programme which is seen as credible by professional groups. Political decision makers will provide resources more readily for health promotion when this accords with community aspirations and where there is overt professional endorsement.

DIOLCH AM BEIDIO SMYGU
PLEASE DO NOT SMOKE
Mae'r Sefydliad hwn yn cefnogi
This Establishment supports HEARTBEAT WALES
CURIAD CALON CYMRU

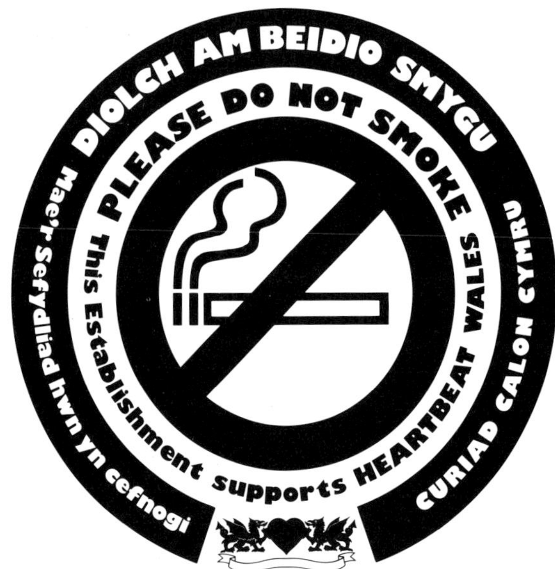

Figure 7.1 The lessons learned from coronary heart disease programmes are highly relevant to cancer prevention.

The Lisbon Colloquium urged the EC Europe Against Cancer project to press for integrated health policy making within the European Community.

Development of policies This includes not only health policies as such, but also all other policies that can affect health. Health policy development should involve informing and consulting the community and those health workers who must deliver the programmes.

Planning Coordinated plans and action are essential where different groups of health professionals have the shared responsibility for achieving a common goal. The Colloquium wished to emphasize the importance of primary prevention. Obviously, it is better to avoid cancers developing in the first place, but with some cancers, early detection with effective treatment that truly extends survival, rather than just lead-in, time must be encouraged. Further research should lead to more effective treatment plans. Since, in screening, a good case can be made for identifying higher risk groups for earlier or additional screening, the hope is that current ongoing research will pinpoint easily identified genetic, biochemical or cellular mishaps, inherited or acquired, whose presence indicates a greater risk, though by no means the inevitability, of developing specific cancers.

Strategies These include not just health education but also 'alternative strategies' that make it easier for people to act on such advice. Implementation of diverse strategies, which together should have a synergistic effect on risk reduction, should be carefully coordinated. The introduction of pricing policies to restrict the supply or demand of products that contribute to ill health, and of subsidies to promote demand for healthier alternatives, certainly pose a challenge requiring sensitive multisectoral negotiation.

2 Delivery as part of health promotion and community development

Cancer prevention can best be delivered and is more acceptable to the public when presented as part of a health promotion programme. Such programmes should aim at enabling individuals and communities to take greater control over the factors affecting their health and be related to existing community groups' interests and actions.

The general principles of health promotion have been well examined in a series of reports of workshops held as part of the WHO European Office Health Promotion Programme. Early workshops considered 'Concepts and Principles of Health Promotion' and 'Research in Health Promotion'. Their 1985 'Health Promotion—The practical aspects of programme implementation: a report of a joint WHO/Welsh Heart Programme Workshop'[1] is of most immediate relevance to this chapter and is highly recommended further reading. This workshop used the Welsh Heart Programme as a case study: the lessons learned are highly relevant and easily transferred to cancer-prevention work within a health-promotion approach.

3 Implementation by multiprofessional teams

> It is all too easy for competition to arise out of changes in working practice. This is detrimental to the health interests of the community and it is important, therefore, to clarify professional roles at the earliest possible opportunity. Credible and respected representatives of the relevant professions should be involved in this process of clarification.[1]

4 Assessment by integrated evaluation

Evaluators, who are seen as part of the development team, should be involved in planning for evaluation from the start of the programme. The team should agree in advance the criteria by which the programme should be judged. Evaluation should be made of the process as well as of the outcomes.

5 Avoidance of 'analysis/paralysis'

Whilst there is a need to understand the rhetoric of integrated action, in practice the reality will fall short of the ideal. Cancer-prevention programmes are about saving lives and reducing ill health so it is better to start a programme in which the shortcomings and barriers have been identified and understood rather than delay too long in the hope of achieving a perfectly coordinated start. Starting 'soon enough' with a 'good enough' programme may be acceptable. But it is not acceptable to plunge in with a project which is:

- ill conceived—because no-one thought through whether the proposed intervention could achieve the desired objective. For example, there is no point in educating people to change to a diet that contains plenty of fresh fruit and vegetables if fresh produce is not available in the local shops or is too expensive for the average budget.
- impossible to evaluate—because the proposed strategies were either not tested in a pilot stage or a system was not devised that would allow collection of the data needed to judge the effectiveness of the intervention. For example, baseline data of dependent variables cannot be collected after the intervention has begun!

The background discussion papers, all of which are available as a three-volume set from the Open University (see footnote on page 7), provided many examples of individual projects from which certain elements could be transferred into a larger integrated programme. The papers chosen for this chapter provide worked examples or models for the development of the types of integrated action outlined above.

The Stockholm Cancer Prevention Programme: an integrated community-based intervention

EC-member countries have much to learn from Sweden in terms of how to organize and evaluate an integrated community intervention model for primary prevention of cancers. This is recognized by the EC cancer group who decided to involve Sweden in its EC's Europe Against Cancer initiative. Holm and Haglund (Paper 7.1) describe The Stockholm Cancer Prevention Programme—Strategies for Primary Prevention of Cancer.

The rest of Europe will follow with interest the continued implementation and evaluation of this programme and further reports will become available from the Karolinska Institute.

A protected programme Perhaps the greatest strength of this programme is that it was founded on a consensus among political parties. This is a very important factor, since it enables health programmes, which by their nature are long term, to span over several electoral periods. The politicians have also participated actively during the planning phase and contributed to the programme design.

Responsibility for planning is at the right level In Sweden, responsibility for cancer education and health promotion rests at county-council level. At this level, health workers may be expected to be able to collect highly relevant health data and to build up a specific knowledge of potential local collaborators.

Community-based intervention They adopted a community-based intervention strategy because:

> ... the majority of those who develop cancer do not belong to the groups having extremely high risk factor values, but rather those having only slightly or moderately elevated risk levels. Prevention must therefore aim at changing the life styles of the entire population. ... The medical profession working together with politicians, administrators, social scientists, and representatives from public and voluntary organizations, focuses activities on the society as a whole. (Paper 7.1)

Intervention and delivery through existing networks The cost of this programme remains reasonable because, on sound health-promotion principles, they decided that: 'The preventive activities will be carried out within the framework of existing organizations and will be financed through their own resources as far as possible.' Indeed, the main emphasis was that the cancer-education programme itself should primarily intervene *indirectly* via existing organizations, rather than mount a mass education programme directly to the public.

Identification of collaborators They used a community diagnosis model and this involved a systematic mapping of potential collaborators. These collaborators included:

- those involved along the food supply chain;
- occupational health organizations;
- health and medical-care organizations;
- municipalities, i.e. the subdivisions of the county holding local responsibility for provision of education, social-welfare services and community care of the elderly;
- voluntary organizations;
- the mass media.

Points of intervention The Stockholm programme seeks to measure reduced risk factors (measurable intermediate variables, rather than changes in morbidity and mortality) within the target population. Of course, this involves individual behavioural change. However, analysis and due attention was given to two areas that affect individual behavioural change: social norms, and the available choice of goods and services. These areas, in turn, can be affected by socio-political issues and also by the laws and regulations that can play a part in determining the supply and demand of goods and services. There is thus a chain of potential points of indirect intervention. The model for the Stockholm programme's intervention policy is explained in detail by

Sanderson and Svanstrom[2]. The next paper in this chapter (Paper 7.2) expands this analysis of alternative points of intervention, with particular reference to the use of tobacco.

Integrated health-promotion strategies

In Paper 7.2 Martin Moreno and Mendoza explain how to calculate epidemiological variables that can be used to monitor progress in cancer-reduction programmes. The data for Spain, even though they are based on several estimated values, serve to raise awareness of the severity of the problem, for example smoking-related cancers, in both the general public and amongst those responsible for developing health policies.

They also acknowledge the value of the base-line data from the EC's Europe Against Cancer Survey, Europeans and the Prevention of Cancer, in planning national and regional-level programmes. They point out that:

> These differences observed between the knowledge and practice of determined patterns of behaviour serve to remind us that the life style of a community is dependent upon a diversity of cultural, geographical, economic, educational and political factors.

Alternative strategies

The paper considers a health-promotion approach to preventing cancers:

> ... combining a wide variety of political measures with educational measures aimed at individuals and communities. ... It is not merely a question of providing information on its origin and how it can be prevented but also making the healthier options (for example, the consumption of low-fat foods) more accessible physically, economically and culturally.

The authors examine in detail the alternative strategies that are the key to a comprehensive tobacco-control policy: measures to decrease tobacco supply and measures to decrease tobacco demand.

A tobacco control policy was urged by almost all participants at the Lisbon Colloquium. There was pressure to demand that all European Community governments legislate against tobacco—and that the EC should add its weight to this argument. It was also agreed that those involved in health-promotion work must also be trained in how to educate, influence and advise politicians and policy makers .

The Andalusian initiative

A comprehensive and integrated policy underlies the Andalusian Tobacco or Health Programme, which was started in 1988. This excellently planned programme includes such diverse elements as education and training for health workers, educators and journalists, the signposting of non-smoking areas in public buildings in line with central government norms, and the drawing up of norms to develop legislation against infringement of anti-tobacco laws. They are fortunate to have the support of an actively involved Ministry of Health and Consumer Affairs. It is hoped that Spain's commitment to tackling issues of health and social welfare policy will be reflected in EC initiatives developed while they currently (1989) hold the EC presidency.

Planned evaluation

Evaluation of the *process* and *outcomes* of educational interventions is a specialist area little known to the general run of medical cancer experts. In any case, their judgement of what constitutes evaluation is coloured by the necessity for the rigorous experimental proof necessary in scientific research.

Acceptable criteria

There seems, at times, to be a hierarchy—which needs to be challenged—of acceptable validation:

- scientific proof of biological oncogenic processes;
- validation of drug interventions and comparison of treatment plans;
- collection, calculation and interpretation of epidemiological variables to establish the risk factors for cancers;

- measurement of 'hard data' outcomes (morbidity and mortality figures) of health programmes, which are usually required to have a quasi-experimental basis;
- monitoring intermediate variables (for example, risk factor reduction, such as serum cholesterol level measurements, or reported behavioural change, such as level of cigarette smoking) which may or may not be entirely attributable to the health-programme interventions;
- evaluation of such educational objectives as increased knowledge or attitudinal change;
- pilot testing the strategies and scrutiny of the process, i.e. how the health intervention programme was planned and delivered.

Evaluation of intermediate outcomes and of the process of planning and delivery can be less valued and therefore difficult to fund. But there is a body of knowledge that can be used to define the criteria by which educational—and most health promotional—programmes can be evaluated.

Planning for evaluation

Evaluation of a programme must be planned from the start. Too often, such planning is not done because funding for it is not part of the planned budget. However, since evaluation can seldom be successfully added on afterwards, it should always be built in at the planning stage. Indeed, the intellectual effort of planning for evaluation can often highlight weaknesses in the planning and strategies for implementation of the programme! It can serve, also, to make clear the constraints—some of which are political—on the proposed intervention. In an ideal world, health promotion planners would refuse, on ethical grounds, to proceed with a programme that did not have funding for evaluation. But, as a minimum, it should be considered ethically unacceptable to develop a plan that does not identify what evaluation could and should be done.

The authors of the papers in this chapter all consider the problems of evaluation. For example, Holm and Haglund acknowledge that the political consensus so vital to the long-term protection of the Stockholm programme has, however, affected the options for evaluation because, as there was a political commitment to offer the programme to the whole population, a quasi-experimental design with a matched control group could not be used. They discuss the options for formative and summative evaluation and justify the pragmatic monitoring of intermediate variables.

Integrated planning within a health authority

Paper 7.3, A District Health Promotion *Plan for Cancer: Developed by the Cancer Education Co-ordinating Group of the United Kingdom and the Republic of Ireland* (McEwen *et al.*) points out that the challenge is for all EC countries to develop plans *at a sufficiently local level* for community specificity to be ensured and where all those working at a local-community level can reasonably be expected to cooperate. Fortunately, at this level of specificity and size, evaluation can more easily be planned. Formative evaluation that, perhaps by pilot studies, establishes the acceptability and effectiveness of the process is particularly important since the interventions must be tailor-made to the needs of the community.

A national policy has to be translated into detailed local plans. Such plans, requiring an integrated intersectoral approach, are difficult to develop and implement. The development of the plan needs the carefully synchronized involvement of all those who must collaborate. The collaboration must be in the development as well as the delivery if the programme is not to be discarded as a 'top-down' imposition. It takes time to involve key people from the professions and the community so that they can feel they 'own' the plan, to provide education for all those involved, to clarify professional roles and to provide additional training where necessary. There has to be ample lead-in time before the programme is launched publicly.

Three key precepts are therefore:

- Don't start public education too soon.
- Get the superstructure in place first.

- Walk alongside collaborators rather than pushing or pulling them along.

Paper 7.3 provides a model of how to develop such a plan.

A part of Health Promotion Paper 7.3 emphasizes in its title that cancer prevention must be presented within a *health promotion* plan. The paper quotes, from the WHO European Regional Office (1984), a summary of the key principles of health promotion:

> At a general level, health promotion has come to represent a unifying concept for those who recognize the need for change in the ways and conditions of living, in order to promote health. Health promotion represents a mediating strategy between people and their environments, synthesizing personal choice and social responsibility in health to create a healthier future.

An educational task Education must first be directed to generating at district level an 'awareness of need' amongst the general public and amongst those who determine health-related policies.

Existing health-promotion activities First, find out what is already going on; not all cancer-education work has to go under a cancer project label. So look at 'whole health' promotion programmes, coronary heart disease-prevention programmes, and anti-smoking and healthy diet campaigns. Many of the points in the European Code Against Cancer are already built into 'whole health' programmes. They may even be getting the message across about the behavioural changes needed to reduce cancer risks without even mentioning the word cancer.

Cost-effectiveness Paper 7.3 addresses the difficult question of whether the cost-effectiveness of cancer *education* can be proved. What data would be needed? Should one seek to justify this educational intervention on the grounds of cost-effectiveness? Are there basic humanitarian grounds for doing this? One can also make comparative cost-effectiveness analyses.

NÃO FUME
PELA SUA SAÚDE!
Conselho de Prevenção do Tabagismo

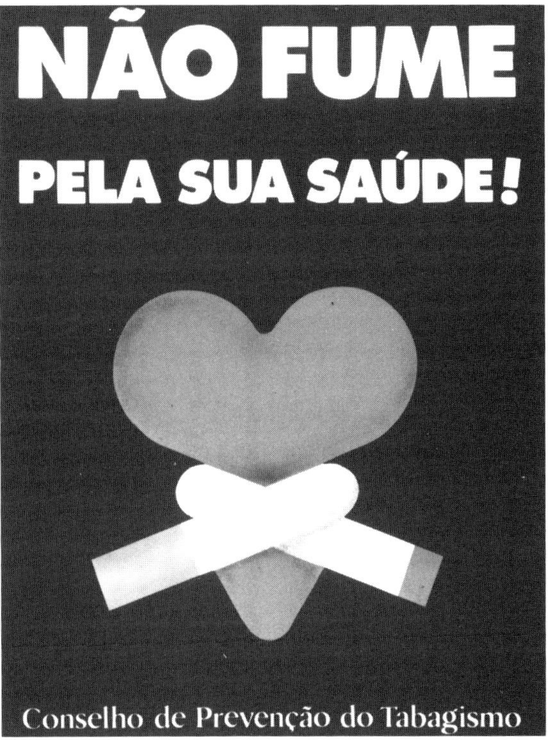

Figure 7.2 Anti-smoking campaigns reduce the risk of heart disease (and chronic respiratory diseases) as well as the risk of cancer.

A challenge for Europe?

At a district-equivalent level throughout Europe, policy makers and planners could use the model plan provided in Paper 7.3 to:

- review what is already being done;
- determine what needs to be done;
- decide who could do it;
- work out what it would cost;
- specify the criteria for success;
- set a timetable for its implementation.

What a challenge! But who makes the challenge? Whose responsibility is it to respond to it? And who does the work? If the rhetoric of the Colloquium is to be turned into action, those who know the potential progress that can be made in cancer control—and this includes informed members of the general public as well as cancer experts—must put pressure on health policy makers at a national level to take action to reduce the risks of cancers. And this pressure should be reinforced by the action of the European Community.

Getting the message across (the title of the Colloquium), whilst at first sight focusing on 'what shall we tell the people?', in reality involves getting the message across to politicians and policy makers. Participants at the Colloquium were all key people in their own countries in the field of cancer and cancer education and by a discussion process similar to that modelled at the Colloquium could educate the multi-professional group of people concerned with developing health policies within their own countries. Establishing a high-level multi-professional cancer-education coordination group plays a key part in educating those who could, once convinced of the need, commit resources to cancer-control programmes. Once there is a policy of commitment to reducing the risks of cancers, there are good models of planning and project implementation that can be adapted to culturally specific programmes.

Educational implications The working groups at the Lisbon Colloquium drew attention on many occasions to the wide range of educational interventions that are needed to 'get the message across' to the right people. The full discussion notes will inform the development of additional education and training materials by the Open University (see below).

Integration within Europe The three-year action programme of the Commission of the European Community's Europe Against Cancer Division contained some 75 objectives, with an emphasis on health information to promote the prevention of cancer. The programmes culminated in 1989 as Europe Against Cancer Year. As part of this Year's activities, the Open University (UK) organized, and the Commission financed, the Lisbon Colloquium and its products—three volumes of background papers especially commissioned for the Colloquium from key cancer experts and educationists in Europe; this book; and a video programme that was mainly recorded at the Colloquium, which illustrates the actions required at many levels to reduce the risks of tobacco-related cancers.

In May 1989, as this book went to press, the Commission put forward proposals for a second action programme against cancer for 1990 to 1994 that will build on the substantial outcomes of the first programme. The priorities will be cancer prevention, information and health education, training of the health professionals, and research on cancer. This programme should also prove to be a model for concerted European action to protect Europe's greatest asset: the health of the people.

This book has identified the wide-ranging target audience for education about the need and possibilities for reducing the risk of cancers. It has also surveyed the many levels of integrated planning and action that are required for effective implementation of cancer-prevention programmes. The difficulties that face those involved in such work could be appreciated if the principles and recommendations in this book were applied to the suggestion that Europe should adopt the Australian skin-cancer prevention campaign. Those involved in integrated action across Europe will have to face the types of complex problems that this case poses:

Australia has very effective education projects on malignant melanoma prevention, which are carried out on the beaches—where the risk population is concentrated! The two main education projects are:

- 'Slip! Slap! Slop!' (Slip on a vest, slap on a hat and slop on some sunscreen.)
- 'Stay under a tree from eleven to three.' (Stay out of the midday sun.)

This type of education is needed on the beaches of the Mediterranean for fair-skinned holiday-makers from the northern European countries. What might be involved in developing and gaining acceptance for a similar European policy and in delivering the programme? Who needs to be educated about melanoma prevention to achieve commitment to and implementation of this programme? What alternative strategies might be needed to ensure this programme could be put into practice? '

DON'T FORGET KIDS
SLIP! on a shirt.
SLOP! on a sunscreen.
SLAP! on a hat.
And have a nice day!
ANTI-CANCER FOUNDATION TEL. (08) 267 5222

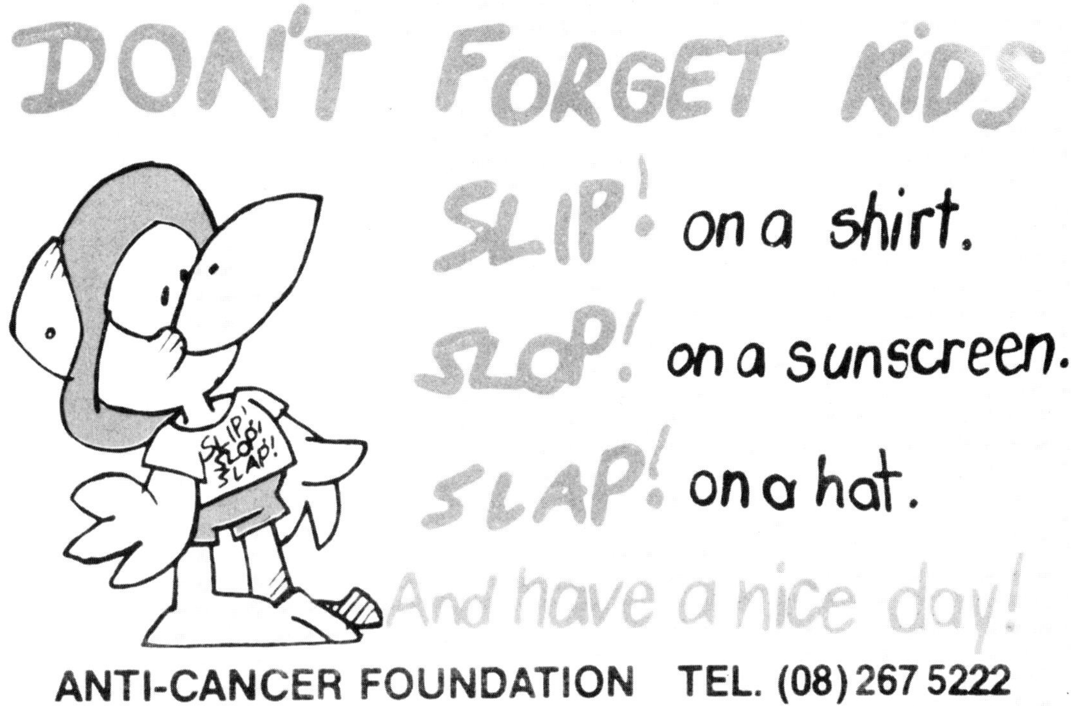

Figure 7.3 Australian campaign slogan for reducing the risk of cancers. A similar campaign in Europe would require carefully integrated plans.

Education and training for health workers

Overcoming negative or depressed attitudes Fundamentally, all of this planning could be wasted if the general public still does not accept that many cancers can be cured and are more likely to be cured if they are detected early. Where fear of cancers is too high, even advice on how to avoid getting one may not be heard.

Even well intentioned cancer-prevention programmes can raise fears, but these can be minimized if the key message about cure and early detection is included with the advice on how to reduce the risks. The programmes should also educate all workers with whom the general public may come into contact on how to answer questions from the general public about cancers and their treatments—including pain management. Worried people all too often ask the first person they come across, and may be put off by evasive or simplistic answers.

Is isn't only members of the general public who hold negative or depressed attitudes to cancer prevention. Ironically, many health workers may also be pessimistic about the value of cancer-prevention programmes. Medical students[3] and cancer-ward nurses, who may never have worked in out-patients where the survivors show up, or otherwise have encountered former cancer patients, are particularly likely to be negative. Contact, as part of their training, with former patients who work in cancer support groups might change these attitudes as well as provide feedback on the difficulties of doctor–cancer patient communication[4].

New ways of working The Colloquium recognized that there is a need for additional training of some health professionals so that they can combine both a good knowledge of cancers (the risk factors, detection, prognosis and treatment options) and the theory and practice of health education and promotion.

Working within an integrated team in health promotion can raise anxieties about professional boundaries and personal competency, which the provision of programme-specific education and training can help to minimize:

> Just as health promotion should seek to minimize anxiety about health in the public at large, it is also important to ensure that programmes in health promotion do not generate concern among those professionals who are called upon to change their working practices. Health promotion is a dynamic process and one consequence for health practitioners and other professionals is that they should be prepared regularly to review their practices and adopt new methods of working. The intention of many programmes is to assimilate a centrally coordinated activity into the everyday work of certain professionals at the local level. The mechanism for transferring knowledge and skills should be made explicit in programme plans. It is necessary, however, to ensure that expectations of professionals' involvement are realistic in the light of their knowledge, skills and other commitments. Further education and training may be necessary prior to any change in role or practice. This has implications for Professional Associations in that there may be a need to devise new courses for professional development.[1]

An Open University contribution

The Open University (UK) is planning to produce courses for health workers and for the general public on the prevention of cancers. It is planned to include this book as a course reader to support the study programme. As well as the origins of cancers, their risk factors and what behavioural changes are needed to minimize these risks, the courses will explore the policy making and planning of health-promotion initiatives within the EC and its member countries.

References

1 Report of a joint WHO/Welsh Heart Programme Workshop (1985) *Health Promotion: the practical aspects of programme implementation*, WHO Europe, Copenhagen.

2 Sanderson, C. and Svanstrom, L. (1988) Contributions of social medicine and systems analysis to formulating objectives for a community-based cancer prevention programme, *Scand. J. Soc.Med.* **16**, 35–40.

3 Polyzos,A., Daskalopoulou, E., Koletti, E., Sfikakis, P. (1989) Clinical experience and style of life in undergraduate medicine, *J. of Cancer Ed.* **4**, supp. 1.

4 Buitenhuis, E. C., van der Ploeg-Aarnout, A. J., Jongsma-Ebbelink, M., Haagedoorn, E. M. L. (1989) A result of student interaction with volunteers of a reach-to-recovery group, *J. of Cancer Ed.* **4**, supp. 1.

Paper 7.1

STRATEGIES FOR PRIMARY PREVENTION OF CANCERS: THE STOCKHOLM CANCER PREVENTION PROGRAMME

Dr. Lars-Erik Holm
Department of Cancer Prevention, Karolinska Hospital, Stockholm, Sweden

Dr. Bo J. A. Haglund
Department of Social Medicine, Karolinska Institute, Sundbyberg, Sweden

Introduction

The incidence of specific cancers varies from one part of the world to another. Cancer of the breast, prostate, colon and rectum are common in the western hemisphere and uncommon in Africa and Asia. Epidemiological and experimental studies have shown that the majority of all cancers are influenced by extrinsic factors, some of which could be avoided once identified. Environmental and life-style factors are believed to play an important role in 70 to 90 per cent of all cancers[1,2]. Many of these factors are not unique to cancers but are risk factors for other chronic diseases, for example cardiovascular diseases, as well.

If the increase in the annual number of cancer cases were to continue at its current rate, one Swede in three would get cancer at some time during his or her lifetime by the year 2000. Furthermore, by the year 2050, every other Swede would be stricken with cancer if this trend were to continue. We can better understand the impact of such a forecast if we realize that we are discussing our present generation of children.

Our situation is similar to the situation in the rest of Europe and in the United States, and demands new means for combating cancer. The American National Cancer Institute states as its objective a 25 to 50 per cent reduction in the 1980 mortality rate[3]. The achievement of this goal depends, to a great degree, on primary prevention, such as reducing tobacco smoking and the adoption of a low-fat, high-fibre diet by all Americans.

The World Health Organization's target with regard to cancer mortality in Europe is a 15 per cent reduction by the year 2000. One of the objectives is to minimize the difference in the distribution of cancer among different socio-economic groups.

The Commission of the European Communities, in its action programme for combating cancer, emphasizes the importance of primary prevention, for example reducing tobacco consumption[4]. The Commission anticipates a decline in cancer mortality by 15 per cent if individuals are prepared to adopt healthier behaviours, and if legislation can be passed to improve the environment where they reside. These two strategies would result in the greatest possible benefit from existing knowledge about cancer prevention. The Council of the Nordic Countries (Nordiska Ministerrådet) also supports comprehensive action programmes aimed at cancer, with a focus on prevention.

The purpose of this paper is to report on a community-based strategy for cancer prevention in Stockholm county, Sweden.

Background to the project

Cancer is the second most common cause of death in Sweden and accounts for approximately 20 per cent of all deaths. The corresponding figure for Stockholm county is 24 per cent. The annual number of new cancer cases reported to the Stockholm Cancer Register has increased in Stockholm county by

86 per cent from 1958, the year the register was established. In 1986, 6900 new cases were reported. The age-standardized incidence has increased at a slower rate and in 1986 was 480 cases per 100 000 males and 386 per 100 000 females in 1986 (see Figure 7.4). Thirty-seven per cent of the cancer patients were less than 65 years at the time of diagnosis.

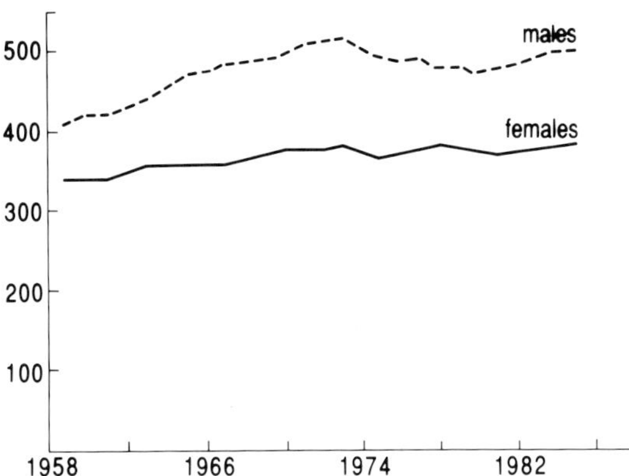

Figure 7.4 Age-standardized cancer incidence per 100 000 in the Stockholm county, Sweden, for the period 1958 to 1986.

The ten most common tumour sites for Stockholm men and women are shown in Table 7.1. Together these comprise 70 per cent of all tumours in males and 68 per cent of all tumours in women. The age-standardized incidence of stomach cancer in both sexes and cervical cancer in women has decreased by approximately 50 per cent since 1958. A rapid increase has, on the other hand, been observed for lung cancer in women (4 per cent per year) and malignant melanoma in both sexes (6 per cent per year).

In 1984, the Swedish Cancer Committee published its report on the causes of cancer in Sweden[2]. The committee's estimates, as shown in Table 7.2, are similar to those made by Doll and Peto for the USA[1]. Tobacco accounts for approximately 15 per cent of all cancer cases. Smoking control is therefore regarded as the most important measure for reducing risks for cancer. Dietary habits are estimated to play a major role in about 30 per cent of all cancers in Sweden with fat consumption believed to be the most significant single factor.

Table 7.1 The ten most common types of cancer in Stockholm county in 1986 in relation to sex

Males Type	%	Females Type	%
Prostate	20.6	Breast	25.1
Lung	13.0	Colon	7.8
Urinary bladder	7.1	Corpus uteri	5.3
Colon	6.5	Lung	5.3
Stomach	4.7	Ovary	4.9
Malignant melanoma	4.3	Malignant melanoma	4.0
Kidney	4.1	Rectum	3.8
Skin excluding melanoma	4.1	Stomach	3.3
Rectum	4.0	Pancreas	3.3
Pancreas	3.8	Skin excluding melanoma	4.1

The Swedish Cancer Committee has recommended a reduction in dietary fat intake from today's rate of 39 per cent of energy source, to 30 per cent. These guidelines coincide with those set up by the National Cancer Institute, USA, as well as by several other international bodies[5].

Current knowledge supports the notion that cancer is to a large extent preventable. The two most important causative factors for cancer are tobacco and dietary fat, which are in addition major risk factors for the development of heart disease and other chronic diseases found in western societies.

Table 7.2 Estimated importance of various risk factors for cancer incidence in Sweden (1983) according to the Swedish Cancer Committee[6]

Risk factor	Estimated % of total cancer incidence in Sweden
Tobacco smoking	15 (12–29)
Dietary factors	30
Other lifestyle factors	10
Infections	>2
Air pollution	1
Work environment	2
Physical factors	
Ionizing radiation excluding radon in homes	2
Radon in homes	<1
Ultraviolet radiation	5

In 1983, a new Swedish Health and Medical Services Act was passed. This Act endows the county councils with the responsibility for promoting health and providing equitable medical care for its residents. The Stockholm County Council is responsible for health and medical care in an area encompassing 25 municipalities with a total of 1.6 million inhabitants. The county's health plan includes a health-action programme addressing major public health issues. Highest priority was given to cancer prevention by the county politicians.

Also in 1983, plans were set in motion for a cancer-prevention programme when the Stockholm Cancer Prevention Programme (SCPP) was established in close cooperation with the county council's Department of Health Promotion and a number of scientific experts from the Karolinska Institute. The SCPP, following the traditions in Finland and the USA, utilizes community-based intervention as its strategy, the rationale being that the majority of those who develop cancer do not belong to groups having extremely high risk factor values, but rather to those that have only slightly or moderately elevated risk levels. Prevention must, therefore, aim at changing the life styles of the entire population[6]. In this type of preventive programme, the participation of the whole community in a process of behavioural change is expected to result in improved health for everyone. The medical profession, working together with politicians, administrators, social scientists and representatives from public and voluntary organizations, focuses its activities on the society as a whole.

The SCPP is the first community-based, health-action programme in Stockholm county and will serve as a model for other programmes in the county. In contrast to the American community-based programmes, but similar to the North Karelia programme in Finland, SCPP was initiated by regional and local politicians and was founded on a consensus among political parties. This is a very important factor as it enables health programmes, which by their nature are long term, to span over several electoral periods. The politicians also participated actively during the planning phase and contributed to the programme design.

The Stockholm Cancer Prevention Programme (SCPP)

The main objective of the SCPP is to reduce cancer incidence and mortality by reducing the risk factors related to life style. At present, SCPP focuses on three issues: tobacco, dietary habits, and sunbathing habits. Tobacco is the major single avoidable cause of cancer, whereas dietary factors together may affect a larger proportion of the cancer cases in Sweden[2]. The incidence of malignant melanoma has increased rapidly in Sweden during the past decades. Today scientists are gathering knowledge which points to the role of ultraviolet rays in the aetiology of this tumour.

The underlying philosophy of the SCPP is to stimulate organizations to take action that will influence the life styles of the people of Stockholm. This influence will be mediated through direct contact with people. In order to facilitate this contact, collaboration with a wide range of regional and nationwide organizations has been initiated. The preventive activities will be carried out within the framework of existing organizations and will be financed through their own resources as far as is possible.

The overall intervention model makes a clear distinction between three types of intervention activities:

- indirect activities involving the organizations themselves;
- direct contact by organizations with individuals to encourage them to alter their life styles;
- direct action by organizations to alter the environment, for example with respect to food supply, smoke-free areas, etc.

The community diagnosis model is a useful tool for developing implementation strategies in community intervention programmes. Methods such as interviewing key people, group interviews and also focus group methods have been used in the development of SCPP.

Since 1985 a systematic mapping has been made of potential collaborators. The following criteria have been used for selecting collaborators: potential impact in quantitative terms, potential impact in qualitative terms, feasibility and cost of implementation.

Based on these criteria, the following collaborators have been approached:

1 Food supply chains
These include producers, wholesalers, retailers, caterers and test kitchens. The food supply chain offers immense potential for influencing a large number of people at the point of purchase. This can be done at a relatively low cost to the project.

2 Occupational health organizations
There are approximately 200 occupational health centres in Stockholm county which serve 620 000 employees. More than half are affiliated to the county's five largest employers—the national government, the county council, the city of Stockholm, the building trade workers collective, and the consumers' cooperative. Each organization is run by a board made up of employees and employers. The present occupational health-care system has the potential to reach people in the workforce and more importantly, to teach them on the work site.

3 Health and medical care organizations
Stockholm County Council is one of the largest employers in Sweden with more than 75 000 employees, the majority of whom work in the health and medical services field. Medical care in Stockholm county accounts for 3.8 million outpatient contacts annually. There are 110 primary health-care centres in 42 primary health care districts. In accordance with the new Health and Medical Services Act, from 1983 each health centre is to be responsible for the health of the population within its own geographic area.

4 Municipalities
The 25 municipalities, which have populations ranging from 6000 to 600 000 inhabitants, are responsible for primary and secondary education, social services, child welfare and community care of the elderly. Our contacts with the local communities have focused on the catering services to schools, pre-schools, and homes for the elderly, as well as on health-promotion programmes in schools. The Swedish school system has enormous potential for reaching students, their parents and teachers. Such programmes can have a positive effect on children for their entire life.

5 Voluntary organizations
Voluntary organizations have been well integrated into Swedish society since the end of the 19th century. They include organizations that are built up around adult educational issues, such as sports and recreation, medical/social problems, church/ethnic affiliation, trade unions, retirement, and politics. A large proportion of the Stockholm population belongs to one or more voluntary organizations. Health promotion is already well established in a number of these organizations.

6 **Pharmacies**
Pharmacies in Sweden are state owned. The 123 pharmacies in the Stockholm county have 14 million visits annually. In addition, there are ten pharmacists responsible for health education and health promotion.

7 Mass media
Experience from other community intervention programmes has shown that the mass media is an important factor in supporting other activities, for example those to do with food supply or occupational health services.

The results of our work are documented in reports presented at conferences and seminars for potential collaborators. These meetings have served to increase awareness of the possibilities for preventing cancer, and have offered opportunities to organizations to become involved in the current health action programme for combating cancer. Interested collaborators have, in this way, been able to become engaged in the programme's planning phase.

Specific projects

Diet

Target Health (Hälsomålet) is a project aimed at reducing the incidence of diet-related cancer in Stockholm county. Its goal is to achieve a 25 per cent reduction in fat intake and an increase in fibre intake to 3g/MJ by the year 2000.

Target Health has contacted ten major food-producing companies whose combined sales is more than 5 billion US dollars. Among them are three major wholesalers and one dairy producer. Six of these companies represent nearly 75 per cent of the total retail market in the Stockholm county.

The catering establishments can be divided into the public sector, i.e. schools, day-care centres, hospitals etc, and the commercial sector. A large number of lunches are served every day in staff canteens and restaurants by the county's approximately 6000 catering establishments. More than half of them are associated with the public sector.

Several of the collaborating test kitchens are located in the Stockholm county. Their main task is to educate people working in catering, and people in general, about food and food preparation. The test kitchens also develop recipes for magazines and recipe books. Some examples of collaboration with the test kitchens are: publishing a recipe book for caterers, producing a video film to describe the dietary change in simple practical terms, and developing a menu labelling system for staff canteens and restaurants.

Food fairs are used to encourage the food industry to develop new products and to increase awareness among its own people, as well as the general population, of healthy food alternatives. In conjunction with the food fairs, conferences are held which deal with various subjects related to diet and health policies.

Several types of independent organizations are capable of, and willing to, collaborate actively to promote good dietary habits, such as occupational health organizations, the county's own health-care organization, and the municipalities themselves.

Tobacco

A community-based project for tobacco control in the county has also been initiated. Its objectives are to reduce tobacco use (including snuff) to 20% of the population by year 2000, and to promote smoke-free environments.

Since autumn 1988, a mass media campaign, aimed at encouraging people to stop smoking and using snuff, was carried out in cooperation with occupational health centres, voluntary organizations and pharmacies. Even the national insurance company and several well known private companies supported the campaign, called 'Fimpa till varje Pris' (Quit and Win). More than 13 000 people registered for and participated in the campaign, which took the form of a contest. First prize was a vacation for two in Hawaii. 'Fimpa till varje Pris' is the first step in a long-term action programme for reducing tobacco use in the county.

Malignant melanoma

A project for reducing malignant melanoma through health education which deals with hazards connected with overexposure to ultraviolet rays is also in the planning phase. It is aimed at the general public.

All of these projects employ a multidisciplinary approach and incorporate collaboration with experts in the fields of oncology, community nutrition, community health, health promotion, sociology, and others.

Evaluation of the SCPP

The overall planning of SCPP has implications for the future evaluation. In 1985, an *ad hoc* evaluation committee was set up with the task of developing methods for evaluating the impact of community intervention programmes.

The committee pointed out that there are two principal models for evaluating community-based programmes: **summative evaluation** measures, for example, cancer incidence and the degree to which certain life styles change at specified time intervals or at the conclusion of a study; and **formative evaluation**, which makes use of results from an evaluation to further develop the programme's strategy, design and activities.

In addition, complementary types of studies are required to obtain knowledge that enhances both summative and formative evaluations. A population-based approach monitors changes in the population with respect to knowledge, attitudes, awareness, and behaviour. Another approach takes into account different programme activities, and uses them as the basis for evaluation studies.

The summative evaluation requires knowledge concerning changes in the population, and this can be obtained through epidemiological studies. These can also provide information as to how participation in, and exposure to, programme activities are distributed in the population or parts thereof. Such studies can be utilized as part of formative evaluations. In a similar manner, action-oriented studies within the formative evaluation can provide data for the interpretation and understanding of changes that can be observed during the summative evaluation.

Primary preventive programmes often use a quasi-experimental design because they can seldom be designed as controlled experiments. The fact that SCPP is founded on a political decision also makes the experimental design impossible. A complete evaluation of all aspects and effects of SCPP is neither feasible nor desirable. It is therefore necessary to define what kind of information is of value for the programme, what can be measured, and with what degree of precision.

There are some general points about the SCPP which suggest an overall evaluation strategy. The first one is that the time lag between intervention and detectable changes in disease incidence is expected to be more than a decade. During this period, programme activities or parallel and independent activities will not be constant. Diverse preventive activities, in addition to changes in medical care, will affect cancer mortality. Furthermore, screening programmes will influence cancer incidence statistically.

In 1986, representatives from the SCPP and from the National Cancer Institute met to discuss evaluation methods. The meeting concluded that, since the proportion of the Stockholm population developing preventable cancers in any one year is relatively small, long-term studies with very large samples would be required to relate for example dietary changes with changes in incidence with any reliability.

The meeting proposed instead to focus evaluation efforts on 'intermediate' variables, such as changes in attitudes and behaviour. SCPP has initiated county-wide base-line studies relating to dietary and smoking habits, which will be the starting point for formative and summative evaluations.

SCPP will involve a variety of interventions and activities via many different organizations. Data must be gathered on strategic outcomes, such as how successful the intervention has been in stimulating activity by other organizations, or what the changes have been concerning risk factor behaviour, as well as changes in access to healthy food or other environmental changes. By integrating the evaluation into SCPP the evaluation can be a tool in the future development of the programme.

References

1 Doll, R. and Peto, R. (1981) *The Causes of Cancer. Quantitative Estimates of Avoidable Risks of Cancer in the United States Today*, Oxford University Press, Oxford.

2 The Swedish Government Cancer Committee (1984) *Cancer—causes, prevention*, Liber Press, Stockholm, SOU 1984:67 (in Swedish).

3 Division of Cancer Prevention and Control, National Cancer Institute (1986), *Cancer Control. Objectives for the Nation: 1985–2000*, P. Greenwald and E. Sondik (eds.), NCI Monographs 2.

4 Europe Against Cancer Programme—Proposal for a Plan of Action, 1987–1989 (1987) *Official Journal of the European Communities* **30**, February 26.

5 O'Connor, T. P. and Campbell, T. C. (1986) Dietary Guidelines. *Dietary Fat and Cancer*, 731–71.

6 Wilhelmsen, L., Berglund, D., Elmfeldt, G., Pennert, K., Vedin, A. *et al.* (1986) The multifactor primary prevention trial in Gothenburg, Sweden, *European Heart Journal* **7**, 279–88.

Paper 7.2

EPIDEMIOLOGICAL EVIDENCE AND THE ROLE OF HEALTH PROMOTION FOR THE PREVENTION OF CANCERS

Professor Jose M. Martin Moreno and Dr. Ramon Mendoza
Andalusia School of Public Health, Granada, Spain

Introduction

There is reasonable evidence to be able to claim that many of the different types of cancer are substantially avoidable. Life style and other environmental determinants have been identified as risk factors. Data from animal studies and other laboratory research, as well as epidemiological observation, suggests that we could identify most risk factors which might lead to the development of cancers and take the appropriate steps to avoid them. This is the main aim of the *primary prevention approach.*

Reviewing the existing epidemiological data, Doll and Peto estimated the risk attributable to different classes of environmental agents[1]. By far the largest proportion related to tobacco and diet. The point estimate for the proportion of cancer deaths attributable to smoking was 30%, while the proportion of all cancer deaths that was estimated to be due to dietary factors was 35%. Wynder and Gori[2] described similar proportions for cancer cases (instead of cancer deaths) and equally consistent conclusions were made by Higginson and Muir[3], even though in their article they used a wider category called 'life style' in which they included diet, instead of estimating specifically the role of diet. The message of these estimates, based on many other studies, is clear the door to avoiding many cases of cancer is open. In addition there are ways to avoid other specific types of cancer, through a better control of occupational hazards, restricting radiation exposure, reducing the excessive exposure to sunlight (especially important in Spain) or controlling the effects of certain drugs, like oestrogen in postmenopausal women. Nevertheless, the major burden of cancers could potentially be avoided by well thought-out action against smoking and negative dietary habits.

The background of the problem in Spain

Smoking and cancer in Spain

Smoking is one of the largest health problems of our time, and in Spain this statement is especially true. Spain is among the European countries with the highest prevalence of the smoking habit. Recently, we have estimated the attributable deaths due to smoking in our country[4]. Here, we are going to describe this work only briefly, focusing our attention on cancer mortality. For the appraisal we used mortality data from the latest figures published by the *Instituto Nacional de Estadistica* (for the year 1983)[5].

The three factors used for our calculations were:

(a) Estimates of the relative risk, taken frongitudinal studies with the highest precision and accepted validity[6-24]

(b) Measures of proportion of the population exposed to tobacco during the decade 1970 to 1979 in Spain [25-28]. Conservative estimates indicate that over 60% of males and 15% of females were smokers during that period.

(c) Number of deaths by different types of cancer[5] according to the classification described on the 9th revision of the *International Classification of Diseases*[29].

In order to calculate the population attributable proportion (PAP) that is, the proportion of cases occurring in the whole population (where we have exposed and unexposed individuals) that is attributable to smoking, we used the following formula[30]:

$$PAP = \frac{RR - 1}{RR + 1/P_e - 1}$$

where RR is the relative risk and P_e represents the proportion of the total population exposed.

The PAP is going to provide us with a measure of how much of the disease in the entire population can be prevented by blocking the effect of the exposure or eradicating the exposure (to tobacco in this case). The number of deaths attributable to smoking was obtained multiplying the number of deaths from each type of cancer by the appropriate PAP for each sex.

In this study, overall, 32.55% of the total number of deaths caused by tobacco were cancer deaths (versus 48.63% cardiovascular deaths and 18.77% deaths from obstructed airways disease). In 1987 we had over 13 000 cancer deaths (8377 of them were deaths from lung cancer) for which tobacco was the main cause.

Potential limitations of these estimates are discussed in the original paper. Residual confounding, unknown effect modifications, uncertain knowledge of the real induction period or lack of perfect reliability of Spanish mortality statistics could be a problem. Moreover, there is an inconsistency or lack of precision across studies of certain estimates of the relative risk and estimates of prevalence of smoking habits.

We are currently reanalyzing the same data following meta-analytical approaches31. The previous estimates seem—if anything—conservative. The frequency of exposure to tobacco has increased since 197032, and we have not arrived at the plateau or the declining trends of other countries. The main goal of this recent study was to sensitize Spanish smokers, and provide potentially useful information to Spanish health planners and administrators. This is the motivation needed for designing and implementing health promotion programs with appropriate vigour.

Approaches to using health promotion to prevent cancer

Both primary and secondary cancer prevention require the adoption of individual and collective measures aimed at modifying the factors which cause cancer, or those which slow down or impede suitable treatment.

Just as in other fields, health promotion has an important role to play in cancer prevention, by making it easy for people to choose these healthier options in their daily life. Their ability to do this depends on whether the physical and social environment in which they live makes it easier to choose these healthy options. And this in turn depends on the existence of healthy public policies within their society, policies designed to take public health into account as an important criterion when it comes to making political decisions.

Health promotion implies the encouragement of factors which help to maintain a healthy life style and the reduction of factors which cause disease, combining a wide variety of political measures with educational measures aimed at individuals and communities[33-36]. This can be applied literally to cancer prevention: it is not merely a question of providing information on its origin and how it can be prevented, but also making the healthier options (for example, the consumption of low-fat foods) more accessible physically, economically and culturally.

Health education and cancer prevention

Health education, if efficiently carried out, can be used not only to inform the general public about individual measures to be applied, but also to show what kind of political or community measures are necessary to promote a healthy life style and prevent cancer.

The Commission of the European Community recently carried out a survey throughout the twelve Member States to investigate the general public's concept of cancer prevention, and to discover the extent of the knowledge and application of the most important individual preventive measures[37]. This is the first international comparative study to be carried out on the subject. Its results are extremely useful in planning health-education programmes relating to primary and secondary cancer prevention, both at a European and at a national and regional level.

The following data are of special importance:

- Of those interviewed, 10% (weighted average for the whole European Community) believe that three-quarters of cancer cases can be prevented. Another 28% believe that half of such cases can be prevented and 23% think that only a quarter of cancer cases can be prevented. The remaining 39% consider that an even smaller proportion of cases can be prevented, or else give no answer. Spain stands out from the other countries of the Community for having a greater proportion (56%) of interviewees in this last category. These data demonstrate how imperative it is to explain to Europeans (and especially to Spaniards) that most cases of cancer are avoidable, in the light of the results of epidemiological studies on causative factors. The public will take an interest in applying the appropriate preventive measures and ensuring their application only if they see cancer as a disease that can be prevented.

- The only preventive measure known to almost all the interviewees is that of not smoking (88%). Preventive measures connected with diet are known to only a third of the people in the survey; eating enough fresh fruit and vegetables (34%), eating sufficient high-fibre cereals (30%), avoiding overweight (35%), and eating foods which are low in fat (30%). Half of the people surveyed were unaware of the need to cut down on alcohol consumption (49%) or to avoid excessive exposure to sun (52%). The educational implications of this set of data are obvious.

- There is a certain discrepancy between the degree of *knowledge* and the degree of *application* of the ten individual preventive measures laid down in the European Code for Cancer Prevention, as the results of the study show, although the nature of this discrepancy varies according to the measure concerned. In the case of some of these measures, more people know of them than practise them. This occurs in the case of not smoking or avoiding excessive exposure to sun, practised by only 63% and 33% respectively of EC citizens. In contrast, as regards the eating of sufficient fruit and vegetables, more people say that they do this frequently (73%) than recognize its preventive value (34%). In the other measures whose application has been studied, this discrepancy does not seem to be significant, although this may be due to the methodology of the study rather than to the real situation.

These differences observed between the knowledge and practice of determined patterns of behaviour serve to remind us that the life style of any community is dependent upon a diversity of cultural, geographical, economic, educational and political factors. Health education, beyond its direct influence on individual or group behaviour, can be used to publicize what community measures are necessary to facilitate healthier options within a certain environment. The case of tobacco is a clear illustration of what the role of health education can be, in the context of the measures to be adopted in health promotion or disease prevention.

Measures to reduce tobacco supply and demand

The rapid changes observed in tobacco consumption trends in many countries suggest that it is other kinds of factors, such as the price of tobacco, its commercial promotion, or its social acceptability which are decisive in determining the per capita consumption level of tobacco products[38-40]. There is no other way of explaining the rapid increase observed in countries where tobacco is freely promoted by the industry, where it is sold at low prices and where social awareness of the problems connected with tobacco is virtually non-existent. The rapid decrease which is seen when these factors are altered cannot be accounted for otherwise, as seen in Norway[41-43] and other countries[44,45].

Tobacco is a product which can be bought and its commerce is therefore governed by the law of supply and demand. It is not quite like any other commercial product, given that it is a drug and, as such, is liable to produce dependence and other health and economic problems. But the fact that we are dealing with a drug is no impediment to our analysis of the product from the point of view of supply and demand, and this can prove highly enlightening. In any place and at any time, the higher and more closely matched the supply and demand of tobacco, the greater the sales and subsequent consumption. Accordingly, the reduction of the consumption of any type of tobacco product requires the adoption of measures which aim to reduce supply and demand.

There are abundant publications by committees of experts which offer guidelines for the drawing up of national programmes aimed at the reduction of tobacco consumption and there is considerable agreement between the different proposals[46-48]. Table 7.3 classifies the most important measures, according to whether they reduce supply and demand or are concerned with support or coordination. These measures are more effective if they are not applied in isolation but rather in a coordinated fashion in the context of a national programme to reduce tobacco consumption. The experiences of Norway and Iceland are illuminating in this respect[41,43,49].

Table 7.3 Comprehensive tobacco control policy

Measures to decrease tobacco supply

- Reduction of national tobacco production
- Reduction of legal and illegal tobacco importation
- Control and reduction of exportation
- Reduction of the number of sales points
- Prohibition of sales to minors
- Reduction of harmful substances in tobacco
- Control of 'new' tobacco products
- Prohibition of free distribution of tobacco

Measures to decrease tobacco demand

- Prohibition of any kind of tobacco promotion
- Price policy
- Health education and information
- Restriction of smoking in public places and places of work
- Help in stopping smoking
- Exemplary role of key people

Support Measures

- Coordination
- Funding
- Data collection
- Training
- Research
- Dissemination of information
- Support to voluntary organizations
- International cooperation

For obvious reasons, the tobacco industry has an interest in denying that tobacco addiction is a problem and that, in any case, the measures detailed in Table 7.3 constitute the solution to the problem. All over the world this industry maintains strong opposition to measures designed to control tobacco production and consumption, using arguments which have been resumed and analyzed in different studies and which basically run as follows:

1. denial of the evidence on smoking and disease;
2. claims that other, more urgent problems should be attended to instead;
3. claims that smoking is a matter of personal choice and that smoking control is an infringement of essential human freedom;
4. claims that any proposed action would be ineffective;
5. claims that economic benefits outweigh health issues;
6. claims that the tobacco industry can be relied upon to act responsibly;
7. claims that tobacco advertising is aimed only at brand-switching and not at increasing overall sales.

In health-education activities relating to the prevention of cancer or other tobacco-linked diseases, it is important to neutralize the arguments put out by the tobacco industry using the powerful means at its disposal. The 1983 report of the World Health Organization's Expert Committee on Smoking offers a simple retort to these arguments[47].

It is of prime importance to publicize the need for *legislative measures* to serve as a key point in the reduction of the supply and demand of tobacco products, given that the example of countries where voluntary agreements between the industry and the government are applied demonstrates that these are insufficient and rarely fulfilled[47,50-54]. Legislation is specially necessary to avoid all forms of tobacco promotion, and is also the most efficient way of ensuring that the packets carry clear health warnings and indicate the tar and nicotine levels so that these do not exceed certain limits, that the non-smoker's right to breathe pure air in his place of work and in public places is respected, that tobacco prices rise sufficiently and that the sales points of this drug are restricted. There are many countries in Europe[52] and other continents[50,51] which have adopted strong legislative measures to control the tobacco industry and to protect citizens from its commercial strategies.

The study *Europeans and the Prevention of Cancer*[37] also shows that the majority of the EC public is in favour of applying various legislative measures to control tobacco production and consumption, such as increased taxes on tobacco (71%), prohibition of tobacco advertising (73%), prohibition of smoking in public places (77%), banning the sale of tobacco in duty-free shops (54%), or its sale to children under 16 (84%).

Legislation is also necessary to kill off the promotion and production of smokeless tobacco in countries where its consumption had previously disappeared or was insignificant. The relation between the consumption of moist snuff and other forms of smokeless tobacco and oral cancer has been clearly established both epidemiologically and experimentally, and as a result of this, various countries have wasted no time in banning the production and sale of this 'new' type of tobacco[55,56]. The absence of this type of legislation can lead to situations like that of the United States and Sweden, where a dramatic increase in the juvenile consumption of smokeless tobacco has been observed since the early seventies[55,57].

The same EC study quoted above[37] makes it clear that there is a negative correlation between tobacco consumption and its price (especially marked in the case of young people and greater in the case of men than that of women). As regards this tendency, it is enlightening to note that the four countries in the EC which have the lowest taxes on tobacco are the very ones which have the highest incidence of smoking amongst young people Spain (55.4%), France (51.1%), Greece (48.4%) and Portugal (45.2%). A *periodic increase in the price of tobacco*, using a progressive rate of taxation, is one of the most important preventive measures that can be adopted, judging by international experience[38,44]. If prices increase more than the rate of inflation and change in income, government revenue is greater and tobacco consumption decreases. If, on the contrary, prices are permitted to grow at a slower rate than that of inflation, consumption tends to increase, even in countries which have been pioneers in adopting measures against tobacco addiction, as is the case of Finland[58-60]. In any case, as the Finnish Advisory Committee on Health Education says: 'Every tobacco price decision is also a health-policy decision: a decision as to the amount of tobacco-related illness and premature deaths in the future.'[58]

Health education is another of the essential components of a comprehensive programme to control tobacco dependence. At the present time, there is overwhelming evidence to show that health education programmes, if they are properly planned and developed, can be efficient in preventing initial dependence or encouraging people to abandon the habit[61,62]. The school is the ideal place to carry out education activities relating to tobacco within broader programmes of health education[63-65]. These activities are also highly cost-effective if carried out by health workers as a part of primary health care[66-68]. The place of work is another environment which offers excellent possibilities for health education, beyond merely banning smoking in certain areas[69].

The Andalusian *Tobacco or Health* programme

1983 saw the beginning of the reform of the health system in the Autonomous Region of Andalusia which was mainly inspired by the conclusions of the Alma Ata Conference (1978). Health education was one of the work areas which the newly formed regional health department (The Andalusian Department of Health and Consumer Affairs) considered to be high priority. From that date on, units to support health education within the health system began to be set up within the coordinating structure of primary health care at central, provincial and district level.

Activities related to tobacco began in 1984 with the launching of a health education journal with a wide distribution called *Salud entre todos* (Health for All). This journal has gradually and systematically increased the awareness of journalists, educators, health workers and people in charge of institutions in the whole of Andalusia[70]. *A Practical Guide to Giving up Smoking,* published by the journal in 1985, met with great success and has had to be republished twice. Since 1984 health education in schools and maternal education have also been promoted, and both of these have included information on tobacco.

In 1987 the Andalusian Minister of Health and Consumer Affairs presented a report to the Andalusian parliament on the adoption of specific measures to combat tobacco dependence in Andalusia. A survey carried out at the end of that year showed figures similar to those in the rest of Spain (44% daily smokers and 7% occasional smokers in the population over 15)[71]. The Department of Health gave the go-ahead to the *Tobacco or Health* Programme at the beginning of 1988. The first campaign to increase the awareness of the Andalusian population, with the slogan '*Let's stop smoking*' was carried out by the Council in April 1988, coinciding with the World Health Organization's first World *No Smoking Day* (April 7th).

The *Tobacco or Health* programme, which is run by the General Direction of Primary Health Care and Health Promotion in the Andalusian Health Service, includes the following lines of action:

- Training of professional people (health workers, educators and journalists) in matters connected with the prevention of tobacco dependence and helping people to give up smoking.
- Publishing technical materials designed for professional people and those in charge of institutions in Andalusia.
- Publishing and wide-scale distribution of informative material, such as the *Practical Guide to Giving up Smoking*, more than 400 000 copies of which were inserted in Andalusian press publications in December 1988 to coincide with the end of the year.
- Effective sign-posting of smoking and non-smoking areas in public buildings in Andalusia, following the norms published by the central Government in March 1988[72].
- The drawing up of a set of norms for the Autonomous Region to develop the national legislation with respect to the steps to be taken in cases of infringement of anti-tobacco laws.
- The carrying out of regular publicity campaigns aimed at the general population or certain sectors, such as young people.
- Development of aspects of health education programmes dealing with tobacco in the School Health Education Programme, the Health Education in Health Centres Programme, and the Health Information in the Media Programme.
- Creation of a small number of units to help smokers to break the habit within the Andalusian health system (the priority is that the focus should be on giving daily help to the smoker in primary health care centres and hospitals).
- Carrying out of regular surveys to assess the evolution of the problem within the Autonomous Region, as well as a study of various indicators of the progress of the programme, its acceptance by and impact on the general public.

It is not yet a year since this programme began, so it is too early to attempt an evaluation of its achievements. However, it should be stressed that various international plans, such as the WHO's plan of action, *Smoke-free Europe*[73], the EC's *European Programme Against Cancer* and, at national level, the new tobacco legislation in Spain[72], together with other activities carried out by the Ministry of Health and Consumer Affairs[74], will interact with the Andalusian programme and help it to achieve its aims.

References

1 Doll, R., Peto, R., (1981) The causes of cancer quantitative estimates of avoidable risks of cancer in the United States today, *JNCI* **66**,1191-1308.

2 Wynder, E. L., Gori, G. B. (1977) Contribution of the environment to cancer incidence An epidemiologic exercise. *JNCI* **58,**825–832.

3 Higginson, J., Muir, C. S. (1979) Environmental carcinogenesis misconceptions and limitations to cancer control, *JNCI* **63**, 1291–1298.

4 Gonzalez, E. J., Rodriguez, A. F., Martin Moreno, J. M., Banegas, J. R, Villar, F. (1989) Meurtes atribuibles a consumo de tabaco en Espana, *Med Clin* (Barc) (in press).

5 Instituto Nacional de Estadistica (1983) Movimiento Natural de la Poblacion Espanola. Tomo III. Defunciones segun causa de muerte.

6 Doll, R., Peto R. (1976) Mortality in relation to smoking 20 years observations on male British doctors. *Br. Med. J.* **2**, 1525–1536.

7 Doll, R., Hill, A. B. (1956) Lung cancer and other causes of death in relation to smoking a second report on the mortality of British doctors. *Br. Med. J.* **2**, 1071–1081.

8 Surgeon General (1979) Smoking and Health: a report of the Surgeons General. Washington, DC: US Department of Health, Education and Welfare; DHEW publication (PHS) 79-50066.

9 Department of Health and Human Services (1982) The health consequences of smoking. Cancer. A report of the surgeon general, Rockville, Md.

10 Department of Health and Human Services (1983) The health consequences of smoking: cardiovascular disease. A report of the surgeon general, Rockville, Md.

11 Department of Health and Human Services (1984) The health consequences of smoking: chronic obstructive lung disease. A report of the surgeon general, Rockville, Md.

12 Hammond, E. C., Horn, D. (1958) Smoking and death rates: report on forty four months of follow-up of 187.783 men. I. Total mortality *JAMA* **166**, 1159–1172.

13 Hammond, E.C., Horn, D. (1958) Smoking and death rates: report on forty four months of follow-up of 187.783 men. II. Death rates by cause. *JAMA* **166**, 1294–1308.

14 Hammond, E. C., Seiman, H. (1980) Smoking and cancer in the United States. *Preventive Medicine* **9**, 169–173.

15 Rogot, E., Murray, J. L. (1980) Smoking and causes of death among U.S. veterans: 10 years observation. *Public Health Rep.* **95**, 213–222.

16 Carstensen, J. M., *et al.* Mortality in relation to cigarette and pipe smoking: 16 years observation of 25.000 Swedish men.

17 Kahn, H.A. (1966) The Dom study of smoking and mortality among United States veterans report on 81/2 years of observation, in W. Haenszel (ed.) Epidemiologic approaches to the study of cancer and other chronic diseases. Bethesda Md.: National Cancer Institute 1, 125. (National Cancer Institute Monograph 19).

18 Dean, G. *et al.* (1977) Report on a second retrospective mortality study in north-east England. Part I: Factors relating to mortality from lung cancer, bronchitis, heart disease and stroke in Cleveland County with particular emphasis on the relative risks associated with smoking filter and plain cigarettes. London, Tobacco Research Council (Research paper 14).

19 Wigle, D.T., Mao, Y., Grace, M. (1980) Relative importance of smoking as a risk factor for selected cancers. *Can. J. Public Health* **71**, 269–275.

20 Hoover, R., Cole, P. (1971) Population trends in cigarette smoking and bladder cancer. *Am. J. Epidemiol.* **94**, 409–481.

21 Moller, Jensen. *et al.* (1987) The Copenhagen case-control study of bladder cancer: the role of smoking in invasive and non-invasive bladder tumours. *J. Epidemiol. Com. Health* **41**, 30–36.

22 Weis, W., Bernarde, M. A. (1983) The temporal relation between cigarette smoking and pancreatic cancer. *Am. J. Public Health* **73**, 1403–1404.

23 The Pooling Project Research Group (1978) Relationship of blood pressure, serum cholesterol, smoking habit, relative weight, and ECG abnormalities to incidence of major coronary events: final report of the Pooling Project. *J. Chronic Dis.* **31**, 201–306.

24 Wolf, P.A. *et al.* (1978) Epidemiologic assessment of chronic atrial fibrillation and risk of stroke The Framingham Study. *Neurology* (Minneap) **28**, 973–977.

25 Ministerio de Sanidad y Consumo (1987) Encuesta Nacional de Salud (in press)

26 Centro de Investigaciones Sociologicas (CIS) (1985) Actividades y comportamientos de los espanoles ante el tabaco, el alcohol y las drogas. Estudio 1.487.

27 Tabacalera, S.A. (1978) Estudio General de Base.

28 Salleras, L. *et al.* (1985) Epidemiologia del tabaquismo en la problacion adulta de Cataluna. I. Prevalencia del habito. *Medicina Clinica* (Barcelona) **85**, 525–528.

29 Organizacion Mundial de la Salud (1975) Clasificacion Internacional de Enfermedades y causas de meurte. 9 Revision.

30 Rothman, K. J. (1987) *Epidemiologia moderna.* Ediciones Diaz de Santos SA.

31 Walker, A. M., Martin Moreno, J. M., Artalejo, F. R. (1988) Odd Man Out: A Graphical Approach to Meta-analysis. *Am. J. Public Health* **78**, 961–966.

32 Tabacalera, S. A., Memoira (1986).

33 Milio, N. (1986) Promoting health through public policy. Ottawa, Canadian Public Health Association.

34 Organisation Mondiale de la Sante (1986) Charte d'Ottawa pour la Promotion de la Sante. Ottawa, Association canadienne de sante publique.

35 World Health Organization/Australian Department of Community Services and Health (1988) Report on the Adelaide Conference: Healthy Public Policy: 2nd International Conference on Health Promotion (April 5–9, 1988, Adelaide, South Australia). Copenhagen/Adelaide, 1988.

36 Nutbeam, D. (1986) Health promotion glossary. *Health Promotion*:**1** (1) 113–127.

37 Commission of the European Communities, Survey: Europeans and the prevention of cancer. Brussels, October 8, 1987 (working document of the services of the European Commission).

38 Townsend, J. (1988) (Advisory Committee on the Health Education, National Board of Health Finland). Tobacco price and the smoking epidemic. Copenhagen/Brussels, World Health Organization/Commission of the European Communities.

39 Chapman, S. (1985) Cigarette advertising and smoking: a review of the evidence. BMA, London.

40 Chapman, S., White, P. (1988) *Pushing smoke: tobacco advertising and promotion.* Copenhagen/Brussels, World Health Organization/Commission of the European Communities.

41 Norwegian National Council on Smoking and Health (1985) *Trends in tobacco consumption and smoking habits in Norway.* Oslo, National Council on Smoking and Health.

42 Norwegian National Council on Smoking and Health (1985) The act relating to restrictive measures for the marketing of tobacco products etc. (no. 14 of 9 March 1973). Oslo, National Council on Smoking and Health.

43 Bjartveit, K., Lund, K. E. (1987) *Smoking control in Norway.* Oslo, National Council on Smoking and Health, 1987.

44 Reid, D., Smith., N. (1988) Cuales son las principales causas del descenso del consumo de cigarrillos en los paises industrializados? document presented at First European Conference on Tobacco Policy, Madrid, 7–11 November 1988.

45 Van Reek, J., Adriaanse, H., Smoking cessation patterns in seven Western countries. *Health Ed. Res.* **2** (3), 267–273.

46 WHO Expert Committee (1979) *Controlling the smoking epidemic: report of the WHO expert committee on smoking control.* Geneva, World Health Organization. (Technical Report Series, 636).

47 WHO Expert Committee (1983) Smoking control strategies in developing countries: report of a WHO expert committee. Geneva, World Health Organization. (Technical Report Series, 695).

48 Gray, N., Daube, M. (eds.) (1980) Guidelines for smoking control. Geneva, International Union Against Cancer.

49 Bjartveit, K. (1988) Some examples of successful measures in tobacco control. First European Conference on Tobacco Policy, Madrid, 7–11 November.

50 Roemer, R. (1982) Legislative action to combat the world smoking epidemic. Geneva, WHO.

51 Roemer, R. (1986) *Recent developments in legislation to combat the world smoking epidemic.* Geneva, WHO (WHO/SMO/HLE/86.1).

52 Roemer, R. (1988) *Legislative strategies for a smoke-free Europe.* Copenhagen/Brussels, World Health Organization/Commission of the European Communities.

53 Amos, A., Robertson, G., Hillhouse, A. (1987) Tobacco advertising and children: widespread breaches in the voluntary agreement. *Health Ed. Res.* **2**(3), 207–214.

54 Roberts, J. L. (1986) Codebusting by tobacco companies: a case against the existing voluntary agreements. Manchester, Project Smoke Free.

55 Connolly, G. N. *et al.* (1986) The reemergence of smokeless tobacco. *N. Engl. J. Med.* **314**, 1020–1027.

56 WHO (1988) Smokeless tobacco control: report of a WHO study group. Geneva, World Health Organization. (Technical Report Series, 773).

57 National Board of Health and Welfare (1987) Tobacco Control in Sweden, p. 16, Stockholm.

58 Advisory Committee on Health Education (1985) An evaluation of the effects of an increase in the price of tobacco and a proposal for the tobacco price policy in Finland in 1985–1987. Helsinki, National Board of Health.

59 Leppo, K., Vertio, H. (1986) Smoking control in Finland: a case study in policy formulation and implementation. *Health Promotion* **1**, 5–16.

60 Rimpela, M. *et al.* (1987). Changes in health habits of young people in Finland in 1977–1987. Helsinki, National Board of Health.

61 Catford, J. C., Nutbeam, D., Woolaway, M. C. (1984) Effectiveness and cost-benefits of smoking education. *Community Medicine* **6**, 264–272.

62 Engleman, S. (1987) The impact of mass media anti-smoking publicity. *Health Promotion* **2**(1) 63–74.

63 Comite Europeen de la Sante (1984) *Education pour la sante visant a prevenir les toxicomanies.* Strasbourg, European Council.

64 Mendoza, R., Vilarrasa, A., Ferrer, X. (1986) *La educacion sobre las drogas en el circlo superior de la EGB: propuesta de programa.* Madrid, Ministerio de Educacion y Ciencia.

65 Nutbeam, D., Mendoza, R., Newman, R. (1988) *Planning for a smoke-free generation.* Copenhagen/ Brussels, World Health Organization/Commission of the European Communities.

66 Ramstrom, L., Raw, M., Wood, M. (1988) *Guidelines on smoking cessation for the primary health care team,* Geneva, World Health Organization/International Union Against Cancer.

67 Raw, M. (1988) *Helping smokers stop,* Copenhagen/ Brussels/London: WHO/EC/British Medical Association.

68 Raw, M. (1988) *The physician's role,* Copenhagen/ Brussels: WHO/EC.

69 King's College School of Medicine and Dentistry, Academic Department of Community Medicine (1985) Action on smoking at work: a guide to good practice, London.

70 Mendoza, R. (1988) Health promotion and intersectoral information: the case of the journal *Salud entre todos.* 2nd International Conference on Health Promotion, Adelaide, Australia, 5–9 April 1988.

71 Junta de Andalucia, Comisionado para la droga (1988) Los andaluces ante las drogas. Sevilla, Consejeria de Salud y Servicios Sociales.

72 Boletin Oficial del Estado de Espana (1988) Real decreto 192/1988, de 4 de marzo, sobre limitaciones en la venta y uso del tabaco para proteccion de la salud de la poblacion. BOE.

73 World Health Organization/Regional Office for Europe (1988) A 5 year action plan: smoke free Europe, Copen-hagen.

74 Ministerio de Sanidad y Consumo de Espana (1988) Actuaciones sanitarias en relacion al tabaquismo en Espana. First European Conference on Tobacco Policy, Madrid.

Paper 7.3

A DISTRICT HEALTH PROMOTION PLAN FOR CANCER: developed by the Cancer Education Co-ordinating Group of the United Kingdom and the Republic of Ireland

Convenor: Professor James McEwen,
Department of Community Medicine, King's College, University of London

Introduction to the plan

The lack of a framework and a co-ordinating group at local level has been a major problem in developing an integrated approach to health promotion for cancer. The attached document, which has been prepared by the Cancer Education Co-ordinating Group of the United Kingdom and the Republic of Ireland, is seen as one way of achieving such co-ordination within these countries.

Whilst it is recognized that the approach outlined is directly linked to the structure of the health and related services within these countries, it is hoped that the framework might be of value in encouraging other countries to develop such a local approach to planning.

The District Plan is a guideline and as such meets the WHO criteria for care programmes. WHO define a care programme as a set of written guidelines which state agreed policy containing recommendations on components of cancer care; it requires the contribution of each of the disciplines involved in cancer care. Health education of the public is one of these. There are several reasons why the concept of care programmes in cancer is expected to benefit both patients and their communities.

These are:

Ethical In any area or region of a country the aim of the health services for cancer patients is to obtain for them access to the best care that area can provide. The care programme approach (district plan) provides a structure for this. The right to protection against unproven and inappropriate messages is a further ethical justification.

Economic Now, more than ever before, economic reality intrudes on every aspect of cancer care and both medical and administrative decision-makers seek the most cost effective means of prevention, diagnosis and therapy. As the district plan identifies optional policies for health promotion it benefits the application of economic considerations.

Educational A wide range of professional groups is involved in the discussion, planning, implementation and evaluation of the district plan. Thus the preparation of the district plan care programmes is in itself an important educational exercise in interdisciplinary thought and collaboration.

Scientific The prospect of introducing the outcome of applied scientific research to a population quickly is a specially good reason for having a district plan.

Administrative The specification of a defined set of cancer control objectives and the identification and allocation of responsibilities at all levels of the health care administrators and would thus benefit the programme.

Evaluation The introduction of the district plan would be of benefit to evaluation strategies as it would require the application of a variety of techniques in order to interpret the impact of the programme on a defined population and to monitor the outcome of the programme. It would be unethical to implement the programme without introducing the evaluation strategy from the beginning.

A District Health Promotion Plan for Cancer[1]

The Cancer Education Co-ordinating Group of the United Kingdom and the Republic of Ireland, 1988

Contents

The purpose of this document is to encourage district health authorities[3] to develop their own plan.

[1] This Plan has been slightly shortened due to constraints on space.

[2] These appendices, which include an extensive collection of resource material, could not be included in this book. The full Plan is obtainable from the Cancer Education Co-ordinating Group of the United Kingdom and the Republic of Ireland.

[3] The term 'district health authority' is used throughout this document for simplicity. It is recognized that in different parts of the UK and the Republic of Ireland, different terminology is used. The intention is to identify an appropriately sized locality which functions as an entity for health care.

The district plan seeks to identify the existing activities and then to encourage the district to concentrate on the areas relevant to cancer education which have in the past received less attention; the aim being to produce a co-ordinated and comprehensive local strategy. To encourage more balanced and realistic views of cancers in general is educationally desirable, not only because education to reduce needless anxiety is worthwhile in its own right, but also to introduce positive knowledge of certain aspects and to place cancers in the perspective of society.

Introduction

This document is intended for all those individuals or organizations who have responsibility for health education, health promotion, development of screening services, provision of care and support for those with cancer or those who care for people with cancer. The hope is that district health authorities will be encouraged to review the importance of cancer as a cause of premature mortality and morbidity and to examine the potential for improvement through health promotion, screening and care.

An overall aim might be to seek 'to change the impact cancer has on society' in the context of Europe Against Cancer which has set the target of 15 per cent fewer cancer deaths by the year 2000. This in turn is set in the wider context of Health For All By The Year 2000, as proposed by the World Health Organization.

The intention is that each district should begin from its current position with regard to the widest aspects of cancer and health. This document is neither a formal plan nor a blueprint, but could perhaps be best described as a practical checklist which will assist districts in the preparation of their own plan. There is no universal approach to cancer education that is uniquely 'right'; nor is there any one successful way of introducing proposals to key personnel and gaining their collaboration.

Many health professionals are uncertain about 'the facts' relating to cancer and feel unable to contribute fully to public or patient education; thus, a major commitment in the first instance must be to assist health professionals to work together in this field.

Background

Over the past decade, cancer has become a topic of increasing interest to the general public. From being mentioned in hushed whispers it has suddenly progressed to being a subject of dinner table interest. This remarkable change owes its origins to a number of factors and whilst the effect is not all good, at last there is now scope for consideration of the topic in terms not before envisaged. The main agents of change have been:

1 An increasing awareness among the public of the individual's responsibility for their own health and well-being.

2 Wide media coverage, especially on television, of new research findings on potential causes and methods of treatment.

3 Progress in research which has popular appeal and is neither too esoteric nor too scientifically based to catch the public's attention.

4 Development of national cancer-screening programmes.

5 European Cancer Week in 1988 and the prospect of European Cancer Year in 1989.

Whilst people are now much more willing, and even eager, to discuss the causes of cancer, recent surveys of attitudes and beliefs have shown that these have changed less than might be expected. Media messages are being misunderstood or misinterpreted, such that a smoker will refuse to buy a sunbed on the grounds that it could cause cancer whilst failing to appreciate the greater risk of smoking. Clarification of knowledge of causes, so far as they are at present known, is needed, as is specific advice and help on what action to take and how to take it.

Screening services will be under-used unless people are aware of them, of their purpose and nature, and where and how to obtain them. New treatments risk being ineffective if people delay in seeking medical advice. Knowledge has increased but sometimes imperfectly and, as is so well known, has not necessarily been accompanied by changes in either attitude or behaviour. In making a decision to take health action, a series of steps are needed. Accurate knowledge of the seriousness of the risk and that the risk is personal is needed first. After learning and accepting these facts, the person must weigh up what will be lost and what will be gained by making a decision to take specific action.

The current state of awareness about cancers needs an educational input at both stages—first, to clarify knowledge, secondly, to help a person through the decision-making process, which is a far more complex activity than imparting knowledge. When these educational steps are worked through, a means must be provided to facilitate action being taken as quickly and as simply as possible. Screening services with a good call and recall system, sited in easily accessible places, open at convenient times or visiting workplaces are good examples. Likewise, readily available 'stop smoking' clinics can provide another opportunity to put a decision quickly and easily into practice.

Cancer education does not end with education, but must encompass a process of health promotion so that when education has been given, action can be taken. Nor is this process exclusive to cancer. Overall health programmes can encompass it, together with heart disease and other health risks in programmes which are not orientated to a specific disease, but to a healthy life style, decision-making and increase in self esteem. An education programme is doomed to failure if factors in the environment appear to negate or prevent the action which is being encouraged. The whole environment and ethos in which the education is undertaken needs to be taken into account.

Health districts are in an ideal position to facilitate cancer education with the necessary back-up of screening and treatment to enable action to be taken, and to influence the environment with regard to safety at work, dietary policy and tobacco advertising, to name but a few.

Europe Against Cancer

The 'Europe Against Cancer' campaign stems from a decision by the Heads of State of the EC in 1986 to launch a European Programme Against Cancer. This is a broad based programme, with two key themes :

- Public Information;
- Training of Members of the Health Professions.

The campaign aims to encourage people to take action to reduce the number of deaths from cancer by 15 per cent. Countries in the European Community are publicizing a 10 point code (see Chapter 1).

Health promotion

In 1978, in the Declaration of Alma Ata, the World Health Organization issued a challenge to the countries of the world to attain 'health for all by the year 2000'. The European Region of WHO has developed a common health policy for all European countries. This calls for an international programme of change and development having three main elements:

- the promotion and facilitation of healthy life styles;
- a re-orientation of health care systems;
- a reduction in the burden of preventable ill health.

In 1984, the European Regional Office of WHO identified the key principles of health promotion which were summarized in a useful definition:

> At a general level, health promotion has come to represent a unifying concept for those who recognize the need for change in the ways and conditions of living, in order to promote health. Health promotion represents a mediating strategy between people and their environments, synthesizing personal choice and social responsibility in health to create a healthier future.

In all discussions on 'health for all' the importance of intersectoral collaboration is emphasized and the Faculty of Community Medicine of the Royal Colleges of Physicians of the United Kingdom in 1986 in its Charter for Action identified the differing responsibilities of central government, local government, health authorities and all health professionals, training organizations, industry, trades unions and professional bodies and individuals.

Inevitably, a special responsibility for health promotion must rest with health authorities and health professionals, especially for initiating and co-ordinating strategies and programmes. Within the health service, at different levels, health promotion teams or groups are active, frequently involving colleagues from other sectors and from voluntary organizations. It is against the background of these important developments that this District Health Promotion Plan for Cancer Control is offered. Whatever approach may be adopted at a local level, it is hoped that the framework provided by this plan will assist with co-ordination of activities and ensure a comprehensive approach.

Cost effectiveness of district health promotion for cancer

A vast range of cancer treatment services, ranging from drug treatment to terminal care, are provided in districts. Treatment services for cancer may produce a cure implying the disappearance of all clinical evidence of the tumour, allowing the patient to enjoy normal longevity and a normal quality of life. Unfortunately, more often, the main benefit of cancer treatment arises from palliation of symptoms with an improvement in the quality, but not necessarily the quantity, of life. As such, the contribution of treatment services to tackling this major health problem appears to be severely limited.

The extent of the health problem posed by cancer can be illustrated by data obtained from Hospital Activity Analysis. For example, within the North West RHA in 1985, patients with a main diagnosis of neoplasm accounted for 9.4% of all occupied bed days. Approximately 85% of these bed days devoted to cancer patients were provided in district-based services outside the regional centre at Christie Hospital. Further, the district-based workload associated with cancer is on the increase, as are the cost implications of treatment provision for cancer patients. Bed throughput for cancer patients has increased significantly, as has the cost of drugs and (due to the greater toxic effects of such drugs) the intensive nursing care required by such patients.

Again, taking the North West Region as an example, a recent review of regional specialities (NWRHA, 1988) provides a conservative estimate of the cost of hospital care for cancer of £38 million per annum. In addition to this massive resource commitment, the cost in terms of human misery is equally enormous. Cancer caused 57 000 deaths in NWRHA between 1982 and 1986. Over 3000 people die annually from lung cancer and 1000 die from breast, stomach and colon cancer within NWRHA. Survival rates for many of these cancers are low—less than 10 per cent of patients with lung cancer can be expected to survive for over 5 years.

Perhaps the greatest tragedy is that there would be virtually no deaths from lung cancer in the absence of cigarette smoking. As such, the most effective approach to this, our most common cancer, is undoubtedly to emphasize its prevention. Perhaps the primary role of health education is to inform the public of how to recognize and act upon significant symptoms promptly. Such knowledge, together with an active health promotional strategy, provides a potentially very valuable process by which to reduce the incidence of cancer. Perhaps the most impressive example of health education is the reduction in smoking prevalence at a time when cost, relative to income, was decreasing.

A detailed analysis would be required to analyze the expected impact of a district health promotion plan upon cancer deaths. In such an analysis the impact of the discount rate (the extent to which we value future health/resources in comparison to current health/resources) would be crucial, given that much of the impact of health promotion may occur over the long term. The potential gains in health, however, are enormous, as are the potential savings in resources arising from an effective district-based health promotion strategy for cancer. In summary, at present, it is still not possible to answer the question 'Is cancer education cost effective?' In many areas, epidemiology is still limited, outcome information is incomplete and cost data are poor. It is hoped that this document might encourage the development of new approaches and projects which might result in improved data to answer this question.

The local setting

Why a Plan for Cancer?

If there is to be any successful development then the initial prerequisite must be an awareness of need and a commitment to action. This may either be from an individual or from a group and may relate to any part of the spectrum related to cancer, for example:

- concern over passive smoking;
- uncertainty as to the reasons for poor uptake of screening;
- complaints about inadequate services;
- lack of health education in schools.

Such concerns may result from the threat of reduction in an existing service from financial constraints, or the impact of new service developments or new staff members. Whatever the cause, they tend to lead to a review of what is being done locally, and how this relates to need. This may be the first step in the development of an information base which is essential for any plan.

At this stage work is required to obtain such information; this may be carried out by the individuals themselves or through an existing health promotion group or cancer oncology group. If no group exists, such information is likely to be necessary before there will be commitment from others to form such a group.

There are existing activities and programmes in every district—some defined by age group, for example, schoolchildren, some by disease, for example, cervical cancer, some by an issue, for example, smoking. Many programmes, such as a healthy eating policy, although not directly related to cancer, clearly have an impact. But there is no overall framework; there are few links between those with responsibility for prevention and those who provide care. There is no overall co-ordinating plan or strategy at either district or regional levels.

The aim is for each district to develop its own local, relevant and living plan—encouraging diverse and appropriate approaches.

Review of existing provision

Any new health promotion activity for cancer must not only be set in the context of existing health service provision, facilities and staff and directly related to other existing or planned health promotional activities, but should also draw upon the experience and resources of voluntary agencies active in the field of cancer education and/or care.

While existing activities may not have been described specifically or exclusively as cancer education, it is clear that they contribute to a reduction in cancer incidence and must be included in the planning stage. This is not to suggest that existing policies, such as a healthy eating policy, should be relabelled a cancer-prevention policy. The public discussion of a healthy diet and moderation in the use of alcohol without a heavy emphasis on cancer risk may be more appropriate.

Similarly, through the World Health Organization's Healthy Cities Project, attention is being paid to many of the adverse environmental issues that affect our deprived inner city areas. Here again, there is the opportunity to identify the links between the initiative and the potential for reducing the risk of cancer and improving attitudes to early detection and care.

The introduction nationally of a call-recall programme for breast and cervical cancer provides an excellent basis for health promotion in relation to two important cancers, and indeed, if these programmes are to achieve the target of a 70% uptake, there is a need for local educational approaches for both health professionals and the public.

A data base

Although there are national and local statistics readily available, particularly for mortality, these have been less often used at both local and national levels for planning and policy with regard to health promotion. Good examples are 'The Big Kill' and 'Broken Hearts', where the impact of smoking and heart disease has been made available widely and used to support health promotion activities. It is suggested that a similar approach might be developed for this initiative, with districts and regions co-operating to produce a national picture.

Locally, through district information officers, health education/promotion departments, community medicine departments and cancer registries, it will be possible to build up information about cancer deaths, registrations, survival, geographical variations, siting of services, staffing, waiting times, etc.

It might be possible to develop a 'newsletter', based on such information which, along with articles on health promotion, could be a regular feature of the district's activities in the field of health prevention of cancer.

Starting the process

There are two likely starting points (see Figure 7.5). The first would be the progressive development of activities from existing ones, into a more comprehensive and co-ordinated plan, or the recognition of the need for a plan and the establishment of a local implementation group which would then review existing activities and develop the plan.

From the beginning, it will be possible to develop a wider framework for health promotion, which may include the organizations identified in Figure 7.6.

Establishing an Implementation Group

An Implementation Group which oversees the planning, monitoring and servicing of such policies related to the control of cancer throughout the Authority is the model proposed in the current strategy. A well-balanced multidisciplinary group of senior representatives drawn from inside and outside the Health Authority is likely to be particularly important where cancer education is concerned. This group should be directly related to the existing or proposed district system of health promotion.

A district-wide strategy must take into account the huge variation in backgrounds and levels of education of health professionals, as well as the various clients or target groups. Cancer health education is frequently most concerned with clients at high risk of cancer, who characteristically do not avail themselves of screening or medical services. The Implementation Group should also include members who are in day-to-day contact with all sections of the community. The General Manager is responsible for ensuring that decisions are taken by the organization to plan, act on, control and measure its decisions and actions, thus providing a more effective and efficient service, so relevant managers, in hospital and in the community, must be members of the Advisory Group.

The size of the Working Group will vary according to local needs and interests. Working members might

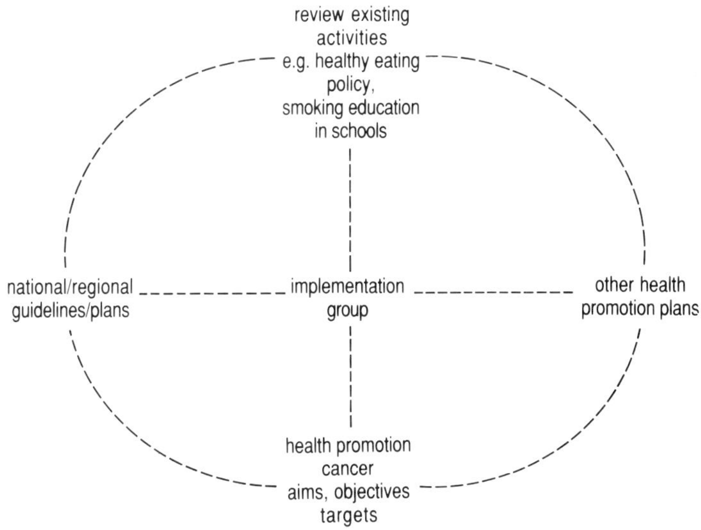

Figure 7.5 Starting points for planning

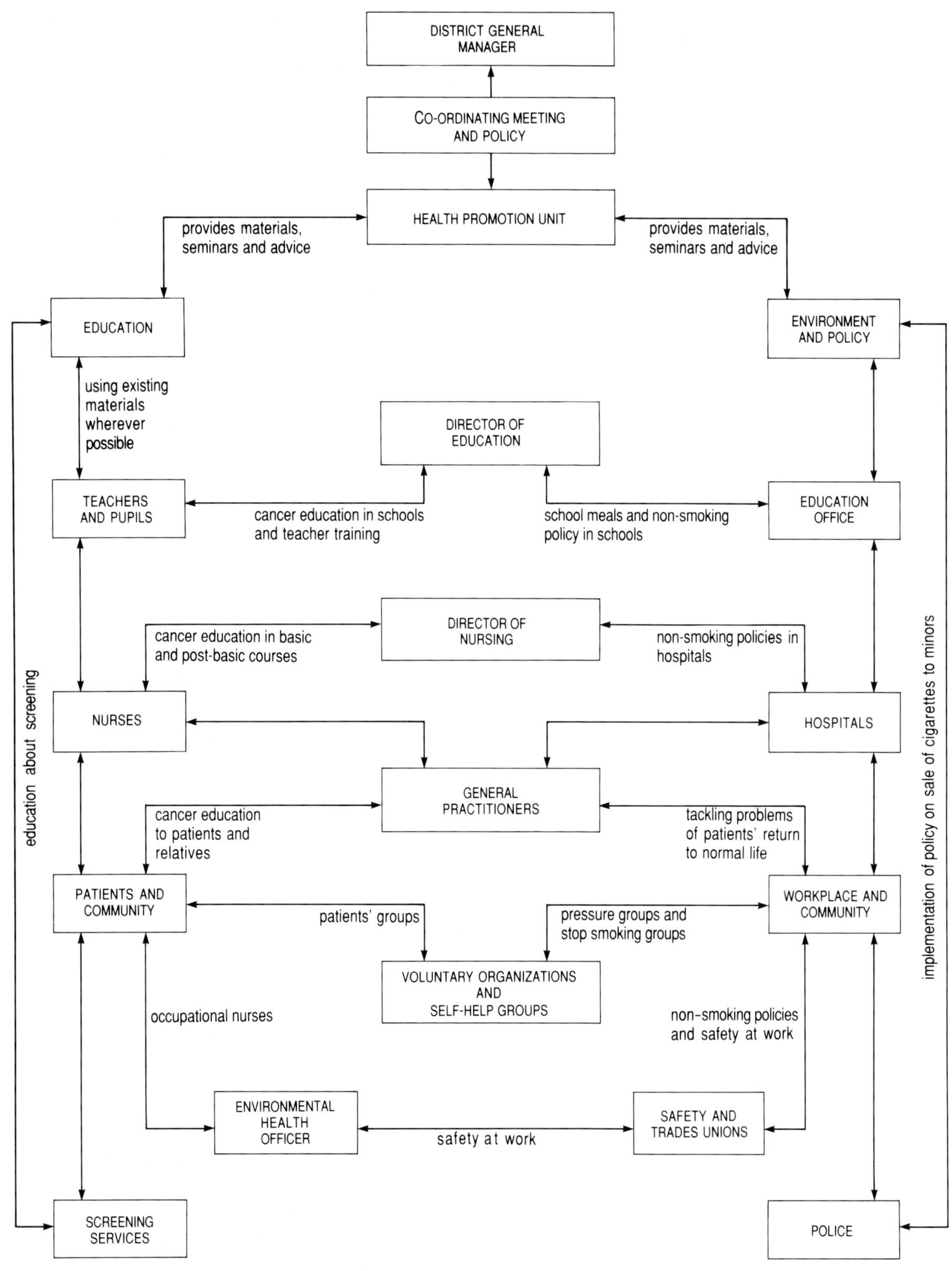

Figure 7.6 Framework for a District Health Promotion Plan for Cancer

be drawn from the following, others being co-opted for specific tasks (exact titles vary in different health authorities):

- Unit Manager (community)—representing the DGM
- Unit Managers (hospital)—representing the DGM
- Director of Nursing Services (community) (this is assuming they
- Director of Nursing Services (hospital) are not Unit Managers)
- District Health Promotion/Education Officer
- Consultants in general medicine/physician/psychiatry
- Consultants from oncology specialty—from large radiotherapy centre, if possible
- Representatives of the Local Authority
  - (a) Advisor for school health education
  - (b) Advisor for adult education
  - (c) Public Relations Officer
  - (d) Community workers
- GP representative of the LMC
- Specialists in Community Medicine
- Director of the School of Nursing
- District Dietitian (nutrition policy)
- Director of Planning and Information
- Market research analyst/statistician (academic department)
- Voluntary agencies that can collaborate, advise, and help recruit voluntary helpers as appropriate
- Representative of the Council for Voluntary Organizations
- Secretary of the Community Health Council
- Educational psychologist
- Representative of the Treasurer's Dept (costings).

Preparing the District Plan

Although reference throughout is to the district plan, as with all other health promotion activities, the health authority services as a co-ordinating agency. To be successful it is essential that the plan is not seen as belonging to any one constituency—hospital or community, medical or educational, nursing or health education. Special emphasis needs to be laid on the participation of all members of the primary care team, the various sections of the local community and the workplace. The group will be able to identify existing mechanisms of collaboration with local authorities, for example joint planning teams, and voluntary organizations to ensure maximum dissemination of information and full use of resources.

Locally, the group will have a key role in identifying what local materials are required and how these can best be utilized in the different ethnic and community groups. At the same time, it will be able to ensure communication with the regional focus for health promotion and support development of regional policies and plans.

Aims

The main aim of the Strategy is to help create a climate of professional and public knowledge, opinion and attitudes, which will allow the cancer services to achieve their full potential for:

1 primary prevention
2 early detection
3 management and care of those with cancer and their families

This is a strategy which is heavily committed to collaborating with interested groups of many kinds, voluntary and statutory, and addresses itself to health professionals, to the community at large, and to specific at-risk and patient groups; and it therefore implies subsidiary aims such as:

(a) to foster more realistic attitudes among all health staff. To help develop their educational and counselling skills. This requires developments in professional education.
(b) to provide information among the community at large about the prevention and cure of cancer.
(c) to encourage at-risk groups to take appropriate preventive action.
(d) to provide additional support for workers engaged in rehabilitation services.
(e) to provide information about help available for terminal care.
(f) to advise and support self-help groups.

Identification of areas for action and priorities

This is likely to include current areas of activity and new ones for action, and could result from a local workshop to launch the concept of A District Plan.

Topics might include the following:

- smoking policies within the district;
- smoking education in schools;
- education related to breast and cervical screening programmes;
- nutrition policies;
- women's health;
- men's health—testicular cancer;
- encourage prompt response to symptoms;
- health and safety at work issues;
- environmental health;
- training of professionals;
- improve efficiency of health services related to cancer, etc.

A subsequent seminar could then be used, with available local data, to identify priorities for action and to group the provisional list of actions within an overall framework of aims and objectives.

At the same time, detailed objectives can be defined. If, for example, an aim is to improve lay education on cancer, this might include:

- role of GP and primary care team;
- opportunities in hospital;
- school education—policies, curriculum, catering;
- mass media;
- leisure and recreation.

Objectives

Indicators to measure progress in cancer control can be medical (e.g. reduction in cervical cancer); educational (e.g. changes in knowledge and attitudes); behavioural (e.g. attendance for screening following an invitation); service (e.g. the provision of a night nursing service for terminally ill patients); or policy (e.g. the extent of the implementation of a health authority smoking policy).

Data bases of knowledge, opinion and behaviour in the community before any education is attempted should be established so that measurement of change may be possible. Therefore research and evaluation are of great importance as an integral part of a district plan.

Each authority will wish to draw up its own objectives based on the booklet 'Can you Avoid Cancer?' and the related Ten Point European Code. Ideally, each authority should identify its present baseline and set its own targets from the appropriate periods of the Plan's initial Five Year Programme.

Targets, evaluation and resources

Based on the defined objectives, targets can be set for each activity.

For example, in the field of smoking, there might be the following targets:

- to increase the number of workplaces in the district with an effective smoking policy from ... % to ... %.
- to ensure that stopping smoking clinics are available to all who want them.
- to reduce the prevalence of cigarette smoking in schoolchildren from ... % to ... %.

This in turn can be related to an overall timetable—possibly an initial 5-year period, allowing development of aims, identification of priorities, clarification of objectives and establishment of targets and methods of evaluation.

The implementation group in its deliberations will need to identify what can be achieved though co-ordination of existing resources, including expertise and funds for evaluation and what requires additional resources, which may exist, for example community and voluntary groups (although not linked to the district effectively) or where requests to health authority, charities, industry etc. may be required for new initiatives. Realism as to what can be achieved and what may be obtained are obviously essential. It might be helpful to draw up a table indicating objective, target and actions to be taken by various organizations necessary to achieve the target.

Timetable

The plan envisages a sustained programme of activities over a specified time period, initially five years. It is a blueprint only. Each district will adapt and develop details according to local needs and services. The plan should have 'depth' in that it should not be a one-off campaign or a short-term publicity burst, but a series of progressive and developing interrelated activities.

Future developments

As mentioned at the beginning of this document, the intention is that district health authorities should be encouraged to use the ideas to develop their own plan. It is hoped that this will be the beginning of a new approach to Health Promotion For Cancer.

As well as local outcomes, it would be of great benefit if, through regional and national co-ordination, a wider body of knowledge could be developed which in turn would enrich local activities.

This information could include:

- sources of data;
- agreement on a core data base;
- priorities for action;
- a list of local, national and international resources;
- regular up-to-date review of organizations;
- examples of good practice;
- summaries of support, research etc. by national health promotion organizations.

The CECG would be pleased to hear from those who receive this document and would welcome proposals for future developments, as well as reports on local action taken.

Acknowledgements

The initial district plan was prepared by a working party (members listed below) of the Cancer Education Co-ordinating Group and was issued as a draft in 1985.

Working Party Members

Group Convenor: Mr. R. L. Davison

Members: Mr. P. A. Gardner, Dr. C. R. Gillis, Mrs R. Hewertson, Miss J. M. Waghorn, Mr. M. A. Wood.

The following editorial group revised the draft in the light of developments particularly associated with Europe Against Cancer; the Cancer Education Co-ordinating Group have issued this document as a contribution to European Cancer Year 1989.

Editorial Group: Dr. Anne Charlton, Dr. C. R. Gillis, Mr. M. A. Wood, Professor J. McEwen (Convenor).

The section on Cost Effectiveness was prepared by Dr. Alan Haycox.

Those attending the Annual Study Day of CECG in November 1988, who contributed to the revision of this document.

Appendix 1

PARTICIPANTS AT THE COLLOQUIUM, LISBON, FEBRUARY 1989

Professor Mario Bernardo
Associate Professor of Oncology
Centro de Lisboa
Instituto Portugues de Oncologia de
Francisco Gentil
Rua Prof. Lima Basto
1093 Lisboa
Portugal

Dr. Franco Berrino
Director
Lombardy Cancer Registry
Instituto Nazionale per lo Studio e la
Cura dei Tumori
Via Venezian, 1
20133 Milano
Italy

Dr. Jose Calheiros
Instituto Nacional de Saude
Largo 1 de Dezembro
4000 Porto
Portugal

Dr. J. Cardoso da Silva
President
Liga Portuguesa Contra o Cancro
Centro do Porto do Instituto Portugues de
Oncologia de Francisco Gentil
Asprela
4200 Porto
Portugal

Professor L. Cayolla da Motta
Professor de Epidemiologia
Escola Nacional de Saude Publica
Av. Padre Cruz
Lisboa
Portugal

Professor Jocelyn Chamberlain
DHSS Cancer Screening Evaluation Unit
Institute of Cancer Research
Royal Cancer Hospital
15 Cotswold Road
Belmont
Sutton
Surrey SM2 5PT
England

Dr. Anne Charlton
Director
Cancer Research Campaign
Education and Child Studies Research Group
University of Manchester
Kinnaird Road
Manchester M20 9QL
England

Professor José Condé
Director
Instituto Portuguese de Oncologie
Universidade Nova de Lisboa
Lisbon
Portugal

Dr. Nick Day
Director
Bio-statistics Units
Medical Research Council
5 Shaftesbury Road
Cambridge CB2 2BW
England

Professor Sir Richard Doll and Lady Doll
International Cancer Research Foundation
Cancer Epidemiology Unit
Gibson Building
Radcliffe Infirmary
Oxford OX2 6HE
England

Dr. Gerard Dubois
ENSM-CNAMTS
66 Av. du Maine
75694 Paris Cedex 14
France

Professor Anna Efremidis
Associate Professor and Director of
Medical Oncology
Hellenic Cancer Institute
St. Savas Hospital
171 Alexandras Avenue
11522 - Athens
Greece

Professor Robert Flamant
Director
Institut Gustave Roussy
Rue Camille Desmoulins
94805 Villejuif Cedex
France

Dr. Jose Guimares Dos Santos
Portuguese Coordinator of the Year of
Cancer Information
Instituto Portugues de Oncologia
Asprela
4200 Porto
Portugal

Dr. E. Milly L. Haagedoorn
Director
Cancer Education Programme
University Hospital Groningen
Division of Surgical Oncology
Box 30.001
9700 RB Groningen
The Netherlands

Dr. Lars-Erik Holm
Cancer Prevention Unit
Radiumhemmet
Karolinska Hospital
S-104 01 Stockholm
Sweden

Professor Jozef V. Joossens
Division of Epidemiology
Sint-Rafael University Hospital
Capucijenvoer 33
B-3000 Leuven
Belgium

Dr. John Kaldor
IARC
150 Cours Albert Thomas
69372 Lyon Cedex 8
France

Professor Gerjo Kok
Department of Health Education
University of Limburg
Postbus 616
6200 MD Maastricht
Holland

Professor Michael Kunze
Institut für Sozialmedizin der
Universität Wien
Alser Strasse 21
1080 Vienna
Austria

Dr. Beverley Littlepage
36 Orchard Street
Swansea SA1 1PM
South Wales

Dr. Elsebeth Lynge
Danish Cancer Registry
Institute of Cancer Epidemiology
Rosenvangets Hovedvej 35
2100 Kobenhavn Ø
Denmark

Professor Jose M. Martin Moreno
Professor of Epidemiology
Escuela Andaluza De Salud Publica
Avda. del sur, 11
18014 Granada
Spain

Professor James McEwen
Director
Department of Community Medicine
Kings College School of Medicine and
Dentistry
Denmark Hill
London SE5 8RX
England

Professor Maria Antonia Modolo
Director
Experimental Centre for Health
Education
University of Perugia
Via del Giochetto 6
Perugia
Italy 06100

Dr. Gabriella Morasso
Insituto Nazionale per la Richerca
do Cancro
Viale Benedetto XV No 10
16132 Genoa
Italy

Dr. Calum Muir
Deputy Director
International Agency for Research on
Cancer
150 Cours Albert Thomas
69372 Lyon
France

Dr. Donatella Pagliacci
Experimental Centre for Health Education
Via del Giochetto 6
Perugia
Italy 06100

Dr. J. M. Pereiz Miguel
Cadeira de Medicina Preventiva
Faculdade de Medecina de Lisboa
Av. Egas Moniz
1600 Lisbon
Portugal

Dr. J. G. da Rocha Alves
Director Centro de Coimbra
Instituto Portugues de Oncologia de
Francisco Gentil
Rua Prof. Bissaya Barreto
3003 Coimbra
Portugal

Professor Armando Rocha Trindade
AEDTU representative
Universidade Aberda
Rua da Escola Politecnica, 147
1200 Lisboa
Portugal

Dr. Nicole Rotmensz
Scientific Assistant
European School of Oncology
Via g. Venezian 1
20133 Milano
Italy

Dr. Helena Saldanha de Oliveira
Coimbra University Hospital
Coimbra
Portugal

Mme Manuela Santos Pardal
Head of Health Education Division
General Directorate of Primary Health Care
Ministry of Health
Al. Afonso Hennigues, 75-3
1056 Lisboa
Portugal

Mme Anne Marie Schoelcher
Chargee D'Etudes Epidemiologiques
Assistance Publique Hopitaux de Paris
3 Avenue Victoria
75100 - Paris
France

Dr. Emer Shelley
Project Leader
Kilkenny Health Project
Dean Street
Kilkenny
Republic of Ireland

Dr. Luis da Silveira Botelho
Director
Centro do Lisboa
Instituto Portugues de Oncologia de Francisco Gentil
Rua Prof. Lima Basto
1093 Lisboa
Portugal

Dr. Maurice Slevin
Imperial Cancer Research Fund
St. Bartholomews Hospital
West Smithfield
London EC1A 7BE
England

Dr. Hans Henrik Storm
Chief of the Section of Cancer Registration
Danish Cancer Registry
Rosenvaengets Hovedvej 35
2100 Kobenhavn Ø
Denmark

David Sweet
Europe Contre le Cancer
Commission of the European Communities
Rue de la Loi 200
B1049 Brussels
Belgium

Dr. Eyvind Thorling
Danish Cancer Society
Department of Nutrition and Cancer
Norrebrogade 44
DK-8000 Århus C
Denmark

Professor Antonia Trichopoulou
Director
Department of Nutrition and Biochemistry
Athens School of Public Health
Leoforos Alexandras 196
11521 Athens
Greece

Professor Stamatis Vassilaros
Director
Breast Cancer Screening Centre
Marika Eliadi Hospital
36 Evrialis Street
Kifissia
14562 Athens
Greece

Professor Andre Wambersie
Head of Radiobiology and Radiation Protection Dept.
Universite Catholique de Louvain
Cliniques Universitaires St-Luc
1200 Brussels
Belgium

Dr. Jack Winkler
Food and Health Policy Research
28 St Paul's Street
London N1 7AB
England

Michael Wood
Director
The Ulster Cancer Foundation
40–42 Eglantive Avenue
Belfast BT9 6DX
Northern Ireland